T0213275

Informatik aktuell

Herausgegeben
im Auftrag der Gesellschaft für Informatik (GI)

Heinz Handels · Thomas M. Deserno
Andreas Maier · Klaus H. Maier-Hein
Christoph Palm · Thomas Tolxdorff
Herausgeber

Bildverarbeitung für die Medizin 2019

Algorithmen – Systeme – Anwendungen

Proceedings des Workshops
vom 17. bis 19. März 2019 in Lübeck

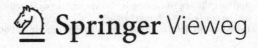

Herausgeber

Heinz Handels
Universität zu Lübeck
Institut für Medizinische Informatik
Ratzeburger Allee 160, 23562 Lübeck

Thomas M. Deserno, geb. Lehmann
Technische Universität Braunschweig
und Medizinische Hochschule Hannover
Peter L. Reichertz Institut für Medizinische
Informatik
Mühlenpfordtstr. 23, 38106 Braunschweig

Andreas Maier
Friedrich-Alexander-Universität
Erlangen-Nürnberg
Lehrstuhl für Mustererkennung
Martensstr. 3, 91058 Erlangen

Klaus H. Maier-Hein, geb. Fritzsche
Deutsches Krebsforschungszentrum (DKFZ)
Medical Image Computing E230
Im Neuenheimer Feld 581, 69120 Heidelberg

Christoph Palm
Ostbayerische Technische Hochschule
Regensburg
Fakultät für Informatik und Mathematik
Galgenbergstr. 32, 93053 Regensburg

Thomas Tolxdorff
Charité – Universitätsmedizin Berlin
Institut für Medizinische Informatik
Hindenburgdamm 30, 12200 Berlin

ISSN 1431-472X
Informatik aktuell
ISBN 978-3-658-25325-7   ISBN 978-3-658-25326-4   (eBook)
https://doi.org/10.1007/978-3-658-25326-4

Die Deutsche Nationalbibliothek verzeichnet diese Publikation in der Deutschen Nationalbibliografie;
detaillierte bibliografische Daten sind im Internet über http://dnb.d-nb.de abrufbar.

CR Subject Classification (1998): A.0, H.3, I.4, I.5, J.3, H.3.1, I.2.10, I.3.3, I.3.5, I.3.7, I.3.8, I.6.3

Springer Vieweg
© Springer Fachmedien Wiesbaden GmbH, ein Teil von Springer Nature 2019

Springer Vieweg ist Teil von Springer Nature
Springer Vieweg ist ein Imprint der eingetragenen Gesellschaft Springer Fachmedien Wiesbaden GmbH
und ist ein Teil von Springer Nature.
Die Anschrift der Gesellschaft ist: Abraham-Lincoln-Str. 46, 65189 Wiesbaden, Germany

Bildverarbeitung für die Medizin 2019

Veranstalter

IMI   Institut für Medizinische Informatik, Universität zu Lübeck

Unterstützende Fachgesellschaften

BVMI	Berufsverband Medizinischer Informatiker
CURAC	Computer- und Roboterassistierte Chirurgie
DAGM	Deutsche Arbeitsgemeinschaft für Mustererkennung
DGBMT	Fachgruppe Medizinische Informatik der Deutschen Gesellschaft für Biomedizinische Technik im Verband Deutscher Elektrotechniker
GI	Gesellschaft für Informatik – Fachbereich Informatik in den Lebenswissenschaften
GMDS	Gesellschaft für Medizinische Informatik, Biometrie und Epidemiologie
IEEE	Joint Chapter Engineering in Medicine and Biology, German Section

Tagungsvorsitz

Prof. Dr. rer. nat. habil. Heinz Handels
Institut für Medizinische Informatik, Universität zu Lübeck

Tagungssekretariat

Susanne Petersen
Institut für Medizinische Informatik
Ratzeburger Allee 160, Gebäude 64
23562 Lübeck
Tel: +49 451 3101 5601
Fax: +49 451 3101 5604
Email: vm2019@imi.uni-luebeck.de
Web: http://bvm-workshop.org

Lokale BVM-Organisation

Dr. Jan Ehrhardt
Prof. Dr. Heinz Handels (Leitung)
Prof. Dr. Mattias Heinrich
Susanne Petersen
Dr. Jan Wrage
und weitere Mitarbeiterinnen und Mitarbeiter des Instituts für Medizinische Informatik der Universität zu Lübeck

Verteilte BVM-Organisation

Prof. Dr. Thomas M. Deserno, Sven Neumann, Aaron Wiora, Jamie-Céline Heinzig, Noah Maxen, Björn Bajor, Peter Reichert, Aleksej Hecht, Hendrik Griesche – Peter L. Reichertz Institut für Medizinische Informatik, Technische Universität Braunschweig (Tagungsband)

Prof. Dr. Heinz Handels, Dr. Jan-Hinrich Wrage – Institut für Medizinische Informatik, Universität zu Lübeck (Beitragsbegutachtung)

Prof. Dr. Andreas Maier – Pattern Recognition Lab, Technische Fakultät der FAU – Nürnberg (Social Media, Special Issue)

Priv. – Doz. Dr. Klaus Maier – Hein, Jens Petersen – Division of Medical Image Computing, Deutsches Krebsforschungszentrum (DKFZ) (Anmeldung, Mailingliste)

Prof. Dr. Christoph Palm, Dr. Alexander Leis, Leonard Klausmann, Sümeyye R. Yildiran – Regensburg Medical Image Computing (ReMIC), OTH Regensburg (Internetpräsenz, Newsletter, Social Media)

Prof. Dr. Thomas Tolxdorff, Dr. Thorsten Schaaf – Institut für Medizinische Informatik, Charité – Universitätsmedizin Berlin (Internetpräsenz)

BVM-Komitee

Prof. Dr. Thomas M. Deserno, Peter L. Reichertz Institut für Medizinische Informatik, Technische Universität Braunschweig

Prof. Dr. Heinz Handels, Institut für Medizinische Informatik, Universität zu Lübeck

Prof. Dr. Andreas Maier, Pattern Recognition Lab, FAU Erlangen-Nürnberg

Priv.-Doz. Dr. Klaus Maier-Hein, Division of Medical Image Computing, DKFZ

Prof. Dr. Christoph Palm, Regensburg Medical Image Computing, OTH Regensburg

Prof. Dr. Thomas Tolxdorff, Institut für Medizinische Informatik, Charité – Universitätsmedizin Berlin

Programmkommitee

Prof. Dr. Jörg Barkhausen, Universitätsklinikum Schleswig-Holstein Campus Lübeck

Priv.-Doz. Dr. Jürgen Braun, Charité-Universitätsmedizin Berlin

Prof. Dr. Thorsten Buzug, Universität zu Lübeck

Dr. Stefanie Demirci, TU München

Prof. Dr. Thomas Deserno, TU Braunschweig

Prof. Dr. Hartmut Dickhaus, Universität Heidelberg

Dr. Jan Ehrhardt, Universität zu Lübeck

Dr. Ralf Floca, DKFZ Heidelberg

Prof. Dr. Nils Forkert, University of Calgary, Canada

Prof. Dr. Horst Hahn, Fraunhofer MEVIS, Bremen

Prof. Dr. Heinz Handels, Universität zu Lübeck
Dr. Tobias Heimann, Siemens, Erlangen
Prof. Dr. Mattias Heinrich, Universität zu Lübeck
Prof. Dr. Ron Kikinis, Fraunhofer MEVIS, Bremen und Harvard Medical School, Boston, USA
Prof. Dr. Andreas Maier, Universität Erlangen-Nürnberg
Priv.-Doz. Dr. Klaus Maier-Hein, DKFZ Heidelberg
Prof. Dr. Lena Maier-Hein, DKFZ Heidelberg
Prof. Dr. Thomas Martinetz, Universität zu Lübeck
Priv.-Doz. Dr. Andre Mastmeyer, Universität zu Lübeck
Prof. Dr. Hans-Peter Meinzer, DKFZ Heidelberg
Prof. Dr. Dorit Merhof, RWTH Aachen
Prof. Dr. Alfred Mertins, Universität zu Lübeck
Prof. Dr. Jan Modersitzki, Fraunhofer MEVIS Lübeck und Universität zu Lübeck
Prof. Dr. Heinrich Müller, TU Dortmund
Prof. Dr. Nassir Navab, TU München
Dr. Marco Nolden, DKFZ Heidelberg
Prof. Dr. Christoph Palm, OTH Regensburg
Prof. Dr. Bernhard Preim, Universität Magdeburg
Prof. Dr. Martin Reuter, Universität Bonn
Prof. Dr. Karl Rohr, Universität Heidelberg
Prof. Dr. Sylvia Saalfeld, Universität Magdeburg
Prof. Dr. Dennis Säring, FH Wedel
Prof. Dr. Stefanie Speidel, NCT Dresden
Prof. Dr. Thomas Tolxdorff, Charité-Universitätsmedizin Berlin
Prof. Dr. Klaus Tönnies, Universität Magdeburg
Dr. Gudrun Wagenknecht, Forschungszentrum Jülich
Dr. Rene Werner, Universitätsklinikum Hamburg-Eppendorf
Dr. Stefan Wesarg, Fraunhofer IGD Darmstadt
Priv.-Doz. Dr. Thomas Wittenberg, Fraunhofer IIS, Erlangen
Prof. Dr. Ivo Wolf, Hochschule Mannheim
Priv.-Doz. Dr. Stefan Wörz, Universität Heidelberg

Sponsoren des Workshops BVM 2019

Die BVM wäre ohne die finanzielle Unterstützung der Industrie in ihrer erfolgreichen Konzeption nicht durchführbar. Deshalb freuen wir uns sehr über langjährige kontinuierliche Unterstützung mancher Firmen sowie auch über das neue Engagement anderer:

Gold-Sponsoren

Euroimmun AG
Seekamp 31, 23560 Lübeck
www.euroimmun.de

ID GmbH & Co KGaA
Platz vor dem Neuen Tor 2, 10115 Berlin
www.id-berlin.de

VisiConsult X-ray Systems & Solutions GmbH
Brandenbrooker Weg 2-4, 23617 Stockelsdorf
visiconsult.de

Silber-Sponsoren

Agfa HealthCare GmbH
Konrad-Zuse-Platz 1-3, 53185 Bonn
global.agfahealthcare.com

Haption GmbH
Dennewartstraße 25, 52068 Aachen
www.haption.de

Ibeo Automotive Systems GmbH
Merkurring 60-62, 22143 Hamburg
www.ibeo-es.com

Sponsoren

Medneo GmbH
Hausvogteiplatz 12, 10117 Berlin
www.medneo.com

MiE medical imaging electronics GmbH
Hauptstraße 112, 23845 Seth
mie-scintron.com

Beste wissenschaftliche Arbeiten

1. Maximilian Blendowski (Universität zu Lübeck)
   Blendowski M, Heinrich MP: 3D-CNNs for Deep Binary Descriptor Learning in Medical Volume Data

2. Hristina Uzunova (Universität zu Lübeck)
   Uzunova H, Handels H, Ehrhardt J: Unsupervised Pathology Detection in Medical Images using Learning-based Methods

3. Maike Stöve (Friedrich-Alexander-Universität Erlangen)
   Stoeve M, Aubreville M, Oetter N, Knipfer C, Neumann H, Stelzle F, Maier A: Motion Artifact Detection in Confocal Laser Endomicroscopy Images

Beste Präsentationen:

Weilin Fu (Friedrich-Alexander-Universität Erlangen)
Fu W, Breininger K, Schaffert R, Ravikumar N, Würfl T, Fujimoto J, Moult E, Maier A: Frangi-Net

Bestes Poster

André Klein (DKFZ Heidelberg)
Klein A, Warszawski J, Hillengaß J, Maier-Hein KH: Towards Whole-body CT Bone Segmentation

Vorwort

In diesem Jahr wird die Tagung Bildverarbeitung für die Medizin (BVM 2019) vom Institut für Medizinische Informatik an der Universität zu Lübeck ausgerichtet. Nach der erfolgreichen Durchführung der BVM 2001, 2011 und 2015 findet diese zentrale Tagung zu neuen Entwicklungen in der Medizinischen Bildverarbeitung in Deutschland nun zum vierten Mal in der traditionsreichen Hansestadt Lübeck statt.

Die medizinische Bildverarbeitung ist eine Schlüsseltechnologie in verschiedenen medizinischen Bereichen wie der Diagnoseunterstützung, der OP-Planung sowie der bildgeführten Chirurgie und Strahlentherapie. Methodisch haben hierbei in den letzten Jahren insbesondere Deep Neural Networks deutliche Fortschritte in Bezug auf Genauigkeit und Geschwindigkeit der Bildverarbeitungsverfahren ermöglicht, wobei das Potenzial maschineller Lernverfahren und Methoden der künstlichen Intelligenz im Bereich der Medizinischen Bildverarbeitung bei weitem noch nicht ausgeschöpft ist.

An der Universität zu Lübeck bilden die Medizinische Bildgebung und Bildverarbeitung einen zentralen universitären Forschungsschwerpunkt, der in den letzten Jahren systematisch ausgebaut wurde. Zudem bildet die Medizinische Bildverarbeitung in den Bachelor- und Masterstudiengängen Medizinische Informatik, Medizinische Ingenieurwissenschaften und Mathematik in Medizin und Lebenswissenschaften eine wichtige Vertiefungsrichtung. Vor diesem Hintergrund ist es eine besondere Freude, die BVM 2019 in Lübeck ausrichten zu dürfen.

Die BVM hat sich als ein zentrales interdisziplinäres Forum für die Präsentation und Diskussion von Methoden, Systemen und Anwendungen im Bereich der Medizinischen Bildverarbeitung etabliert. Ziel der Tagung ist die Darstellung aktueller Forschungsergebnisse und die Vertiefung der Gespräche zwischen Wissenschaftlern, Industrie und Anwendern. Die BVM richtet sich ausdrücklich auch an Nachwuchswissenschaftler, die über ihre Bachelor-, Master-, Promotions- und Habilitationsprojekte berichten wollen.

Die BVM 2019 wird unter der Federführung von Prof. Dr. rer. nat. habil. Heinz Handels, Direktor des Instituts für Medizinische Informatik der Universität zu Lübeck, ausgerichtet. Die Organisation ist wie in den letzten Jahren auf Fachkollegen aus Berlin, Braunschweig, Erlangen, Heidelberg, Lübeck und Regensburg verteilt, so dass die Organisatoren der vergangenen Jahre ihre Erfahrungen hier mit einfließen lassen können.

Anhand anonymisierter Bewertungen durch jeweils drei Fachgutachter wurden aus 87 eingereichten Beiträgen 28 Vorträge, 45 Poster und 2 Softwaredemonstrationen zur Präsentation ausgewählt. Die Qualität der eingereichten Arbeiten war insgesamt sehr hoch. Die besten Arbeiten werden auch in diesem Jahr mit BVM-Preisen ausgezeichnet. Die schriftlichen Langfassungen der Beiträge sind im Tagungsband zusammengefasst, der auch dieses Jahr wieder im Springer Verlag in der Reihe Informatik aktuell zur BVM erscheint. Das Programm wird durch eingeladene Gastvorträge zu aktuellen Themen des Deep

Learnings in der Medizinischen Bildverarbeitung sowie zur Beleuchtung und Diskussion der Sicht des Radiologen auf die aktuellen Entwicklungen abgerundet.

Die Internetseiten des Workshops bieten ausführliche Informationen über das Programm und organisatorische Details rund um die BVM 2019. Sie sind abrufbar unter der Adresse:

http://www.bvm-workshop.org

Am Tag vor dem wissenschaftlichen Programm werden drei Tutorials angeboten, bei denen in diesem Jahr verschiedene Aspekte der Deep Learnings in der Medizinischen Bildverarbeitung beleuchtet werden: Prof. Dr.-Ing. habil. Andreas Maier von der Friedrich-Alexander-Universität Erlangen-Nürnberg hält gemeinsam mit seinen Mitarbeiterinnen und Mitarbeitern ein Tutorial zum Thema „Deep Learning: Fundamentals" ab. Hier wird eine Einführung in die grundsätzlichen Methoden des Deep Learnings und Ihre Anwendung auf medizinische Bilder gegeben. Fortgeschrittene Methoden des Deep Learnings in der Medizinischen Bildverarbeitung stehen im zweiten Tutorial mit dem Titel „Advanced Deep Learning Methods" im Vordergrund, das von PD Dr. Klaus Maier-Hein und seinem Team vom DKFZ Heidelberg durchgeführt wird. Ergänzt wird dieses Angebot durch das dritte Tutorial „Hands-on Deep Learning in Pytorch", das von Prof. Dr. Mattias Heinrich von der Universität zu Lübeck und seinem Team durchgeführt wird. Hier erhalten die Teilnehmenden Anleitungen zum praktischen Einsatz von neuesten Deep Learning Netzwerken und zur Handhabung der hierzu benötigten Softwarewerkzeuge.

Die Herausgeber dieser Proceedings möchten allen herzlich danken, die zum Gelingen der BVM 2019 beigetragen haben. Den Autoren für die rechtzeitige und formgerechte Einreichung ihrer qualitativ hochwertigen Arbeiten, dem Programmkomitee für die gründliche Begutachtung, den Gastrednern und den Referenten der Tutorials für Ihre aktive Mitgestaltung und inhaltliche Bereicherung der BVM 2019. Unser besonderer Dank gilt dem lokalen Organisationsteam in Lübeck, bestehend aus Dr. Jan Ehrhardt, Prof. Dr. Heinz Handels, Prof. Dr. Mattias Heinrich, Susanne Petersen und Dr. Jan Wrage, sowie den übrigen Mitarbeiterinnen und Mitarbeitern des Instituts für Medizinische Informatik in Lübeck, die durch ihren engagierten Einsatz die Organisation und Durchführung der BVM 2019 in der vorliegenden Form erst möglich gemacht haben. Weiterhin möchten wir den Helferinnen und Helfern an den Instituten in Berlin, Braunschweig, Erlangen, Heidelberg und Regensburg für Ihre Unterstützung bei der Organisation der BVM 2019 in Lübeck danken. Für die finanzielle Unterstützung bedanken wir uns bei den Fachgesellschaften und der Industrie.

Wir wünschen allen Teilnehmerinnen und Teilnehmern der BVM 2019 lehrreiche Tutorials, viele anregende Vorträge, Gespräche an den Postern und in der

Industrieausstellung sowie interessante neue Kontakte zu Kolleginnen und Kollegen aus dem Bereich der Medizinischen Bildverarbeitung.

Januar 2019

Heinz Handels (Lübeck)
Thomas Deserno (Braunschweig)
Andreas Maier (Erlangen)
Klaus Maier-Hein (Heidelberg)
Christoph Palm (Regensburg)
Thomas Tolxdorff (Berlin)

Inhaltsverzeichnis

Die fortlaufende Nummer am linken Seitenrand entspricht den Beitragsnummern, wie sie im endgültigen Programm des Workshops zu finden sind. Dabei steht V für Vortrag, P für Poster und S für Softwaredemonstration.

Session 1: Segmentation and Prediction

Session 2: Deep Learning: Learning Strategies and Adversarial Models

Postersession 1:

Segmentation (Poster)

Denoising and Imange Enhancement (Poster)

Registration and Motion Correction (Poster)

Software-Demonstrationen

Session 3: Image Recontruction and Intra-operative Navigation

Postersession 2:

Classification and Detection (Poster)

Visualization and Virtual Reality (Poster)

Imaging and Intra-operative Tracking (Poster)

Session 4: Virtual Reality and 3D Modeling

Session 5: Registration and Motion Models

Session 6: Visible Light

XXII

Abstract: Anchor-Constrained Plausibility
A Novel Concept for Assessing Tractography and Reducing False-Positives

Peter F. Neher[1], Bram Stieltjes[2], Klaus H. Maier-Hein[1,3]

[1]Division of Medical Image Computing, German Cancer Research Center (DKFZ), Heidelberg, Germany
[2]University Hospital Basel, Radiology & Nuclear Medicine Clinic, Switzerland
[3]Section for Automated Image Analysis, Heidelberg University Hospital, Germany
p.neher@dkfz.de

The problem of false positives in fiber tractography is one of the grand challenges in the research area of diffusion-weighted magnetic resonance imaging (dMRI). Facing fundamental ambiguities especially in bottleneck situations, tractography generates huge numbers of theoretically possible candidate tracts. Only a fraction of these candidates is likely to correspond to the true fiber configuration, posing a difficult sensitivity-specificity trade-off. Current methods address this issue either by focusing exclusively on well-known fiber bundles using prior knowledge or by using tract filtering techniques based on the image signal. Currently, the link between these two choices of purely data driven and prior knowledge based approaches is missing.

We propose a novel concept that rigorously exploits prior knowledge about the existence of anatomically known tracts (anchor tracts) to reduce the degrees of freedom of a successive data-driven filtering of the remaining candidate tracts: anchor-constrained plausibility (ACP). This approach is based on the hypothesis that information about the presence or absence of each anchor influences the plausibility of the candidates and thereby reduces the ambiguities in the problem.

We demonstrate the potential of this concept in a series of phantom experiments: ACP significantly improved the tractography sensitivity-specificity trade-off in such controlled settings (AUC 0.91). The direct assessment of false-positive reduction rates requires a ground truth, which does not exist *in vivo*. *In vivo*, we therefore concentrated on assessing the capabilities of ACP in a structured and objective tractogram analysis of 110 subjects of the Human Connectome Project (HCP) young adult study, providing detailed data-driven insights into what we might be missing when focusing only on anatomically known tracts. This work has previously been published at MICCAI 2018 [1].

References

1. Neher PF, et al. Anchor-constrained plausibility (ACP): a novel concept for assessing tractography and reducing false-positives. Proc MICCAI. 2018;11072:20–27.

Automatic Detection of Blood Vessels in Optical Coherence Tomography Scans

Julia Hofmann[1], Melanie Böge[1], Szymon Gladysz[1], Boris Jutzi[2]

[1]Fraunhofer Institute of Optronics, System Technologies and Image Exploitation (IOSB), Ettlingen
[2]Institute of Photogrammetry and Remote Sensing (IPF), KIT Karlsruhe
julia.hofmann@iosb.fraunhofer.de

Abstract. The aim of this research is to develop a new automated blood vessel (BV) detection algorithm for optical coherence tomography (OCT) scans and corresponding fundus images. The algorithm provides a robust method to detect BV shadows (BVSs) using Radon transformation and other supporting image processing methods. The position of the BVSs is determined in OCT scans and the BV thickness is measured in the fundus images. Additionally, the correlation between BVS thickness and retinal nerve fiber layer (RNFL) thickness is determined. This correlation is of great interest since glaucoma, for example, can be identified by a loss of RNFL thickness.

1 Introduction

Since optical coherence tomography (OCT) offers a noninvasive method for an ophthalmology diagnosis in the fundus area of the eye, this imaging method is of increasing importance. Glaucoma, for example, can be identified by a loss of retinal nerve fiber layer (RNFL) thickness, visible in OCT scans.

The aim of this research is to develop an automated blood vessel (BV) detection algorithm for OCT scans and corresponding fundus images. Recent researches showed reliable results using shadowgraphs to find lateral position and diameter of BVs in 2D OCT-scans. By adding Doppler information, 3D orientation was also obtained [1]. Supervised pixel classification [2] enabled lateral BV detection in OCT 3D volumes. Except manual parameter setting, unsupervised segmentation [3] offered a fully automated segmentation algorithm. Model-based approaches [4, 5] then extended the detection to axial BVs. Efficient automated detection was demonstrated using a deep learning algorithm [6] trained on a specific training data set.

In this research a new automated BV detection algorithm is described without the need of an additional model, training or supplementary data. BVs are visible as vertical shadows in OCT images. This is caused by light absorption through a BV during the OCT procedure. Since the Radon transformation is based on line integrals, vertical lines can be easily reinforced with this method. Together with supporting image processing methods, the approach offers a robust, automated BV shadow (BVS) detection in OCT images. For medical interest a correlation between BV thickness and RNFL thickness is determined to define a new glaucoma metric.

2   Materials and methods

The data consists of OCT images and corresponding fundus images for each eye. They are recorded as circular and linear scans. Besides the recording mode (circular/linear), the recording density of the single scans (B-scan) can be varied. In this study circular scans and sparse linear OCT images (with 37 B-scans) from 16 participants and dense linear OCT images (with 193 B-scans in the recording area and a density of 30 μm) from 12 participants are included.

2.1   Methodology

The different data types are processed with the same operational sequence (Fig. 1) which was developed for 2D data. The processing steps are described in this section. Afterwards, a description of the process in case of 3D data is given.

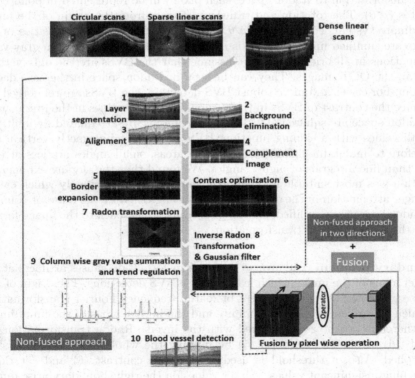

Fig. 1. Flowchart of the proposed approach.

Preparatory steps for the radon transformation The first process step
is the layer segmentation (1). For background elimination (2) all values above
the top layer, Inner Limiting Membrane (ILM), are set to the maximum gray
value to ensure maximum contrast for the BVSs. For alignment (3) each column
(A-scan) in the OCT image is shifted up or down according to the Retinal
Pigment Epithelium layer (RPE) as baseline. This step simplifies cropping of
the image to the area of interest, which suppresses the influence of noise from
surrounding areas. Layer segmentation and alignment are applied with functions
created by Mayer et al. [7]. At this point in the process BVSs have low gray values
which are hard to reinforce. For this reason, a negative image (4) is produced to
enable an amplification of the bright BVSs. Border expansion (5) and contrast
optimization (6) are part of the boundary problem step. They will be explained
after the Radon transformation.

Radon transformation Since the BVSs in OCT scans are vertical lines, a
line detection algorithm is beneficial for this application. The Radon transformation (7) is a linear integral transformation defined by Johann Radon [8]. For
the transformation to Radon space, each pixel will be represented in polar coordinates (ρ, θ). The rotation and translation starts from the origin of the image
coordinate system. For each angle θ and each distance ρ the intensities of the
image are summed up. The result is $r(\rho, \theta)$, consisting of the column gray value
summations in all orientations. We assume that the BVSs are the only vertical
lines in the OCT images. They can be seen in Radon space in the zero degree
column. For easier and more robust BVS detection, the BVSs are reinforced. To
enhance the contrast of BVSs in the original image, all values in the first column
in Radon space are squared. The following columns are attenuated by multiplying all values with a sloping function. BVSs might not be exactly vertical and
therefore to maintain slightly slant shadow areas, small angles are less attenuated than line integrals of higher angles. We found that the sloping exponential
function was most suitable for reinforcement. It falls very steeply which causes
stronger attenuation in the columns of higher angles. After the relevant columns
in Radon space are amplified, the image is transformed back to the image format
with the inverse Radon transformation.

Boundary problem The inverse Radon transformation causes artifacts at the
border areas of the image which leads to false BVS detections. The origin of this
can be explained using the concept of spatial frequency Fourier transformation.
Frequencies are expected to be infinite and the border areas of the finite image
can therefore not be reconstructed with the inverse Radon transformation. To
avoid this, a border expansion (5) by flipping the whole image on both sides
is applied. Also, a threshold is used to optimize contrast (6) and get rid of
disturbing insignificant values. Darker values on the right boundary arise during
the OCT recording and cause falsely detected BVSs. To remove this trend (9) a
15 x 15 pixel window is shifted along the graph. The mean values of the window
values are subtracted from the original summation values.

Blood vessel shadow detection After these image processing steps, the BVSs can be detected in the trend-regulated gray value summation graph. For the BVS detection a quantile threshold is calculated from the graph.

Thickness measurement The BVSs visible in the OCT data do not necessarily correspond to the real BV thickness. Often the scan corresponds to a diagonal cut through the BV. The position of a BVS is therefore transferred to the fundus image. Here, a diameter measurement is performed by generating a BV-filling circle around the detected position.

Pseudo-3D processing - fusion after bidirectional processing The acquisition density of the B-scans corresponding to the dense linear data is too sparse to allow a true 3D processing. For that reason, a pseudo 3D processing (fusion) is applied to approximate a volumetric processing and gain an anisotropic detection. For a volumetric approximation all dense linear scans consecutively are approximated as a cube (Fig. 2). The dense linear scans are concatenated and A-sheets are generated. The A-sheets consist of the same A-scan column in each B-scan. In the x-, y-, z-coordinate system (Fig. 2), they consist of one y-z plane for each x. The pixel size varies between B-scans (4×4 μm) and A-sheets (30×4 μm) according to the acquisition density of 30 μm. After the generation of the A-sheets, the whole non-fused approach is performed separately for all B-scans and all A-sheets. This way the processing is performed for two directions giving two resultant cubes. The cubes are fused with pixel-wise averaging of the pixel values. After the fusion, the BVS detection is applied similarly to the non-fused approach (Fig. 1).

Evaluation A comparison of BVS detections to ground truth is presented. Manual detections by an expert ophthalmologist are used as ground truth in all evaluations. The consistency of the BVS thickness measurements between ground truth and the developed approach was validated using the root mean square error (RSME). This metric defines the deviation between the expected

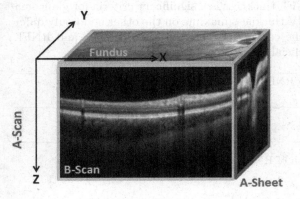

Fig. 2. Coordinate system of the OCT images.

Table 1. Table of results and comparison values.

	Radon approach (all data)	Radon approach (dense scans)		OCTSeg (all data)	OCTSeg (dense scans)
Detection rate	90%	90%	89%	90%	85%
RMSE (pixel)	5.16	5.32	5.44	3.25	8.24

value and the measurement. It provides information about the accuracy of the measurements.

Glaucoma causes RNFL thinning. It might also effect BV thickness. For this reason the correlation of the layer thickness and BV thickness is of interest for ophthalmology. It is tested if the correlation generated from patients suffering from glaucoma shows significant differences in comparison to the correlation obtained from healthy eyes. Only ground truth layer segmentation and BVS detections of sparse OCT scans are used for the correlation estimation to avoid influence of false detections. Correlation can only be determined for detected BVSs without transfer to the fundus image (Sec. Thickness measurement), since for glaucomatous eyes, only OCT scans and not fundus images are available in the data set.

3   Results

The experiments involved sparse linear scans and circular scans from 16 participants and 241 dense linear scans.

The detection rates and thickness accuracies are given in Tab. 1. All detections were compared to the approach of Mayer [7] (OCTSeg). The proposed algorithm is able to achieve the same detection rate as OCTSeg. On the dense linear scans the Radon approach even outperforms the fusion approach and OCTSeg. Regarding all data, OCTSeg achieves the best thickness measurement accuracy. On the dense linear scans the Radon approach performs best. As shown in Tab. 3, the RNFL thickness for the healthy eyes is immensely higher than for glaucomatous eyes. As expected, the RNFL thickness is a significant criteria for glaucoma identification. The measured BV thickness maxima on the other hand only differ 3 μm. The BV thickness or the correlation between BV thickness and RNFL thickness is therefore not beneficial as glaucoma metric.

	Maximum RNFL thickness (μm)	Maximum BV thickness (μm)
Glaucomatous eyes	72	38
Healthy eyes	252	41

Table 2. Correlation of RNFL thickness and BV thickness.

4 Discussion

The advantage of the proposed BV detection algorithm is that no model, training or supplementary data is needed. The results described in this paper show that a sufficient BVS detection rate is enabled with the non-fused, and also the fusion approach. Since the resolution varies according to the recording direction, the fusion detection is not as dense as the radon approach and therefore achieves a lower detection rate. With the transfer to the fundus image (Sec. Thickness measurement) a reliable BV thickness measurement is demonstrated. A metric for glaucomatous eyes could be found, even if the RNFL thickness is more significant for glaucoma than the BV thickness. Here, an additional data acquisition of OCT scans with corresponding fundus images on glaucomatous eyes should be performed to enable a meaningful correlation of layer thickness and BV thickness. Layer segmentation in the approach influences the detection. In the future, a greater independence from the layer segmentation approach (here taken of OCTSeg) will be sought. In further research, the approach could be compared with OCT Angiography to additionally prove the effectiveness.

References

1. Wehbe H, Ruggeri M, Jiao S, et al. Automatic retinal blood vessel parameters calculation in spectral domain optical coherence tomography. Procs SPIE. 2007;6429:6429–1–7.
2. Niemeijer M, Garvin MK, van B Ginneken, et al. Vessel segmentation in 3D spectral OCT scans of the retina. Procs SPIE. 2008;6914:6914–1–8.
3. Annunziata R, Garzelli A, Ballerini L, et al. Leveraging multiscale hessian-based enhancement with a novel exudate inpainting technique for retinal vessel segmentation. IEEE J Biomed Health Inform. 2016;20(4):1129–38.
4. Lee KM. Segmentations of the Intraretinal Surfaces, Optic Disc and Retinal Blood Vessels in 3D-OCT Scans. Iowa: Univ Iowa; 2009.
5. Pilch M, Wenner Y, Strohmayr E, et al. Automated segmentation of retinal blood vessels in spectral domain optical coherence tomography scans. Biomed Opt Expr. 2012;3(7):1478–91.
6. Li Q, Fengi B, Xie L, et al. A cross-modality learning approach for vessel segmentation in retinal images. IEEE Trans Med Imaging. 2016;35(1):109–18.
7. Mayer MA, Hornegger J, Mardin C, et al. Retinal nerve fiber layer segmentation on FD-OCT scans of normal subjects and glaucoma patients. Biomed Opt Expr. 2010;1(5):1358–83.
8. Radon J. Über die Bestimmung von Funktionen durch Ihre Integralwerte Längs Geweisser Mannigfaltigkeiten. Berichte Sächsische Acad Wissenschaft Math Phys, Klass. 1917;69:262.

Prediction of Liver Function Based on DCE-CT

Oliver Rippel[1], Daniel Truhn[2], Johannes Thüring[2], Christoph Haarburger[1],
Christiane K. Kuhl[2], Dorit Merhof[1]

[1]Institute of Imaging & Computer Vision, RWTH Aachen University, Germany
[2]Department of Diagnostic and Interventional Radiology, University Hospital Aachen,
Germany
oliver.rippel@lfb.rwth-aachen.de

Abstract. Liver function analysis is crucial for staging and treating
chronic liver diseases (CLD). Despite CLD being one of the most preva-
lent diseases of our time, research regarding liver in the Medical Image
Computing community is often focused on diagnosing and treating CLD's
long term effects such as the occurance of malignancies, e.g. hepatocellular carcinoma. The Child-Pugh (CP) score is a surrogate for liver function used to quantify liver cirrhosis, a common CLD, and consists of 3
disease progression stages A, B and C. While a correlation between CP
and liver specific contrast agent uptake for dynamic conrast enhanced
(DCE)-MRI has been found, no such correlation has been shown for
DCE-CT scans, which are more commonly used in clinical practice. Using a transfer learning approach, we train a CNN for prediction of CP
based on DCE-CT images of the liver alone. Agreement between the
achieved CNN based scoring and ground truth CP scores is statistically
significant, and a rank correlation of 0.43, similar to what is reported for
DCE-MRI, was found. Subsequently, a statistically significant CP classifier with an overall accuracy of 0.57 was formed by employing clinically
used cutoff values.

1   Introduction

Assessing liver function is crucial for staging and treating chronic liver diseases
(CLD) [1]. Due to its various functions, there exist a multitude of tests to assess
liver state [2], some of them based on imaging. A very common clinical scoring system of liver function is the Child-Pugh score (CP) [3]. It scores several
important indicators such as e.g. ascites and subsequently aggregates them. CP
classes are then gained by applying the following thresholds: CP A 5-6 points,
CP B 7-9 points, and CP C 10-15 points. The CP score is clinically used to
assess the prognosis of liver cirrhosis, a CLD responsible for more than 1 million
deaths annually [4], and monitor its transition to the end stage.

In the Medical Image Computing community, research on CP so far has been
focused on Dynamic Contrast Enhanced-MRI (DCE-MRI). Here, Motosugi et
al. [5] have shown an association between CP score and accumulation of liver
specific contrast agent, as confirmed by further literature [6, 7]. Moreover, a
successful prediction of liver fibrosis was performed by Yasaka et al. [8], again

based on the accumulation of liver specific contrast agent in DCE-MRI. To the best of our knowledge, successful evaluation of liver function based on DCE-CT has not been reported yet, irrespective of the widespread use of DCE-CT in clinical practice as a routine examination.

The main contribution of our work is an approach for predicting CP scores based on DCE-CT imaging alone, using a combination of state-of-the-art convolutional neural networks (CNN) with transfer learning.

2   Methods

2.1   Dataset

In total, the dataset comprises 259 subjects (76 CP score A, 120 CP B, 63 CP C). For each subject, a radiologist with more than 3 years of experience in abdominal imaging reviewed automatic liver delineation in the venous phase generated by Philips Intellispace.

CT imaging was performed by using helical CT scanners (Somatom Definition Flash and Somatom Definiton AS, Siemens Medical Sysems, Forchheim, Germany). The scans were acquired in a craniocaudal direction by using a detector configuration of 128 or 40 x 0.6 mm, a tube current of 120 kVp, quality reference of 240 mAs, and online dose modulation in all phases (pitch 1.0), during a single breath-hold helical acquisition of roughly 10 seconds (slightly varying due to the differing liver sizes). For all imaging, the gantry rotation speed was 2 Hz. The contrast-enhanced images were created with a weight-adjusted application of iodinated contrast material (1.5 mL per kilogram of body weight; Iopramide 370 mg/mL, Ultravist, Shering, Germany) administered at a rate of 3 mL/s by power injector. Subsequently the non-enhanced (native) as well as arterial and venous phases were acquired. The acquisition of the arterial phase started 6 seconds after the automatic detection of peak aortic enhancement at the level of the coeliac trunk with a threshhold of 140 HU; portal venous phase was scanned 55 seconds after the start of the contrast injection. Image reconstruction was performed with axial 1-mm images, an increment of 0.7 mm, and a B30f convolutional kernel for all phases (Fig. 1, representative axial slices).

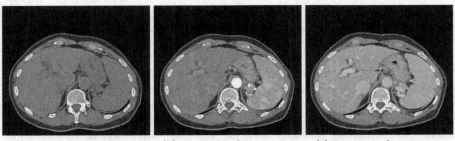

(a) non-contrast enhanced   (b) arterial enhancement   (c) venous enhancement

Fig. 1. Representative images of a contrast enhanced liver CT-scan. Images were reconstructed with a B30f kernel in soft-tissue-window.

2.2 Pre-processing

First, native and arterial phases were registered to the venous phases with a rigid registration algorithm under the assumption that liver shape would be constant in all three phases. Registration itself was performed using SimpleElastix [9] with default parameters. Subsequently, voxel intensities were linearly mapped to a soft tissue window (center 40 HU, width 400 HU).

Next, axial patches of 224x224 in-plane dimension were extracted around the centerpoint of the liver along 20 % to 80 % of its craniocaudal extension. This approach has the advantage of incorporating the context around the liver in a patch, and may thus capture effects such as ascites. Furthermore, it reduces the need for resizing, as axial patch dimensions are concordant with the input shape expected by the pretrained model. In total, 12492 patches were extracted in this manner to be used for model finetuning.

2.3 Model architecture and training

For the model architecture, a ResNet18 [10] pretrained on ImageNet [11] was used in a transfer learning approach [12]. At its core, ResNet consists of residual blocks, where deviations from an identity mapping are learned by the model. This has been shown to sucessfully tackle the problem of vanishing gradients inherent to deep CNNs. While model depth of a ResNet architecture can be arbitrary, we use a depth of 18, minimizing the number of trainable parameters and therefore risk of overfitting.

The output of the pretrained ResNet18 model was adapted to our ordering problem, giving a single continous value for every slice. By stacking the three phases of the CT scan, the number of input channels satisfy the number of channels as required by the pretrained model. While modifications to the axial dimensions are not necessary, on-the-fly data augmentation was used to reduce overfitting of trained models. These consisted of rotation, scaling, as well as elastic deformation and were performed by the batchgenerators framework[1]. Model finetuning on the CT images itself was performed using an L2-regularized Adam optimizer with initial learning rate of 0.0005 and a decay rate of 0.5 every 10 epochs and L2-penalty of 0.001. All layers were trained simultaneously, employing the MeanSquareError (MSE) metric for training and the accuracy metric for validation. MSE was chosen over a classification loss function, such as e.g. CrossEntropy, to reflect the ordinal nature of the CP score. For this, class labels were assigned based on the clinically used thresholds: [5, 6] for CP A, [7, 9] for CP B and [10, 15] for CP C. As the output of the model is continuous, values are rounded to the nearest integer to yield CP class predictions.

The model was trained using 10 fold cross-validation. For each fold, patches are split into training, validation and test set such that patches from a single patient are exclusively included in either training, validation or test set. The splitting ratios were 0.63, 0.27 and 0.1 for training, validation and test sets,

---
[1] https://github.com/MIC-DKFZ/batchgenerators

respectively. Total number of training epochs were 20 epochs per fold, and validation was performed after every epoch. The model state with highest validation score was subsequently used to predict the test set. All experiments were implemented using PyTorch on a workstation equipped with Intel i7-7700K processor and Nvidia GTX 1080 Ti GPU.

2.4 Prediction generation and statistical evaluation

As the CP score is an ordinal score, Kendall's τ statistic was used to quantify rank correlation betweeen CNN-based CP scoring and groundtruth values [13]. Agreement was considered to be statistically significant when $p < 0.05$.

Although the CP score is ordinal in nature, its clinical use corresponds to a classification problem. To yield class predictions, the same clinical thresholds were used for the test set as during model validation. To quantify performance of the classifier, comparison against the No Information Rate (NIR) was performed with a one-sided binomial test. Here, again $p < 0.05$ was considered significicnant.

3 Results

To obtain subject-level classification results from slice-level predictions, slice-level prediction was performed and subsequently averaged. Continuous CP prediction results over all 10 splits are given in Fig. 2a. The computation time for training a single fold was 15 min. Inference for a single subject can be performed in 1.5 s.

In total, a statistically significant agreement could be seen between model and groundtruth values for CP ranking ($p = 3.23 \cdot 10^{-16}$). Correlation denoted

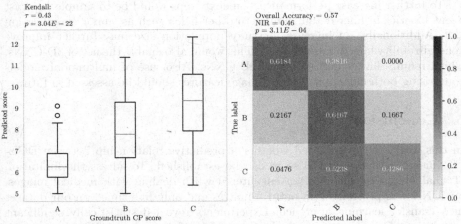

(a) Continuous CP score generated by the CNN.

(b) CP classification gained by thresholding continous score.

Fig. 2. Cross validated prediction of the CP score with a CNN.

by τ was 0.43 (Fig. 2a). Using the cutoff values, an overall classification accuracy of 0.57 was achieved (Fig. 2b). When compared to NIR (0.46), this classification performance is statistically significant ($p = 3.11 \cdot 10^{-4}$).

4   Discussion

We developed and presented a transfer learning based approach to predict CP based on DCE-CT.

When assessing model performance in predicting CP values based on DCE-CT images, a statistically significant agreement was found between CNN predictions and groundtruth scores with a rank correlation of 0.43 (Fig. 2a). Moreover, overall achieved classification accuracy was statistically significant compared to the NIR (Fig. 2b). Motosugi et al. [5] performed a similar analysis in DCE-MRI, but found a statistically significant correlation with insufficient predictive value between CP and contrast agent enrichment in liver parenchym. While predictive models between DCE-MRI and CP have not been established in literature, correlations are well reported [6, 7]. Apart from the connection between CP score and liver CTs/MRIs, CNNs have been used to perform liver fibrosis staging, again based on DCE-MRI [8]. In this study, a Spearman rank correlation of 0.63 was reported between predicted and true fibrosis scores. The authors, however, explicitly state that their model cannot be used to perform liver function analysis, as performed by CP scoring assessed in our work.

Therefore, achieved values are within reason, but further research is required to facilitate clinical use. Nonetheless, to the best of our knowledge, we are the first to report such a correlation in DCE-CT images, with CT being the more frequently used routine diagnostic tool that is more readily available compared to DCE-MRI.

To further increase performance, the next steps would be to sample contrast agent kinetics in finer detail, similar to other fields such as tumor classification [14]. Additionally, an increase in study population size may further improve generalizability of generated models. This would also enable the use of 3D-CNNs, which require larger datasets than 2D-CNNs. Also, use of multimodal models comprising both clinical as well as image features should be assessed in future.

5   Conclusion

In this work, we investigated whether a predictive relationship between DCE-CT image features and CP score can be established. To adress the limitation of small datasets that is often encoutered when dealing with medical images, our CNN was pretrained on natural images and only fine tuned on our dataset in a transfer learning approach. Experiments revealed statistically significant correlation of rankings generated by the model and groundtruth CP scores, which were subsequently used to form a statistically significant classifier of CP score. While the classifier is overall significant, further research is needed to improve discrimination between individual CP classes.

References

1. Suk KT, Kim MY, Baik SK. Alcoholic liver disease: treatment. World J Gastroenterol. 2014;20(36):12934–12944.
2. Kortgen A, Recknagel P, Bauer M. How to assess liver function? Curr Opin Crit Care. 2010;16(2):136–141.
3. Pugh R, Murray-Lyon I, Dawson J, et al. Transection of the oesophagus for bleeding oesophageal varices. Br J Surg. 1973;60(8):646–649.
4. Rowe IA. Lessons from epidemiology: the burden of liver disease. Dig Dis. 2017;35(4):304–309.
5. Motosugi U, Ichikawa T, Sou H, et al. Liver parenchymal enhancement of hepatocyte-phase images in Gd-EOB-DTPA-enhanced MR imaging: which biological markers of the liver function affect the enhancement? J Magn Reson Imaging. 2009;30(5):1042–1046.
6. Verloh N, Haimerl M, Rennert J, et al. Impact of liver cirrhosis on liver enhancement at Gd-EOB-DTPA enhanced MRI at 3 tesla. Eur J Radiol. 2013;82(10):1710–1715.
7. Tamada T, Ito K, Higaki A, et al. Gd-EOB-DTPA-enhanced MR imaging: evaluation of hepatic enhancement effects in normal and cirrhotic livers. Eur J Radiol. 2011;80(3):e311–e316.
8. Yasaka K, Akai H, Kunimatsu A, et al. Liver fibrosis: deep convolutional neural network for staging by using gadoxetic acid-enhanced hepatobiliary phase MR images. Radiol. 2017;287(1):146–155.
9. Marstal K, Berendsen F, Staring M, et al. SimpleElastix: a user-friendly, multilingual library for medical image registration. Proc CVPR. 2016;.
10. He K, Zhang X, Ren S, et al. Deep residual learning for image recognition. Proc CVPR. 2016; p. 770–778.
11. Deng J, Dong W, Socher R, et al. ImageNet: a large-scale hierarchical image database. Proc CVPR. 2009; p. 248–255.
12. Tajbakhsh N, Shin JY, Gurudu SR, et al. Convolutional neural networks for medical image analysis: full training or fine tuning? IEEE Trans Med Imaging. 2016;35(5):1299–1312.
13. Kendall MG. The treatment of ties in ranking problems. Biometrika. 1945;33(3):239–251.
14. Haarburger C, Langenberg P, Truhn D, et al. Transfer learning for breast cancer malignancy classification based on dynamic contrast-enhanced MR images. Proc BVM. 2018; p. 216–221.

Abstract: Adversarial Examples as Benchmark for Medical Imaging Neural Networks

Magdalini Paschali[1], Sailesh Conjeti[2], Fernando Navarro[1], Nassir Navab[1,3]

[1]Computer Aided Medical Procedures, Technische Universität München, Germany
[2] Deutsches Zentrum für Neurodegenerative Erkrankungen (DZNE), Bonn, Germany
[3]Computer Aided Medical Procedures, Johns Hopkins University, USA
magda.paschali@tum.de

Deep learning has been widely adopted as the solution of choice for a plethora of medical imaging applications, due to its state-of-the-art performance and fast deployment. Traditionally, the performance of a deep learning model is evaluated on a test dataset, originating from the same distribution as the training set. This evaluation method provides insight regarding the generalization ability of a model. However, in medical imaging scenarios, especially in cases when a deep learning framework is utilized by a physician for a real-world application, the samples forwarded into the model might belong to a distribution different from the one of the training dataset, or might suffer from noise which cannot usually be modelled by a known distribution, thus raising the need for an evaluation scheme that investigates the robustness of a model, i.e. its performance on data originating from a manifold different from the training one.

To this end, we recently proposed [1] to utilize adversarial examples [2], images that look imperceptibly different from the originals but are consistently missclassified by deep neural networks, as surrogates for extreme test case scenarios, like the ones mentioned above. Extensive evaluation was performed on state-of-the-art classification and segmentation deep neural networks, for the challenging tasks of fine-grained skin lesion classification and whole brain segmentation, leveraging a variety of methods to generate adversarial examples. The results showcased the significant difference in the performance of the utilized networks on clean and on adversarial images. Specifically, networks that performed equally well regarding their generalizability had an astounding 20% difference in robustness, highlighting the need for the proposed, more thorough evaluation technique to uncover which neural network was able to grasp a deeper understanding of the training data and when deployed in real-world applications can showcase a higher robustness to out-of-distribution test samples.

References

1. Paschali M, Conjeti S, Navarro F, et al. Generalizability vs. robustness: investigating medical imaging networks using adversarial examples. Proc MICCAI. 2018; p. 493–501.
2. Szegedy C, Zaremba W, Sutskever I, et al. Intriguing properties of neural networks. Int Conf Learn Representations. 2014;Available from: http://arxiv.org/abs/1312.6199.

Evaluation of Image Processing Methods for Clinical Applications
Mimicking Clinical Data Using Conditional GANs

Hristina Uzunova, Sandra Schultz, Heinz Handels, Jan Ehrhardt

Institut für Medizinische Informatik, Universität zu Lübeck
uzunova@imi.uni-luebeck.de

Abstract. While developing medical image applications, their accuracy is usually evaluated on a validation dataset, that generally differs from the real clinical data. Since clinical data does not contain ground truth annotations, it is impossible to approximate the real accuracy of the method. In this work, a cGAN-based method to generate realistically looking clinical data preserving the topology and thus ground truth of the validation set is presented. On the example of image registration of brain MRIs, we emphasize the necessity for the method and show that it enables evaluation of the accuracy on a clinical dataset. Furthermore, the topology preserving and realistic appearance of the generated images are evaluated and considered to be sufficient.

1 Introduction

The validation of medical image processing algorithms relies on the availability of datasets with a dedicated ground truth, but translation into clinical practice is often significantly hindered by the fact that available validation datasets differ from real clinical data in the acquisition parameters and presence of pathologies, artifacts or noise. For example, a validation using images of healthy subjects possibly underestimates image registration errors for clinical images containing pathologies. On the other hand, the generation of ground truth data is tedious and costly and therefore not feasible for all kinds of clinical data. However, reliable error estimates are crucial for the application of automated image processing in many medical applications, e.g. radiotherapy or surgical planning.

Therefore, we propose to automatically generate realistically looking clinical data with ground truth annotations, based on the validation dataset at hand. With the recent development of image generation methods, especially GANs [1], their application for various medical image processing tasks gets considered more frequently, like image domain translation and denoising [2] or unsupervised detection of anomalies [3]. Works like [4, 5] show that GANs can also be used to translate between image domains. In this work we lay our focus on paired style transfer based on the pix2pix network [5], used to generate realistically looking clinical data constrained on the topology of the validation data and thus preserving ground truth segmentations, achieving the possibility to evaluate the error of algorithms applied on clinical images

2   Materials and methods

GANs are generative models that learn to map a random noise vector $\mathbf{z}$ to an output image y using a generator function $G : \mathbf{z} \rightarrow y$ [1]. An extension of regular GANs are the conditional GANs, that learn the mapping from an observed image x additionally, $G : \{x, \mathbf{z}\} \rightarrow y$ To ensure that the generator produces realistically looking images that cannot be distinguished from real ones, an adversarial discriminator, D, is enclosed in the training process, aiming to perfectly distinguish between real images and generator's fakes.

2.1   Style transfer using conditional generative adversarial networks

One possible application of cGANs is style transfer. In this case the generator takes an image x as input and trains to generate its corresponding style-transferred image $G(x) \approx y$ The discriminator takes a pair of images as input: x and $G(x)$ (fake) or x and y (real) and is trained to determine whether the pair is real of fake. Thus the objective of the fully conditional GAN can be expressed as

$$\mathcal{L}_{cGAN}(G, D) = \mathbb{E}_{x,y}[\log D(x, y)] + \mathbb{E}_{x,\mathbf{z}}[\log(1 - D(x, G(x, \mathbf{z})))] \qquad (1)$$

where G tries to minimize this objective and an adversarial D tries to maximize it. Also to encourage the generator to produce realistic images more directly, it is beneficial to use an L1 loss: $\mathcal{L}_{L1}(G) = \mathbb{E}_{x,y,\mathbf{z}}[||y - G(x, \mathbf{z})||_1]$ The final objective is then

$$G^* = \arg\min_G \max_D \mathcal{L}_{cGAN}(G, D) + \lambda\mathcal{L}_{L1}(G) \qquad (2)$$

One popular style transfer representative is pix2pix [5] and it requires strictly paired data for training. In [5] the authors show that they are able to transfer contours of an object to the photographic image of the object itself. Also if trained on a certain domain A the cGAN will generate images with the style of A even if the contours belong to a different image domain B, however the topology of the contours of B remains. Those properties are interesting for our work, since we seek contour-to-gray-value topology-preserving translation of medical images.

2.2   Medical image style transfer

Assume there is a validation dataset of healthy patients images with ground truth segmentations or landmarks of the anatomically significant parts, V, and a clinical dataset of possibly pathological images containing only segmentations of the pathologies, C. Since the focus of our work lies on applying image registration, pathologies would lead to strongly decreased registration accuracy and ground truth anatomical annotations are crucial for its evaluation. However, the presented method is not restricted to this application.

Aiming to generate realistically looking data from the clinical domain, but preserving the topology and thus the segmentation masks of the healthy validation data, the cGAN described in 2.1 is used as follows. G is trained to generate clinical images $c_i \in C$ conditioned on the edges extracted from the images e.g. by using a Canny filter, such that $G(x_i, \mathbf{z}) \approx c_i \in C$ where $x_i = \text{edges}(c_i)$ Then in test phase only the edges of the validation images $\text{edges}(v_j)$ are inputed and $G(\text{edges}(v_j)) \in C$ outputs an image looking like clinical data but preserving the topology of the validation image v_j and thus the ground truth segmentations apply. Still, $\text{edges}(v_j)$ does not contain any pathologies and the generator would most likely generate a healthy image. However, one can explicitly simulate pathologies on the images, since we assume that their segmentations are available in C.

2.3 Network architecture

Contrary to pix2pix [5], here ResNet blocks [6] are used for the generator, as in our experience, they show better reconstruction abilities. The generator downscales the input image first by using three 2D strided convolutions (conv2D) each followed by batch normalization (BN) and a ReLU, resulting in 256 channels. Then nine ResNet blocks with 256 channels each are applied, and the image is upsampled to the original size using two transposed conv2Ds each followed by a BN and a leaky ReLU (lReLU), and at last a conv2D layer followed by the Tanh function.

The discriminator takes as input a two-channel image composed of a gray value image and its corresponding contour image. The input is then send through the architecture: conv2D $\rightarrow$ lReLU $\rightarrow$ (conv2D $\rightarrow$ BN $\rightarrow$ lReLU)$\times 3 \rightarrow$ lReLU $\rightarrow$ conv2D, that first iteratively downscales the image and produces 512 channels and the last convolution reduces the overall size to one neuron (real/fake).

3 Results

3.1 Data and setup

Our experiments simulate an atlas-to-patient registration scenario for brain MRI images. The LPBA40 data [7] containing 40 healthy whole-head T1 MRIs with 56 labeled anatomic regions is chosen as validation dataset. The clinical data is represented by a subset of the BRATS 2015 challenge data [8], which contains 220 brain MRI T1c images with high-grade glioblastomas. The BRATS data differs from LPBA40 by different gray value ranges as well as the presence of skull stripping artifacts and pathologies (Fig. 1(left)). For both datasets 2D slices on the same positions are extracted and the BRATS images are cropped around the center to a size of 181×217 matching the size and approximate alignment of the LPBA40 images.

The network described in Sec. 2.3 is trained to generate images in the style of BRATS from their corresponding edge images. The edge images are generated using a Canny filter. Our experience showed that better results are achieved when using gradient magnitude weighted edges rather than binary ones. Furthermore, we want to explicitly integrate the tumor structures in the training process, to prevent the network from hallucinating pathologies [9]. Therefore, segmentation masks of the pathologies available to the BRATS data are combined with the edge images. For the test phase, the extracted LPBA40 edge images are combined with 4 different tumor masks picked at random from the BRATS dataset (affine pre-registration undertaken to ensure that the masks are placed inside the brain) resulting in 5 generated images pro input image (4 with tumors and 1 without). The generated images then have the appearance of BRATS with predefined pathology availability but follow the contours of the LPBA40 images.

To validate the atlas-to-patient registration, one subject of the LPBA40 data is selected as atlas and registered to the remaining 39 subjects using the variational registration method presented in [10]. Label overlap measures (Dice) are used as surrogate for registration accuracy. The cGAN-based style transfer now allows for the replicated validation using the generated data.

3.2   Experiments and results

Visual evaluation In first place it is important to determine whether the images generated by the cGAN are realistic for the particular domain at all. Fig. 1 shows a few generated images and in our experience they generally have a realistic appearance.

Topology preservation An important point of the method presented here, is the assumption that the topology of the LPBA40 image is being preserved, allowing for the segmentation labels to be transferred directly (Fig. 1 (right)). To evaluate this quantitatively, the contours of the input LPBA40 images and the contours of the corresponding generated BRATS images are extracted (here

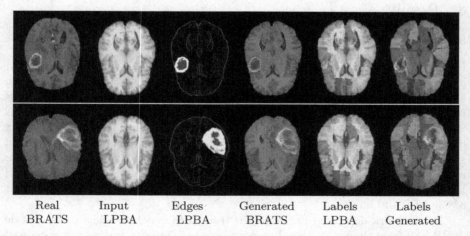

| Real | Input | Edges | Generated | Labels | Labels |
| BRATS | LPBA | LPBA | BRATS | LPBA | Generated |

Fig. 1. Examples of two generated images. From left to right: Real BRATS image containing the tumor; LPBA image; Contours of LPBA image and tumor mask serving as input in test phase; Generated image; LPBA labels overlayed over the real LPBA; LPBA labels overlayed over the generated image (best viewed in color).

Table 1. Mean Dice coefficients ± standard deviation over all labels and reference images before (Initial) and after VarReg (Results comparable to [10]). NN: Normal LPBA atlas to Normal LPBA images; NG: Normal LPBA atlas to generated image without tumors; GG: Generated atlas to generated images without tumors; NGT: Normal LPBA atlas to generated image with tumors; GGT: Normal LPBA atlas to generated image with tumors. AL: All labels; OL: Labels outside the tumors. Subscripts indicate statistical significance in a t-test($p \ll 0.001$): $\star$ – compared to NN; $\diamond$ – compared to GG; †
– compared to GGT.

Initial	NN (AL)	NG (AL)	GG (AL)	NGT (OL)	GGT (OL)
0.610 ± 0.07	0.735 ± 0.02	$0.700 \pm 0.03^{\star\diamond}$	$0.708 \pm 0.03^{\star}$	$0.707 \pm 0.02^{\star\dagger}$	$0.714 \pm 0.02^{\star}$

the contours of the tumor are used for evaluation instead of its mask) and the measured average symmetric contour distance (ACD) reaches 0.58±0.07 mm, indicating sub-pixel accuracy. The worst result with ACD 0.83mm is still in sub-pixel space and is achieved for the image shown in the second row of Fig. 1, still the well aligning labels show that the topology is sufficiently preserved and the relatively large distance occurs caused by the edge extracting method. As baseline serves the ACD between the LPBA40 image contours and their best matching images from the real BRATS dataset yielding 1.75±0.13 mm. This of course cannot be used as a direct comparison, but shows that the ACD values of the generated images are clearly in favor of the topology preserving assumption.

Atlas-to-patient registration scenario To underline the need for an evaluation using realistic clinic-like data, the following registrations are considered: 1) NN: normal LPBA40 atlas to all normal LPBA40 images; 2) NG: normal LPBA40 atlas to all generated images (with the BRATS style) without tumors; 3) GG: First translating the LPBA40 atlas to the BRATS domain and then registering the generated atlas to all the generated images without tumors; 4) and 5) Analogous to 2) and 3) respectively, but with simulated tumors on the generated images.

Tab. 1 shows the Dice overlaps resulting from the registration experiments. When tumors are contained in one of the images, only the labels outside the tumors are evaluated, otherwise all labels are considered. The results strongly emphasize the need to generate ground truth clinical data for error approximation, since the registration results for the validation dataset are significantly better and cannot be generalized to application on clinical data. Unfortunately, it is impossible to determine whether the results on the generated dataset correspond to the registration results on the real BRATS data, since no anatomical annotations are available. Furthermore, we show that, despite histogram normalization, the registration results get significantly better, when the atlas image is also translated to the same image domain. The presented cGAN method is flexible enough in its application to easily transfer the style of the atlas without additional training or optimization, which enables further possibilities like better registration between different image modalities.

4   Discussion and conclusion

We presented a cGAN-based method to combine the topology of validation images and appearance of clinical images, preserving the ground truth segmentations and enabling the evaluation of image processing algorithms on clinic-like data.

The evaluation shows that the presented method indeed generates realistically looking data and the topology of the validation images stays unchanged. The need for such methods is underlined on the example of image registration. On a healthy patients validation dataset containing ground truth segmentations, the registration method works significantly better than on the generated clinical dataset containing pathologies, implying that it is crucial to be able to generate clinical ground truth data for the reliable evaluation of algorithms. Currently this method is limited to 2D images, so future work will consider a computationally feasible extension to 3D images.

References

1. Goodfellow I, Pouget-Abadie J, Mirza M, et al. Generative adversarial nets. Adv Neural Inf Process Syst. 2014;27:2672–2680.
2. Armanious K, Yang C, Fischer M, et al. MedGAN: medical image translation using GANs. CoRR. 2018;abs/1806.06397.
3. Schlegl T, Seeböck P, Waldstein SM, et al. Unsupervised anomaly detection with generative adversarial networks to guide marker discovery. Proc IPMI. 2017; p. 146–157.
4. Zhu JY, Park T, Isola P, et al. Unpaired image-to-image translation using cycle-consistent adversarial networks. Proc ICCV. 2017; p. 2242–2251.
5. Isola P, Zhu JY, Zhou T, et al. Image-to-image translation with vonditional adversarial networks. Proc CVPR. 2017;00:5967–5976.
6. He K, Zhang X, Ren S, et al. Deep residual learning for image recognition. Proc CVPR. 2016; p. 770–778.
7. Shattuck DW, Mirza M, Adisetiyo V, et al. Construction of a 3D probabilistic atlas of human cortical structures. NeuroImage. 2008;39.
8. Menze BH, Jakab A, Bauer S, et al. The multimodal brain tumor image degmentation benchmark (BRATS). IEEE Trans Med Imaging. 2015;34(10):1993–2024.
9. Cohen JP, Luck M, Honari S. Distribution matching losses can hallucinate features in medical image Translation. Proc MICCAI. 2018;11070:529–536.
10. Ehrhardt J, Schmidt-Richberg A, Werner R, et al. Variational registration: a flexible open-source ITK toolbox for nonrigid image registration. Proc BVM. 2015; p. 209–214.

Abstract: Some Investigations on Robustness of Deep Learning in Limited Angle Tomography

Yixing Huang[1], Tobias Würfl[1], Katharina Breininger[1], Ling Liu[1],
GÃ¼nter Lauritsch[2], Andreas Maier[1,3]

[1]Friedrich-Alexander Universität Erlangen-Nürnberg, 91058 Erlangen, Germany
[2]Siemens Healthcare GmbH, 91301 Forchheim, Germany
[3]Erlangen Graduate School in Advanced Optical Technologies (SAOT),
91058 Erlangen, Germany
yixing.yh.huang@fau.de

In computed tomography, image reconstruction from an insufficient angular range of projection data is called limited angle tomography. Due to missing data, reconstructed images suffer from artifacts, which cause boundary distortion, edge blurring, and intensity biases. Recently, deep learning methods have been applied very successfully to this problem in simulation studies. However, the robustness of neural networks for clinical applications is still a concern. It is reported that most neural networks are vulnerable to adversarial examples.

In this paper, we aim to investigate whether some perturbations or noise will mislead a neural network to fail to detect an existing lesion.

Our experiments demonstrate that the trained neural network, specifically the U-Net, is sensitive to Poisson noise. While the observed images appear artifact-free, anatomical structures may be located at wrong positions, e.g. the skin shifted by up to 1 cm. This kind of behavior can be reduced by retraining on data with simulated Poisson noise. However, we demonstrate that the retrained U-Net model is still susceptible to adversarial examples. We conclude the paper with suggestions towards robust deep-learning-based reconstruction [1].

References

1. Huang Y, Würfl T, Breininger K, et al. Some investigations on robustness of deep learning in limited angle tomography. Proc MICCAI. 2018; p. 145–153.

Abstract: nnU-Net: Self-adapting Framework for U-Net-Based Medical Image Segmentation

Fabian Isensee[1], Jens Petersen[1], Andre Klein[1], David Zimmerer[1], Paul F. Jaeger[1], Simon Kohl[1], Jakob Wasserthal[1], Gregor Koehler[1], Tobias Norajitra[1], Sebastian Wirkert[1], Klaus H. Maier-Hein[1]

[1]Department of Medical Image Computing, German Cancer Research Center, Heidelberg, Germany
f.isensee@dkfz-heidelberg.de

The U-Net was presented in 2015. With its straight-forward and successful architecture it quickly evolved to a commonly used benchmark in medical image segmentation. The adaptation of the U-Net to novel problems, however, comprises several degrees of freedom regarding the exact architecture, preprocessing, training and inference. These choices are not independent of each other and substantially impact the overall performance. The present paper [1] introduces the nnU-Net ("no-new-Net"), which refers to a robust and self-adapting framework on the basis of 2D and 3D vanilla U-Nets. We argue the strong case for taking away superfluous bells and whistles of many proposed network designs and instead focus on the remaining aspects that determine the performance and generalizability of a method. We evaluate the nnU-Net in the context of the Medical Segmentation Decathlon challenge, which measures segmentation performance in ten disciplines comprising distinct entities, image modalities, image geometries and dataset sizes. Most importantly though, algorithms submitted to this challenge are required to work out of the box for any of these datasets without manual intervention or fine tuning. The challenge is divided in two distinct phases: phase I comprises seven datasets and is mainly intended for model development while phase II comprises three previously unknown datasets indented for model evaluation. nnUNet successfully adapted itself to all of these datasets without user interaction and, with the sole exceptions being class 1 in the BrainTumour and the Spleen datasets, achieved the highest dice scores out of all participating algorithms (phase I leaderboard: https://decathlon.grand-challenge.org/evaluation/results/). In the final evaluation it won the Medical Segmentation Decathlon challenge with a margin.

References

1. Isensee F, Petersen J, Klein A, et al. nnU-Net: self-adapting framework for U-Net-based medical image segmentation. arXiv:180910486. 2018;.

Deep Multi-Modal Encoder-Decoder Networks for Shape Constrained Segmentation and Joint Representation Learning

Nassim Bouteldja[1], Dorit Merhof[1], Jan Ehrhardt[2], Mattias P. Heinrich[2]

[1]Institute of Imaging and Computer Vision, RWTH Aachen University
[2]Institute of Medical Informatics, University of Luebeck
nassim.bouteldja@rwth-aachen.de

Abstract. Deep learning approaches have been very successful in segmenting cardiac structures from CT and MR volumes. Despite continuous progress, automated segmentation of these structures remains challenging due to highly complex regional characteristics (e.g. homogeneous gray-level transitions) and large anatomical shape variability. To cope with these challenges, the incorporation of shape priors into neural networks for robust segmentation is an important area of current research. We propose a novel approach that leverages shared information across imaging modalities and shape segmentations within a unified multi-modal encoder-decoder network. This jointly end-to-end trainable architecture is advantageous in improving robustness due to strong shape constraints and enables further applications due to smooth transitions in the learned shape space. Despite no skip connections are used and all shape information is encoded in a low-dimensional representation, our approach achieves high-accuracy segmentation and consistent shape interpolation results on the multi-modal whole heart segmentation dataset.

1 Introduction

Accurate multi-organ segmentation is an important prerequisite for image-guided interventions and CAD. Despite its remarkable advances, accurate and robust approaches for segmenting multiple organs with large shape variability, e.g. heart structures, are still scarce. A particular difficulty arises from the complex regional characteristics and large shape variability. To cope with these challenges and enable meaningful analysis of shape variations, model-based approaches, that restrict shape variations to a compact linear shape space, have been frequently used in the past [1]. However, due to its linear nature and decoupling of feature learning and shape fitting, are limited in segmentation accuracy and nonlinear representation-learning abilities of deep networks [1].

Recently, new state-of-the-art segmentation accuracies have been achieved using fully-convolutional architectures that heavily rely on skip connections [2, 3]. While these frameworks are useful for quantifying exact volumetric measurements, their skip connections disconnect the final prediction from the shape space encoding and thus limit prediction smoothness, further physiological analysis and shape retrieval. Some recent work tried to address these shortcomings by incorporating shape priors into deep networks [4, 5, 6]. In particular, [4, 5] trained an additional convolutional auto-encoder (CAE) to project predictions and ground truth labels into its shape space and apply a soft penalty on their discrepancies during training, so that models are guided to follow global anatomical shape properties. However, these models are not end-to-end trainable and still rely on skip connections resulting in the aforementioned limitations.

In this work, we propose a new and more elegant approach inspired by the work in computer vision of Jetley et al. [6], who directly regressed input images to their shape encodings by ℓ_1-distance minimization. In addition, we propose a novel approach for improving image regression into the common shape space by utilizing a fixed decoder to minimize a cross-entropy (CE) loss between predictions and ground truth labels.

2   Materials and methods

Our model (Fig. 1) follows a traditional CAE structure with a contracting encoder and expanding decoder part. CAEs are optimized for an intermediate representation that best reconstructs the input itself. The space of intermediate representations is referred to as shape space (Fig. 1) and is of low-dimensional nature to force the network to capture the most salient features of the underlying anatomy. In our model, the encoder E is of multidomain nature and projects different inputs (CT, MR volumes and segmentations) into a joint 1584 dimensional

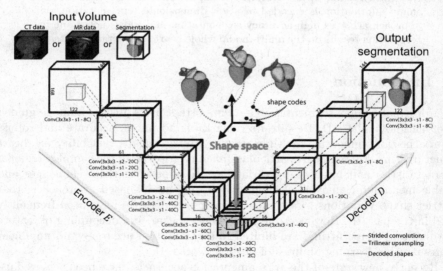

Fig. 1. Our proposed all-convolutional model providing 624K trainable parameters. E projects its input into the $2 \cdot 8 \cdot 9 \cdot 11 = 1584$ dimensional shape space. "Conv(3x3x3 -s1-10C)" stands for a conv layer with $3 \times 3 \times 3$ kernel, stride of 1 and 10 channels.

shape space resulting in very smooth shape predictions (Fig. 2.1 a). The first conv layer of our network is the only one that differs for grayscale images and segmentations since multi-organ integer labels are converted to multi-channel one-hot encodings, while MRI and CT are single-channel inputs and are therefore passed through the same conv layers. Besides, every conv layer is followed by batch norm and LeakyReLU except the last layer being followed by softmax.

2.1 Joint training

Our learning approach alternates between mini-batches of segmentations S_i and grayscale images I_i (MRI and/or CT). When segmentations are seen at the input, the network represents a CAE. Input shapes are encoded in the low-dim. shape space (by E) and mapped through D for reconstruction. E and D are jointly optimized by minimizing the CE-loss between predictions and input shapes.

When CT and MR images are considered as inputs, we do not follow the classical approach (e.g. as in [6]) to directly regress them to the corresponding shape encodings of their manual segmentations by minimizing their ℓ_1-distances $||E(I_i) - E(S_i)||_1$ Instead, we further propagate grayscale encodings $E(I_i)$ through a fixed decoder and then minimize the CE-loss between predictions and ground-truth labels. Despite potential vanishing gradient issues, this procedure provides several advantages: Firstly, the embedding is optimized for the optimal shape code in the current shape space instead of its (suboptimal) shape encoding. Secondly, CE is a more qualitative loss than ℓ_1, and thirdly, it helps to produce balanced updates of E for segmentation and grayscale inputs (rather than ℓ_1- and CE-loss-updates) improving the stability of the model.

On the one hand, E is trained to improve reconstruction quality of segmentations, and on the other hand, E simultaneously learns to transfer shape as well as multi-modal image features into a common shape space trying to yield an equal representation of each domain. Since D is only optimized for reconstruction quality of segmentations and E for extracting domain-invariant, high-level features, we let E provide about three times as many conv layers (and therefore abstractational depth) as D. Interestingly, we found that five conv layers suffice for D to map from the shape space in the segmentation domain with a high representation ability.

Besides, keeping the decoder fixed for grayscale inputs is necessary to avoid two separate feature extraction paths for grayscale images and segmentations throughout the entire network, thus resulting in two different shape spaces (as shown in [7]). Since D is only optimized for segmentation reconstruction yielding one common shape space, close spatial correspondence of shape and image encodings is still achieved through CE-loss minimization despite not being explicitly optimized for that (Fig. 2.1 b).

2.2 Implementation details and experiments

The model is trained using Adam on random mini-batches of size 3 containing either CT and/or MR data, or solely segmentations, in an alternating order for

1000 epochs. Learning rates start at 0.002 for the label and 0.004 for the grayscale optimizer and are reduced by 0.9 every $30th$ epoch. Weight decay and affine transformations for data augmentation were used. It is also important to note that we use instance normalization during evaluation to compensate for the fact that batch statistics differ strongly between label- and grayscale- mini-batches.

We evaluate our approach (referred to as *CE-Reg*) on the MM-WHS training dataset which consists of 40 multi-modality whole heart images (20 CT and 20 MRI). Our preprocessing pipeline starts with data resampling into isotropic voxel sizes of $(1.5mm)^3$ We then crop bounding boxes with sizes of $144 \times 122 \times 168$ around the ROI and finally apply Z-normalization on the cropped patches.

We further compare our approach with the following variants: ℓ_1-*Reg* using ℓ_1-loss between grayscale and shape encodings for image regression into the shape space; *2E-D*: decoupled variant of our approach consisting of two separate encoders (one for segmentation and the other for grayscale image inputs) each with half the number of feature channels in every conv layer; *E-D*: traditional encoder-decoder network being solely trained on MR and CT data, and finally *U-Net*: E-D with skip connections. The models share equal training and architectural properties. To measure the segmentation accuracy, we perform 5-fold cross-validation and report mean Dice scores.

3   Results

Tab. 1 lists quantitative segmentation accuracies of the evaluated models. Our model significantly outperforms ℓ_1-*Reg* underlining improvements to image regression when using the CE-loss. Furthermore, both regression models ℓ_1-*Reg*

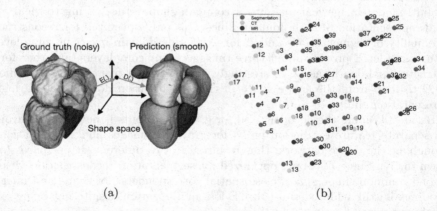

(a)   (b)

Fig. 2. a) shows rather noisy ground-truth labels as well as its satisfyingly smoothed prediction. (b) displays the t-SNE visualization of the embedding after training our model on the MM-WHS dataset (patient no. displayed). b) displays the t-SNE visualization of the embedding (patient no. displayed). As desired, corresponding shape codes lie in close proximity to one another.

Table 1. Dice scores of the evaluated approaches. CE-Reg is our proposed model, ℓ_1-Reg uses ℓ_1-loss between image and corresponding shape encodings for image regression into the shape space. 2E-D is a decoupled variant of CE-Reg with two separate encoders one for segmentation and the other for grayscale image inputs. Besides, E-D is an encoder-decoder model being trained solely on MR and CT volumes and U-Net its variant using skip connections.

	LV	Myo	RV	LA	RA	aorta	PA	∅
CT data								
CE-Reg	0.888	0.822	0.848	0.874	0.848	0.724	0.874	0.840
ℓ_1-Reg	0.877	0.796	0.840	0.846	0.841	0.676	0.863	0.819
2E-D	0.850	0.760	0.846	0.806	0.820	0.602	0.811	0.785
U-Net	0.921	0.824	0.872	0.879	0.885	0.800	0.944	0.875
E-D	0.848	0.746	0.822	0.822	0.792	0.596	0.812	0.777
MR data								
CE-Reg	0.882	0.746	0.832	0.816	0.836	0.704	0.734	0.793
ℓ_1-Reg	0.877	0.722	0.822	0.793	0.831	0.678	0.731	0.779
2E-D	0.866	0.702	0.806	0.768	0.796	0.562	0.718	0.745
U-Net	0.923	0.796	0.881	0.871	0.883	0.778	0.769	0.843
E-D	0.860	0.704	0.784	0.780	0.794	0.622	0.684	0.747

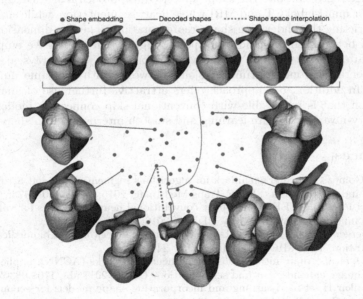

Fig. 3. Visualization of the shape embedding, its decoded shapes and shape interpolations along the dotted line. Note the smoothness of the decoded shapes, the realistic shape deformations as well as the smooth transitions in the compact shape space.

and *CE-Reg* clearly outperform their decoupled variant *2E-D* as well as traditional encoder-decoder networks *E-D*. The former indicates that segmentation performance can greatly benefit from shared information across the domains, whereas the latter shows that, even if these encoder-decoder networks might also learn a qualitative shape space, regressing grayscale images into a learned shape space yields considerably better performance. In comparison, skip connections (*U-Net*) yields performance increases, which are, however, only relevant for pixelwise segmentation and more importantly, lack smoothness of predictions and explainability of shape variations.

Furthermore, Fig. 3 illustrates the learned shape space. It shows plausible shapes decoded from a compact shape space with smooth and realistic transitions. These properties, that can only be achieved without skip connections, enable further applications including object-mask registration or robust multimodal registration by projecting multi-modal data into a common shape space, followed by the sampling of intermediate shape interpolated versions.

4   Conclusion

First, we have presented a novel architecture for deep encoder-decoder networks that jointly learns shared features within a single end-to-end trainable model without skip connections, and second, we introduced a novel approach to improve image regression into the shape space. Our approach reaches excellent accuracies for multi-label CT and MRI whole heart segmentation, while simultaneously restricting the underlying shape representation to be low-dimensional and consistent between shapes and corresponding grayvalue scans. We empirically demonstrate a highly effective use of shared information across grayscale images and segmentations outperforming disjoint networks with the same number of channels. In addition, our approach offers attractive further use of anatomical information that is impossible with conventional skip connection models, such as modality-invariant feature learning and smooth interpolation in shape space.

References

1. Tobon-Gomez C, et al. Benchmark for algorithms segmenting the left atrium from 3D CT and MRI datasets. IEEE Trans Med Imag. 2015;34(7):1460–1473.
2. Milletari F, et al.; IEEE. V-net: fully convolutional neural networks for volumetric medical image segmentation. Proc 3D Vis. 2016; p. 565–571.
3. Ronneberger O, et al.; Springer. U-net: convolutional networks for biomedical image segmentation. Proc MICCAI. 2015; p. 234–241.
4. Oktay O, et al. Anatomically constrained neural networks (ACNN): application to cardiac image enhancement and segmentation. CoRR. 2017;abs/1705.08302.
5. Ravishankar H, et al. Learning and incorporating shape models for semantic segmentation. Proc MICCAI. 2017; p. 203–211.
6. Jetley S, Sapienza M, Golodetz S, et al. Straight to shapes: real-time detection of encoded shapes. CoRR. 2016;abs/1611.07932.
7. Bouteldja N, Heinrich MP. Deep 3D encoder-decoder networks with applications to organ segmentation. Stud Conf. 2018; p. 229–232.

Abstract: Fan-to-Parallel Beam Conversion
Deriving Neural Network Architectures Using Precision Learning

Christopher Syben[1,2], Bernhard Stimpel[1,2], Jonathan Lommen[1,2], Tobias Würfl[1], Arnd Dörfler[2], Andreas Maier[1]

[1]Pattern Recognition Lab, Department of Computer Science,
Friedrich-Alexander-Universität Erlangen-Nürnberg, Germany
[2]Department of Neuroradiology, Universitätsklinikum Erlangen,
Friedrich-Alexander-Universität Erlangen-Nürnberg, Germany
christopher.syben@fau.de

In this paper, we derive a neural network architecture based on an analytical formulation of the parallel-to-fan beam conversion problem following the concept of precision learning [1]. Up to now, this precision learning approach was only used to augment networks with prior knowledge and or to add more flexibility into existing algorithms. We want to extent this approach: we demonstrate that we can drive a mathematical model to tackle a problem under consideration and use deep learning to formulate different hypothesis on efficient solution schemes that are then found as the point of optimality of a deep learning training process. The network allows to learn the unknown operators in this conversion in a data-driven manner avoiding interpolation and potential loss of resolution. The concept is evaluated in the context of Hybrid MRI/X-ray imaging where transformation of the parallel-beam MRI projections to fan-beam X-ray projections is required. The proposed method is compared to a traditional rebinning method. The results demonstrate that the proposed method is superior to ray-by-ray interpolation and is able to deliver sharper images using the same amount of parallel-beam input projections which is crucial for interventional applications. Based on the reconstruction problem and the problem description, we derived a network topology which allows to learn the unknown operators. We believe that this approach forms a basis for further work uniting deep learning, signal processing, physics, and traditional pattern recognition.

References

1. Syben C, Stimpel B, Lommen J, et al. Deriving neural network architectures using precision learning: parallel-to-fan beam conversion. Proc GCPR. 2018; p. 1–15.

Abstract: Tract Orientation Mapping for Bundle-Specific Tractography

Jakob Wasserthal[1,2], Peter F. Neher[1], Klaus H. Maier-Hein[1,3]

[1]Division of Medical Image Computing, German Cancer Research Center (DKFZ), Heidelberg, Germany [2]Medical Faculty, Heidelberg University, Germany [3]Section for Automated Image Analysis, Heidelberg University Hospital, Germany
j.wasserthal@dkfz.de

While the major white matter tracts are of great interest to numerous studies in neuroscience and medicine, their manual dissection in larger cohorts from diffusion MRI tractograms is time-consuming, requires expert knowledge and is hard to reproduce. Tract orientation mapping (TOM) is a novel concept that facilitates bundle-specific tractography based on a learned mapping from the original fiber orientation distribution function (fODF) peaks to a list of tract orientation maps (also abbr. TOM). Each TOM represents one of the known tracts with each voxel containing no more than one orientation vector. TOMs can act as a prior or even as direct input for tractography. We use an encoder-decoder fully-convolutional neural network architecture to learn the required mapping. In comparison to previous concepts for the reconstruction of specific bundles, the presented one avoids various cumbersome processing steps like whole brain tractography, atlas registration or clustering. We compare it to four state of the art bundle recognition methods on 20 different bundles in a total of 105 subjects from the Human Connectome Project. Results are anatomically convincing even for difficult tracts, while reaching low angular errors, unprecedented runtimes and top accuracy values (Dice). Our code and our data are openly available at https://github.com/MIC-DKFZ/TractSeg and https://zenodo.org/record/1285152, respectively. This work has previously been published at MICCAI 2018 [1].

References

1. Wasserthal J, Neher PF, Maier-Hein KH; Springer. Tract orientation mapping for bundle-specific tractography. Proc MICCAI. 2018; p. 36–44.

Segmentation of Vertebral Metastases in MRI Using an U-Net like Convolutional Neural Network

Georg Hille[1], Max Dünnwald[1], Mathias Becker[2], Johannes Steffen[1], Sylvia Saalfeld[1], Klaus Tönnies[1]

[1]Department of and Graphics, University of Magdeburg, Germany
[2]Department of Neuroradiology, University Hospital of Magdeburg, Germany
georg.hille@ovgu.de

Abstract. This study's objective was to segment vertebral metastases in diagnostic MR images by using a deep learning-based approach. Segmentation of such lesions can present a pivotal step towards enhanced therapy planning and implementation of minimally-invasive interventions like radiofrequency ablations. For this purpose, we used a U-Net-like architecture trained with 38 patient-cases. Our proposed method has been evaluated by comparison to expertly annotated lesion segmentations via Dice coefficients, sensitivity and specificity rates. While the experiments with T_1-weighted MRI images yielded promising results (average Dice score of 73.84 %), T_2-weighted images were in average rather insufficient (53.02 %). To our best knowledge, our proposed study is the first to tackle this particular issue, which limits direct comparability with related works. In respect to similar deep learning-based lesion segmentations, e.g. in liver MR images or spinal CT images, our experiments with T_1-weighted MR images show similar or in some respects superior segmentation quality.

1 Introduction

Life expectancy has been steadily increased over the last decades, promoting age-related diseases like cardiovascular diseases, as well as cancer and cancer induced malicious metastases. Beside liver and lungs, osseous metastases are the third most likely and up to two thirds of them are located in the spine [1]. Radio-frequency ablation (RFA) has been used to reduce lower back pain caused by facet osteoarithritis or osteoid osteoma and was introduced more recently to treat osseous spinal metastases [2]. Segmentation of vertebral metastases is a pivotal step towards RFA therapy planning and implementation due to the importance of assessing extent, shape and spatial relations of the metastases with risk structures, as well as to assign state-dependent tissue parameters for numerical heat dissipation simulations [3]. Additionally, pre-interventionally segmented metastases as image overlays onto the intra-operatively acquired images can enhance and speed-up RFA needle placement during interventions and therefore, may have a beneficial effect on the treatment outcome. However, segmentation of spinal metastases is time-consuming and fatiguing considering the number of image slices and sequences acquired per patient. Computer-assisted methods could relieve the workload of radiologists and reduce the time required for the therapy planning. Beside well established segmentation methods like threshold-based, region-based, classification or model-based approaches, deep learning techniques like deep convolutional neural networks (CNN) have been introduced more recently to lesion and metastasis segmentation tasks [4]. The latter focussed mainly on liver [5, 1] and brain [6, 7] lesions, both in CT and MR imaging. Recently, a deep learning-based approach for vertebral metastasis segmentation in CT imaging has been published [8].

The main objective of this work was to develop a deep learning-based method for segmenting vertebral metastases in MR imaging. Since bone tumours and metastases typically replace focal bone marrow, which can be visualized in MR imaging, we focussed on diagnostically acquired MR images of patients who underwent RF ablations of spinal metastases. These metastases are of both, sclerotic or lytic type and therefore, affect vertebrae in their shape and visibility differently. While bony structures emit similar signals in T_1- and T_2-weighted MRI sequences, metastases could differ considerably in image intensities. This tremendously complicates automatic segmentation methods. Due to its widespread applicability in medical image segmentation, we propose a U-Net-like architecture [9] to cope with the huge variety of shape, extent and appeerence of the metastastic lesions.

2   Materials and methods

2.1   Image data and pre-processing

34 patients who underwent RF-ablations of both, single or multiple vertebral metastases, were chosen retrospectively. Overall, 38 metastases were assembled for this work, originating from rena cell, prostate, cervical, kolon, pancreatic, breast, bladder, stomach, lung, caecal, urothelial and spinocellular carcinoma. For diagnostic purposes spine MR imaging was performed pre-interventionally, including sagittal native T_1- and T_2-weighted MRI sequences. The resolution of the scans varied in-plane from 0.47 to 1.25 mm, as well as in depth (3.3 to 4 mm). The acquired MRI data was pre-processed by registering cohesive MR sequences patient-wise to the respective T_1-weighted images via an automatic mutual information-driven rigid transformation, as well as by resampling each image volume to a total number of 64 sagittal slices. This was due to produce a rather isotropic spatial resolution, while maintaining a fixed image matrix size to simplify any further processing. Subsequently, each metastasis has been contoured manually by a field expert trained by neuroradiologists. Starting from the center of each segmentation, a volume of interest (VOI) with the size of $128 \times 128 \times 64$ voxels was set up and extracted from the original MR images as well as the binary ground truth images. Furthermore, every VOI was whitened by subtracting the mean intensity from every voxel value and a subsequent division

by the standard deviation. Since our data set is comparably small for a deep learning-based approach, each of the 38 metastases has been augmented 25 times, yielding in total 950 samples. In detail the images were rotated between $\pm 25°$ around the center of volume in z-direction. Furthermore, each image was enlarged or shrunk within a range of $\pm 30\%$ as well as translated in all directions by a random value between ± 42 pixels in x- and y-direction and ± 21 pixels in z-direction, thus approximately a third of each dimension's extent. Finally, random flips were applied with a 75 % probability overall and 50 % for each direction, i.e. horizontal, vertical and in depth.

2.2   Network architecture

We used a smaller version of the U-Net [9] network architecture with 15 convolutional layers and only 3 instead of 4 poolings (Fig. 3). Furthermore, we replaced up-convolutions by simplified upsampling layers, which have been found to be equally effective, while being less computationally expensive [10]. Each convolution had a kernel size of $3 \times 3 \times 3$ with the exception of last one, which applies an $1 \times 1 \times 1$ kernel to reduce the dimensionality to the desired output size, i.e. the size of the input image. A Rectified Linear Unit (ReLU) was used as the activation function for all convolutional layers, except the last one again, where a sigmoid function was applied to provide values between 0 and 1. Training was done for 25 epochs and a fuzzy Dice coefficient was used as a loss function. Furthermore, we used Adam as an optimizer with a starting learning rate of 0.001 and a mini batch size of 2 samples. Finally, a threshold of 0.5 was applied to produce binary output images. The CNN hyperparameters were set empirically by preliminary experiments.

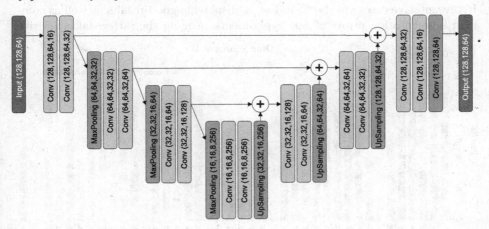

Fig. 1. U-Net-like architecture for segmentation of vertebral metastases in T_1- or T_2-weighted MR images. The dimension of each layer is defined as width, height, depth and channels.

2.3   Evaluation

Expertly annotated lesion segmentations were produced considering both registered MR sequences of each patient within a synchronized viewer. Due to comparability with related segmentation works and the similarity to clinical evaluation methods, we chose Dice coefficients as a volume overlapping measure of automatically segmented structures and expertly contoured lesions, as well as sensitivity and specificity rates. For evaluation purposes 8-fold-cross validation was performed. Each subset contained 4-5 original volumes as well as their patient-wise augmentation. Overall 8 runs with varying subsets were carried out yielding Dice scores, calculated on the original image data.

3   Results

The Dice scores of automatic and expert segmentations were average $73.84 \pm 16.94\%$ for the T_1-weighted and $53.02 \pm 24.33\%$ for the T_2-weighted data, respectively (Fig. 4). Overall the metastases segmentation in T_1-weighted MRI sequences yielded significantly better results with average 20.51% higher Dice scores and only one sample (case 23) with $< 1\%$ lower quality. For the experiments with T_1-weighted image data the average sensitivity rate was $77.8 \pm 16.5\%$ and the specificity rate was $98.5 \pm 1.3\%$, while the results for T_2-weighted images yielded overall more inaccurate results with $65.1 \pm 30.3\%$ (sensitivity rate) and $95.5 \pm 4.7\%$ (specificity rate).

4   Discussion

Representative cases are shown in Fig. 3, displaying good results as well as common segmentation errors of our experiments. Among the latter, false positive

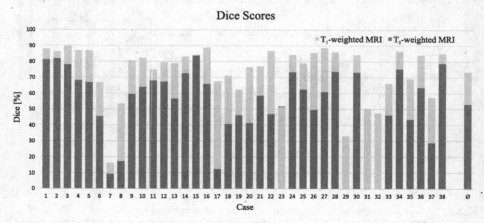

Fig. 2. Dice scores for each patient and MRI sequence. Our data set contained lytic and sclerotic metastases, which influences their appearance, e.g. intensity and texture, especially within T_2-weighted images.

classified pixels, often most prominent in the marginal space, which contains multiple tissues and therefore, varying intensities and inaccurate segmentations at the transverse and spinous processes are the most common. A greater loss of quality was produced by exceptionally shaped metastases, especially if they were not roughly starconvex. This was very likely due to the fact that the required level of shape variance was not represented by the training set. Compared to the network that has been fed with T_1-weighted images, our experiments with T_2-weighted MR data performed worse most of the time. We assume this was caused by the metastases appearances in this particular modality. While in T_1-weighted images the metastases presented themselves hypointense compared with surrounding non-metastatic bone tissue, they appeared either hypo-, iso- or hyperintese and even with mixed intensity and texture distribution in the T_2-weighted sequences. Again, this level of appearance variance may not been represented by our comparatively small training set.

It is rather difficult to compare our results with related works, since there are to our best knowledge no studies regarding vertebral metastases segmentation in MR imaging. Thus, comparison is rather indirect and refers to CNN-based segmentation approaches for instance of liver and brain tumors, as well as a recently published work by Chmelik et al. [8] for spinal CT data. Depending on the used data sets, CNN-based brain tumor segmentations in MR images achieved Dice scores up to 88 % [6] or 84.7 % [7]. Segmented liver tumors in MR images achieved Dice values of 69.7 % [5], in CT images up to 72.2 % [11]. Overall, our results on T_1-weighted spinal MR images are similar to the related segmentation accuracies of liver lesions, although our data base was comparatively small (34 patient cases vs. 200 cases in [11]), which is also reflected in the rather high standard deviation of our results. Chmelik et al. [8] were one of the first to adapt a

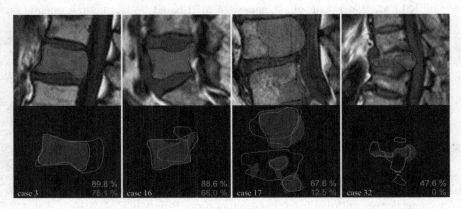

Fig. 3. Comparison of the expertly annotated data (green) with our automatically produced segmentations on T_1- (blue) and T_2-weighted MR images (red) for exemplary cases. Case 3 and 16 represent our best results, which were achieved with T_1-weighted images. Most of our insufficient results (like case 17 and 32) indicated, that the weaker the shape or appearance variance is represented in the training set, the more likely the accuracy of the segmentation decreases.

CNN to vertebral metastases segmentation in CT images. They achieved a voxel-wise sensitivity rate of 74 % for sclerotic and 71 % for lytic lesions as well as a specificity rate of 88 % (sclerotic) and 82 % (lytic). In comparison, our results with the T_1-weighted images are somewhat better, though the experiments with T_2-weighted images lack accuracy. Nevertheless, it is important not to neglect the differences in spatial resolution (slice thickness of 0.67 mm vs. our average 3.50 mm) and the effects of high spatial anisotropy.

To summarize, we presented a CNN-based segmentation approach for metastases of the spine in diagnostic MR images. Although, only an approximate classification of our results with reference to related work is possible, our experiments yielded a quality similar for instance to the state-of-the-art in liver lesion segmentation. Our results with T_1-weighted MR images indicate good potential to automatically segment cancerous structures in spinal MR images, while the results on T_2-weighted MR data were not satisfactory. In further experiments we will investigate the influences of the combination of different MR sequences.

Acknowledgement. This work was supported by the German Ministry of Education and Research (13GW0095A) within the *STIMULATE* research campus.

References

1. Harrington K. Metastatic disease of the spine. JBJS. 1986;68:1110–1115.
2. Dupuy DE, Liu D, Hartfeil D, et al. Percutaneous radiofrequency ablation of painful osseous metastases. Cancer. 2010;116:989–997.
3. Kröger T, Pätz T, Altrogge I, et al. Fast estimation of the vascular cooling in RFA based on numerical simulation. Open Biomed Eng J. 2010;4.
4. Liu J, Li M, Wang J, et al. A survey of MRI-based brain tumor segmentation methods. Tsinghua Sci Technol. 2014;19(6):578–595.
5. Christ PF, Ettlinger F, Grün F, et al. Automatic liver and tumor segmentation of ct and mri volumes using cascaded fully convolutional neural networks. arXiv:170205970. 2017;.
6. Havaei M, Davy A, Warde-Farley D, et al. Brain tumor segmentation with deep neural networks. Med Image Anal. 2017;35:18–31.
7. Kamnitsas K, Ledig C, Newcombe VF, et al. Efficient multi-scale 3D CNN with fully connected CRF for accurate brain lesion segmentation. Med Image Anal. 2017;36:61–78.
8. Chmelik J, Jakubicek R, Walek P, et al. Deep convolutional neural network-based segmentation and classification of difficult to define metastatic spinal lesions in 3D CT data. Med Image Anal. 2018;49:76–88.
9. Çiçek Ö, Abdulkadir A, Lienkamp SS, et al.; Springer. 3D U-Net: learning dense volumetric segmentation from sparse annotation. Proc MICCAI. 2016; p. 424–432.
10. Isensee F, Kickingereder P, Bonekamp D, et al. Brain tumor segmentation using large receptive field deep convolutional neural networks. Proc BVM. 2017; p. 86–91.
11. Li X, Chen H, Qi X, et al. H-DenseUNet: hybrid densely connected UNet for liver and liver tumor segmentation from CT volumes. arXiv:170907330. 2017;.

Synthetic Training with Generative Adversarial Networks for Segmentation of Microscopies

Jens Krauth[1,2], Stefan Gerlach[1], Christian Marzahl[1], Jörn Voigt[1], Heinz Handels[2]

[1]Research Development Projects, EUROIMMUN Medizinische Labordiagnostika AG
[2]Institut für Medizinische Informatik, Universität zu Lübeck
jenskrauth@gmail.com

Abstract. Medical imaging is often burdened with small available annotated data. In case of supervised deep learning algorithms a large amount of data is needed. One common strategy is to augment the given dataset for increasing the amount of training data. Recent researches show that the generation of synthetic images is a possible strategy to expand datasets. Especially, generative adversarial networks (GAN)s are promising candidates for generating new annotated training images. This work combines recent architectures of Generative Adversarial Networks in one pipeline to generate medical original and segmented image pairs for semantic segmentation. Results of training a U-Net with incorporated synthetic images as addition to common data augmentation are showing a performance boost compared to training without synthetic images from 77.99 % to 80.23 % average Jaccard Index.

1 Introduction

In many imaging domains and especially medical imaging only limited number of segmented and annotated data is available. In case of supervised machine learning this often leads to restricted performance of algorithms. Particularly, deep learning algorithms require big training datasets to perform well on unseen data. One effective way for extending a given training dataset is image augmentation, which has given a significant performance boost in deep learning [1]. Recent methods like generative adversarial networks (GANs) [2] for generating new image data become more popular. Frid-Adar et al. [3] have proven that synthetic generated images by GANs can lead to improved accuracy in classification tasks.

The contribution of this work is extending the idea of generating synthetic images for classification by generating an image pair of ground truth segmentation and corresponding image for segmentation tasks. These image pairs can be used as training samples for deep learning algorithms in addition to traditional data augmentation. The used dataset is a dataset of fluorescence microscopy images of esophagus of a monkey containing 137 training and 37 test images. Segmentation of esophagus is defined by segmenting the appearing tissue sections (Fig. 1). The spatial resolution of the images is 4656 times 3692 pixel and is down sampled to 512 times 512 pixel for segmentation.

Fig. 1. Samples of esophagus in first row and corresponding human annotated segmentation in second row. The segments are longitudinal muscle (blue), circular muscle (red), muscularis mucosae (dark green), eptihelium (pink).

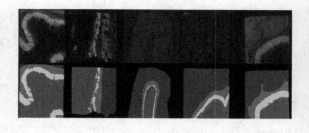

2   Materials and methods

The used pipeline consists of combination of wasserstein GAN [4] and Stack-GAN [5] for creating synthetic microscopy images and ground truth segmentation masks. The last step of the pipeline is a pix2pixHD GAN [6] for Image-to-Image translation of ground truth segmentation to esophagus microscopy images.

2.1   Generative adversarial networks

Goodfellow et al. [2] introduced Generative Adversarial Networks as two networks, namely generator (G) and discriminator (D) which are trained against each other. The generator gets an input noise variable $p_z(z)$ as input and tries to generate samples which are close to the ground truth data distribution p_{data}. The discriminator is a two class classifier which either gets an original or generated image as input and is trained to separate fake and original images. This can mathematically be defined as

$$\min_G \max_D V(D, G) = \mathbb{E}_{x \sim p_{\text{data}}(x)}[\log D(x)] + \mathbb{E}_{z \sim p_z(z)}[\log(1 - D(G(z)))] \quad (1)$$

and states a two-player minimax game. The second term $\mathbb{E}_{z \sim p_z(z)}[\log(1 - D(G(z)))]$ can saturate in early training stages due to high confidence of D while G generates samples near random noise. Therefore instead of minimizing $\log(1 - D(g(z)))$ maximizing $\log(D(G(z)))$ is leading to much stronger gradients in early stages of training.

Wasserstein GANs [4] are an extension to GANs which stabilizing the training procedure of GANs. It can be shown, that the optimal generator is minimizing the Jensen Shannon Divergence [2]. The JSD as divergence function is not a good cost function when learning data distributions supported by low dimensional manifolds [4]. Therefore the wasserstein distance or earthmover distance (EM) $W(\mathbb{P}_r, \mathbb{P}_g) = \inf_{\gamma \in \prod(\mathbb{P}_r, \mathbb{P}_g)} \mathbb{E}_{(x,y) \sim \gamma}[||x - y||]$ can be used instead. With help of the Kantorvich-Rubinstein duality the EM can be derived to Wasserstein loss

$$\max_{||f||_L \leq 1} \mathbb{E}_{x \sim \mathbb{P}_r}[f(x)] - \mathbb{E}_{x \sim \mathbb{P}_\theta}[f(x)] \quad (2)$$

which can be used as loss function for GANs. Notice that now f has to be 1-Lipschitz. To enforce this Lipschitz constraint weight clipping is one possible solution, but can result in long training times or vanishing gradients. The discriminator can be trained without unstable training since the EM is continuous and differentiable always everywhere. Since weight clipping leads also to capacity underuse of parameters and is not the most sufficient way to enforce the Lipschitz constraint, Gulrajani et al. [7] are introducing a gradient penalty term without these major drawbacks.

2.2 StackGAN

StackGAN [5] is a Framework of two separate GANs which operates on two stages. It transforms text descriptions into photo-realistic images. Therefore in the first stage a text embedding of the description is combined with the latent vector and given into the generator. The generator will create a low resolution image of the description. Respectively, the Stage-I discriminator aims to classify fake and real images on low resolution. In Stage-II the Generator will get the low resolution image as input as well as the text embedding and create through down- and upsampling operations a high resolution image. The Stage-II discriminator now aims to distinguish between high resolution fake and real images. The Stage-II helps to refine the low resolution image and leads to much finer details.

2.3 Pix2pixHD GAN

Pix2pixHD GAN [6] is a GAN for image-to-image translation tasks. Therefore the generator of this GAN does not need a latent vector $p_z(z)$, instead it is conditioned on an input image. The generator is trained to transfer an image from one domain to another, such as label maps of segmentations to photo-realistic images. The generator consists of two networks, one which operates on full input resolution, called the local enhancer network, and one which operates on half input resolution, called the global generator network. Both networks are built of a convolutional front-end, residual blocks, and a convolutional back end. The input of the residual blocks of the local enhancer network is the element-wise sum of the last feature map of the global generator network and the feature map of the local enhancer network. The discriminator now gets two images as input, one from source domain and one from target domain. The image from target domain can either be fake or real which has to be discriminated. Also, multi-scale discriminator is used, therefore three separate discriminators which have the same architecture are operating on different image scales.

3   Results

Generating synthetic training data for semantic segmentation requires label maps, with 6 labels in our case, and corresponding real world domain images. Therefore a pipeline of two sequential networks was build. The first network is a StackGAN-like network which generates synthetic label maps. The second network is the pix2pixHD GAN which is trained to generate esophagus microscopy images from label maps.

Fig. 2. StackGAN results with
the low resolution image and
refined high resolution image.

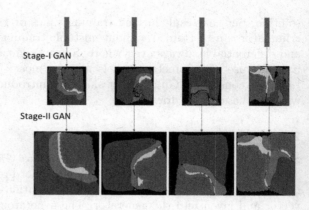

3.1 Generating label maps for esophagus

The Stage-I generator gets an 100 dimensional latent vector $p_z(z)$ as input and upsamples the spatial resolution by repeating convolutional blocks consisting of Transposed Convolutional Layer, Batchnorm and ReLU activation. The initial filter size is 2048 which is halfed in every convolutional block. The result of the first convolutional block has spatial resolution of 4x4 pixel. Every other convolutional block doubles the spatial dimension until 256x256 pixel are reached. Hence, 7 convolutional blocks were used. The activation function of the last block is tanh. The discriminator is a classical deep convolutional network with convolutional layer and LeakyReLU as activation function.

The generated 256x256 pixel label map serves as input for the Stage-II generator. The input image is down sampled by four convolutional blocks of Convolutional Layer, Batchnorm and LeakyReLU as activation to a spatial size of 16x16 pixels. The result will be processed by four residual blocks and up sampled by 4 convolutional blocks consisting of transposed convolutional layer, batchnorm and ReLU activation followed by a last transposed convolution with tanh as activation. All down sampling operations are resulting in halved spatial dimension and doubled filter size, all up sampling operations in double spatial resolution and halved filter size. The result is a 512x512 pixel label map representating the ground truth label maps of the dataset (Fig. 2). Also, the discriminator of the Stage-II is a classical deep convolutional network.

Both networks were trained separately on the 137 training images, first the Stage-I GAN was trained until convergence. Afterwards, the Stage-II GAN was trained, as it uses the results of the first GAN as input. The wasserstein loss [2] with gradient penalty [7] was used as loss function.

3.2 Transfer of label maps to esophagus microscopy images

To create training data for semantic segmentation the label maps have to be transferred into real world domain, in this case to esophagus microscopy images. Therefore the reference implementation of pix2pixHD GAN [6] was used to train the image-to-image translation network on the 137 training images which were augmented by flipping, zooming and affine transformations. The result is corresponding pairs of generated ground truth label maps and microscopy image which can be used for training (Fig. 3).

3.3 Training a U-Net with synthetic image pairs

Since the synthetic image pairs shall be used as an addition to standard image augmentation, the images are used as additional training images for a neural network for semantic segmentation. Therefore a U-Net [1] was trained to segment the 6 classes (Fig. 1) only on the original data with augmentation and separately with original data with augmentation combined with synthetic data. The batch size was set to four and for each experiment, a prior rate of synthetic images per batch was set, namely 0 %, 25 %, 50 %, 75 % and 100 %. The original data got online augmented in all experiments, as well as the synthetic images are generated online if used.

For comparing the segmentation the average Jaccard Index on the 37 test images is evaluated over several training runs for each rate of synthetic images in a batch. The average Jaccard Index is defined as

$$\text{avgJC} = \frac{1}{n} \sum_{i=1}^{n} \frac{\text{true positive}_i}{\text{true positive}_i + \text{false positive}_i + \text{false negative}_i} \quad (3)$$

for each class. The results are given in (Fig. 4). Training the U-Net with traditional image augmentation (0% synthetic rate) leads to an average Jaccard Index of 77.99%. Additionally adding synthetic image pairs (25% and 50% synthetic rate) improve the segmentation performance to 80.23% and 79.75% respectively. Too many synthetic images (75% and 100% synthetic rate) are leading too much poorer segmentation results.

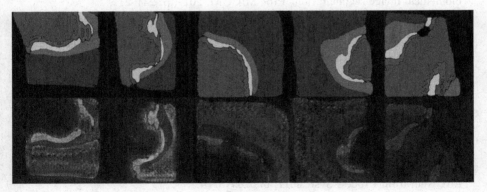

Fig. 3. Synthetic training image pairs of semantic label maps and corresponding microscopy images of esophagus.

Fig. 4. Results of average Jaccard Index of a U-Net trained on different rates of original and synthetic training images for semantic segmentation.

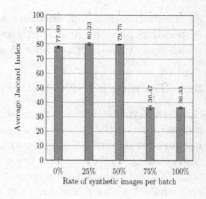

4 Discussion

We presented a pipeline for synthesizing image pairs in a medical domain for improving the data amount of small datasets for supervised learning. Comparing the synthetic (Fig. 1) and real (Fig. 3) images reveal that the label maps are generated with valid topology of tissue and characteristic shapes. The generated fluorescence microscopy images contain artifacts, but also contain typical structural features but are clearly distinguishable for human eyes. Incorporating the image pairs into training of neural networks results in improved performance. However, using too many synthetic images results in poorer performance than training without synthetic images.

References

1. Ronneberger O, Fischer P, Brox T; Springer. U-net: convolutional networks for biomedical image segmentation. Proc MICCAI. 2015; p. 234–241.
2. Goodfellow I, Pouget-Abadie J, Mirza M, et al. Generative adversarial nets. Adv Neural Inf Process Syst. 2014; p. 2672–2680.
3. Frid-Adar M, Diamant I, Klang E, et al. GAN-based synthetic medical image augmentation for increased CNN Performance in Liver Lesion Classification. CoRR. 2018;abs/1803.01229.
4. Arjovsky M, Chintala S, Bottou L. Wasserstein generative adversarial networks. Proc 34th Int Conf Mach Learn. 2017;70:214–223.
5. Zhang H, Xu T, Li H, et al. StackGAN: text to photo-realistic image synthesis with stacked generative adversarial networks. CoRR. 2016;abs/1612.03242.
6. Wang T, Liu M, Zhu J, et al. High-resolution image synthesis and semantic manipulation with conditional GANs. CoRR. 2017;abs/1711.11585.
7. Gulrajani I, Ahmed F, Arjovsky M, et al. Improved training of Wasserstein gans. Adv Neural Inf Process Syst. 2017; p. 5769–5779.

Gradient-Based Expanding Spherical Appearance Models for Femoral Model Initialization in MRI

Duc Duy Pham[1], Gurbandurdy Dovletov[1], Sebastian Warwas[2],
Stefan Landgraeber[2], Marcus Jäger[2], Josef Pauli[1]

[1]Intelligent Systems, Faculty of Engineering, University of Duisburg-Essen, Germany
[2]Department of Orthopedics and Trauma Surgery, University Hospital Essen,
University of Duisburg-Essen, Germany
duc.duy.pham@uni-due.de

Abstract. While deep learning strategies for semantic segmentation increasingly take center stage, traditional approaches seem to take a backseat. However, in the domain of medical image processing, labeled training data is rare and expensive to acquire. Thus, traditional methods may still be preferable to deep learning approaches. Many of these conventional approaches often require initial localization of the structure of interest (SOI) to provide satisfactory results. In this work we present a fully automatic model initialization approach in MRI, that is applicable for anatomical structures that contain a near-spherical component. We propose a model, that encapsulates the difference between intensity distribution within the SOI's spherical component and its proximity. We present our approach on the example of femoral model initialization and compare our initialization results to a diffeomorphic demons registration approach.

1 Introduction

In modern medicine, especially in the domain of orthopedics and trauma surgery, 3D models are helpful tools to aid in preoperative planning and to design prosthetics, tailored specifically to the patient's needs. The human hip joint in particular is a structure of interest, as it carries a major portion of the body weight, therefore being naturally prone to physical deterioration. Patient-specific models allow simulations of joint movements and the detection of possible points of friction. For these kind of simulations, first the 3D models need to be generated by segmenting the anatomical structures of interest (SOI). While deep learning approaches are current topics of research, usually a large amount of training data is required to train them. Even in the context of transfer learning, one needs to consider the availability of pretrained models and the additional amount of fine tuning data. Therefore we argue, that Active Shape Models, Active Appearance Models, and Active Contours such as Snakes and Level Set methods are still relevant traditional approaches for solving the segmentation problem.

The segmentation quality of these methods, however, heavily depends on their initialization. While these methods have been extended for better segmentation results in numerous ways, research regarding model initialization has been receiving reasonably less attention. Li et al. [1] propose a Poisson inverse gradient approach, which is however restricted to the initialization of Active Contours. Younes et al.'s approach [2] in first detecting the SOI by primitive shapes recognition in 3D CT data to apply deformable shape models afterwards, is similar to our requirement of the SOI containing a spherical component. Pham et al. [3] propose an appearance model, in which the intensity distribution of the SOI in the euclidean space is combined with the boundary appearance in polar space in an axial slice-wise manner. In this work we present a 3D localization strategy, taking into account the highly correlated nature of the 2D slices, and propose an appearance model based initialization approach, applicable for anatomical structures that contain a near-spherical component.

2   Materials and methods

In the following, our proposed initialization approach by means of the based Expanding Spherical Appearance Model (GESAM) is described. Afterwards, the evaluation details are outlined.

2.1   GESAM

We propose a three stage model initialization method, that robustly approximates the location of the SOI's near-spherical component and expands to the SOI's remaining area, estimating the orientation of the SOI. The first stage consists of training the based Expanding Spherical Appearance Model (GESAM) in a Principal Component Analysis manner, whereas the second stage uses the trained model to robustly localize the near-spherical component of the SOI. In the final stage, the estimated location is used as the initial region to expand to the remaining SOI by a simple Level Set approach, which is, however, restricted by the MRI's gradient information.

Training Let $\mathcal{A}_1, \ldots \mathcal{A}_N$ denote N atlases, where the i-th atlas consists of a MRI volume $\mathcal{I}_i$ with voxel size $(1 \times 1 \times 1)\text{mm}^3$ and a label volume $\mathcal{L}_i$, i.e. $\mathcal{A}_i := (\mathcal{I}_i, \mathcal{L}_i)$ For each atlas the near-spherical component is approximated by a sphere. Let r_i be the radius of the fitted sphere in $\mathcal{L}_i$, then an encapsulating spherical outer neighborhood of the sphere can be extracted, such that the volume of the outer neighborhood is equal to the sphere volume. The outer neighborhood can be visualized as the volume difference between a larger sphere, surrounding the fitted smaller sphere. With this outer boundary, the normalized intensity distributions with a fixed amount of n_{bins} intensity values inside and outside of the sphere can be modeled by means of two vectors $w_i^{in}, w_i^{out} \in [0, 1]^{n_{bins}}$ To reduce the effects of global intensity changes, the derivatives of inner and outer intensity distributions are considered and concatenated to a joint feature vector $\tilde{w}_i$ of length $2(n_{bins} - 1)$ With the feature vectors of all training data, dimensionality reduction by means of Principal Component Analysis (PCA) yields a matrix $\mathcal{E}_{\tilde{v}} := (\tilde{v}_1, \ldots, \tilde{v}_{n_{PCA}})$ containing $n_{PCA} < n_{bins}$ eigenvectors and a set with the corresponding eigenvalues $\mathcal{S}_\lambda := \{\lambda_1, \ldots, \lambda_{n_{PCA}}\}$ With the mean inner and outer derivative intensity distribution $\overline{w} := \frac{1}{N} \sum_i^N \tilde{w}_i$, the maximal and minimal radius r_{max}, r_{min} in mm of the fitted spheres, and the standard deviation σ_r of the sphere radii, the Spherical Appearance Model is defined as

$$\mathcal{M} := (\mathcal{E}_{\tilde{v}}, \mathcal{S}_\lambda, \overline{w}, r_{\max}, r_{\min}, \sigma_r)$$

Localization The next stage of our proposed method deals with the initial localization of the near-spherical component. We propose a RANSAC like fitting scheme, i.e. a hypothesis-verification strategy, in which the number of samples, which generate the hypothesis, is kept minimal. In this case the hypothesis is a distinct sphere candidate, specified by a minimal sample set of four image coordinates. For computational efficiency we constrain the sample domain to those voxels with a feasible gradient magnitude, after regularizing with a simple Gaussian filter. Let $\mathcal{I}$ denote the 3D MRI, then the constrained sample domain is implied by the binary volume

$$\mathcal{I}_\nabla := \begin{cases} 1, & \text{if } |\nabla\{\mathcal{I} * \mathcal{G}\}| \geq m \\ 0, & \text{else} \end{cases}$$

where ∇ is the gradient operator, $\mathcal{G}$ denotes a Gaussian kernel, and m represents the mean value of all positive values in $|\nabla\{\mathcal{I} * \mathcal{G}\}|$ Since anatomical structures that contain spherical components are the objects of interest, it is possible to further restrict the sampling domain, by only keeping those image points, that are most likely part of the SOI's spherical component. We propose applying 2D Hough transforms on each axial, frontal, and sagital image slice to extract the $n_{circles}$ most probable circles, respectively. The intersection of circles with different spatial orientation yields voxel coordinates that presumably address spherical structures. For the 2D circle detections the minimal and maximal radii, and the standard deviation $r_{min}, r_{max}, \sigma_r$ from the GESAM can be used to limit the radius range of the 2D Hough transforms to $[r_{min} - \frac{\sigma_r}{2}, r_{max} + \frac{\sigma_r}{2}]$ Let $\mathcal{I}_\circ$ denote the binary volume, containing the most probable aforementioned intersections. Then the Hadamard product $\mathcal{I}_{\nabla,\circ} := \mathcal{I}_\nabla \cdot \mathcal{I}_\circ$ contains image points that both have a strong gradient and also probably contribute to a feasible sphere hypothesis. We will refer to any image point p in $\mathcal{I}_{\nabla,\circ}$ that has value $\mathcal{I}_{\nabla,\circ}(p) = 1$ as *feasible sample point*. With the drastically reduced sample set in $\mathcal{I}_{\nabla,\circ}$, we propose a structured sampling approach, to ensure the suggestion of promising sphere candidates. For each k_{sample}-th feasible sample point p, with $k_{\text{sample}} \geq 1$, a 3D sampling cube with width $r_{max} + \frac{\sigma_r}{2}$ is spanned around p. From this restricted sampling cube three additional feasible sample points are randomly chosen to propose a sphere candidate. This process is repeated until at least a minimal number of spheres $n_{sp} \geq 1$ with a radius within the range $[r_{min} - \frac{\sigma_r}{2}, r_{max} + \frac{\sigma_r}{2}]$ is proposed. If this is not possible, a maximum number of subsequent non-sufficient proposals $n_{nsp} \geq 1$ ensures termination. In the same manner as for the GESAM, a feature vector w can be computed by means of concatenating the derivatives of inner and outer intensity distributions for each of the sphere proposals. Instead of only using the feasible sample points within an ϵ-environment of the sphere (inliers) as selection criterion, we propose utilizing the weighted distance s of the feature vector w to $\overline{w}$ in eigenspace, i.e. $s := \sum_{i=1}^{n_{PCA}} \frac{1}{\lambda_i} \left(\tilde{v}_i^T \cdot (w - \overline{w}) \right)^2$ This distance can be incorporated into a weighted cost function, which may also consider additional features such as homogeneity, variance and further statistics of the volume intensities within the sphere. However, the distance s in eigenspace should be strongly weighted to exploit the discriminative property of the GESAM for multiple near-spherical objects within the image. In our experiments we use homogeneity and variance and weight s with a factor of 10. The sphere with minimal cost is finally selected as the localization approximation of the SOI's near-spherical component.

Expansion The third stage deals with the expansion of the detected near-spherical component into the remaining SOI to determine its spatial orientation. This is achieved by a simplified region based Level Set approach [4], in which gradient information of the volume is used to heavily restrict the expansion to stay within the SOI. Instead of applying the standard Chan Vese Level Set approach on the original MRI data set, we propose utilizing a dilated version of $\mathcal{I}_\nabla$. This simplification of the image volume ensures the expanded area to stay within the bounds of the SOI. Thus, strong gradients serve as boundaries of the expansion, strengthened by the previous dilation. The located sphere from the localization stage serves as initial contour of the Level Set approach. To increase computational efficiency, $\mathcal{I}_\nabla$ can be resized to a smaller resolution and reducing the initial contour's radius ensures initialization within the SOI.

2.2   Evaluation

We evaluated our method on the example of femoral model initialization and compared our results to the initializations achieved by a 3D multi-atlas diffeomorphic demons registration (MADDR) [5] implementation in MATLAB. The respective ground truths have been validated by clinical experts. In the T1-weighted MR images only the proximal part of the femur is captured with partly very different field of views (FOVs). We denote the data sets as P1,...,P6 and label the post operative data sets as P1PO and P2PO. In a leave-one-out cross validation manner for each patient data set, the atlases of the respective other patients were used for training the GESAM and for the multi-atlas approach. We use the Dice Similarity Coefficient (DSC) to measure and compare the localization quality. In the multi-atlas approach simple majority voting was conducted on the normalized summation of the transformed label images. For each data set, the threshold $t \in \{0.1, 0.2, \ldots, 1.0\}$ resulting in the best DSC was chosen to compare to our GESAM results. In the training stage, we set n_{bins} to 20. For preprocessing in the localization stage we set $n_{circles}$ to 10 circles in each slice.

Table 1. DSCs from multi-atlas initialization method (MADDR) compared to the proposed GESAM approach before (GESAM$_1$) and after expansion (GESAM$_2$).

	P1	P1PO	P2	P2PO	P3	P4	P5	P6	$\emptyset$
DSC [%]									
MADDR	30.99	28.99	30.35	26.11	29.67	27.99	21.98	28.84	28.11±2.06
GESAM$_1$	42.05	45.83	49.89	46.74	43.35	48.90	40.68	38.05	44.44±3.40
GESAM$_2$	73.34	74.76	76.87	75.10	76.34	76.26	72.82	75.10	75.07±1.08
Time [s]									
MADDR	638.35	729.52	801.42	954.86	798.38	798.45	960.68	961.78	830.43±96.51
GESAM$_2$	96.87	109.18	101.75	122.81	115.36	112.83	125.47	109.30	111.69±7.42

For the proposed structured sampling method we determined k_{sample}, such that about 500 feasible sample points remain in $\mathcal{I}_{\nabla,\circ}$ and we found $n_{sp} = 10$ and $n_{nsp} = 10$ to be sufficient termination parameters. In the expansion stage we reduced the volume resolution to a factor of 0.5 in each dimension for the Level Set approach, and initialized with the located sphere reduced to half of the estimated radius.

3   Results

Tab. 1 shows the resulting DSCs and the measured computation time for each data set, comparing the multi-atlas localization quality with the achieved results of our proposed GESAM approach before and after the expansion stage. An average DSC of 28.11 ± 2.89% is achieved by the multi-atlas approach, which is surpassed by the GESAM with a mean DSC of 44.44±4.12% before the expansion stage and 75.07±1.08% after expansion. It is noticeable that in all data sets the multi-atlas approach is already outperformed by our proposed GESAM method before expansion. We measured an average computation time of 830.43±119.32s for the multi-atlas approach and a mean computation time of 111.69 ± 9.70s for the complete GESAM including expansion stage. It can be observed that while the registrations show a high variance in computation time, depending on the data set, the GESAM approach's localization time is comparatively consistent.

4   Discussion

The results show a significant improvement regarding computation time and initialization quality, as can be also observed in the exemplary initialization results in Fig. 1. While the initialization region of the registration approach fails to approximate the location of the proximal femur (Fig. 1(a)), the localization stage of our method already proposes a close estimation of the femur's spherical component (Fig. 1(b)). The following expansion stage gives additional information about the spatial orientation of the femoral bone (Fig. 1(c)). Using gradient information to restrict the expansion area to stay within the SOI boundary,

Fig. 1. From left to right: Exemplary initialization results of the multi-atlas approach (blue) and the GESAM approach before (yellow) and after (orange) expansion stage, each overlayed with ground truth (green).

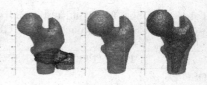

however, results in the SOI never being completely captured by the expansion stage. Nevertheless, since the aim is merely a rough approximation of the femur location, not capturing the whole SOI is preferred to leaking into other anatomical structures. The multi-atlas method's poor performance may be due to the different FOVs of the MRI data sets. This hypothesis is supported by Fig. 1(a), in which it is clearly visible that the registration result still resembles the femoral bone, which is missing a large portion of the femur shaft, as the inconsistency of the FOV might increase the difficulty of the registration problem. In this contribution, we present an appearance model approach, namely the GESAM, that incorporates modeling the normalized intensity distributions of the SOI's spherical component and its proximity. After locating the spherical component with a structured sampling strategy, a Level Set based expansion stage, restricted by the MRI's gradient information, is finally applied to estimate the remaining area of the SOI. The resulting area can then be used to fit a model template into the 3D MRI. The fitted template can be utilized for subsequent segmentation techniques, e.g. Active Contours. On the example of femoral model initialization, we validated that our proposed method outperforms a non-rigid multi-atlas demons registration approach on whole MRI volumes, especially in the context of strongly varying FOVs. In the future, we would like to investigate our approach on the application of other anatomical structures that show near-spherical components, such as humerus, bladder, spleen or prostate. We are aiming to improve the robustness of the localization stage by incorporating more expert knowledge into the structured sampling process and involving a learning based cost function for the localization stage.

References

1. Li B, Acton ST. Automatic active model initialization via poisson inverse gradient. IEEE Trans Image Process. 2008;17(8):1406–1420.
2. Younes LB, Nakajima Y, Saito T. Fully automatic segmentation of the femur from 3D-CT images using primitive shape recognition and statistical shape models. Int J Comput Assist Radiol Surg. 2014;9(2):189–196.
3. Pham DD, Morariu CA, , et al. Polar appearance models: a fully automatic approach for femoral model initialization in MRI. Proc ISBI. 2018;.
4. Chan TF, Vese LA. Active contours without edges. IEEE Trans Image Process. 2001;10(2):266–277.
5. Vercauteren T, Pennec X, Perchant A, et al. Diffeomorphic demons: efficient non-parametric image registration. NeuroImage. 2009;45(1):S61–S72.

Deep Segmentation Refinement with Result-Dependent Learning
A Double U-Net for Hip Joint Segmentation in MRI

Duc Duy Pham[1], Gurbandurdy Dovletov[1], Sebastian Warwas[2],
Stefan Landgraeber[2], Marcus Jäger[2], Josef Pauli[1]

[1]Intelligent Systems, Faculty of Engineering, University of Duisburg-Essen, Germany
[2]Department of Orthopedics and Trauma Surgery, University Hospital Essen,
University of Duisburg-Essen, Germany
duc.duy.pham@uni-due.de

Abstract. In this contribution, we propose a 2D deep segmentation refinement approach, that is inspired by the U-Net architecture and incorporates result-dependent loss adaptation. The performance of our method regarding segmentation quality is evaluated on the example of hip joint segmentation in T1-weighted MRI data sets. The results are compared to an ordinary U-Net implementation. While the segmentation quality of the proximal femur does not significantly change, our proposed method shows promising improvements for the segmentation of the pelvic bone complex, which shows more shape variability in the 2D image slices along the longitudinal axis.

1 Introduction

In orthopedics and trauma surgery, bone segmentations can aid in diagnosis, preoperative planning, and patient-specific prosthetics design. Although bones are often more distinguishable from their background in CT scans, segmentation approaches in MR images need to be further investigated, as CT scans require patients to be exposed to radiation, which can be harmful, especially for young patients. The human hip joint is a particular structure of interest, as it carries a major portion of the body and is at risk to physical deformations, such as femoroacetabular impingements. As manual segmentation is usually a tedious and time consuming task, where expert knowledge is required, automated approaches are a fast and cost-efficient alternative. Regarding hip joint segmentation there have already been several contributions. Chu et al. [1] employ random forests for landmark detection, and multi-atlantes and articulated statistical shape models for segmentation, yielding a fully automatic hip joint segmentation approach for CT scans. Xia et al. [2] compare multi-atlas-based methods to Active Shape Model based approaches for hip joint segmentation from MR images, and Chandra et al. [3] extend Active Shape Models to Focused Shape Models. This is a weighted shape learning approach, in which predefined areas of importance are weighted more heavily than unimportant shape regions, ordering the shape representation towards these relevant areas, in order to segment the hip joint with focus on cartilage from 3D MR images. With the success of deep learning approaches in the biomedical domain, Klein et al. [4] take a broader approach and investigate the general bone segmentation capabilities of deep learning methodologies by slightly modifying Ronneberger et al.'s U-Net architecture [5] for whole body segmentations in CT images. Regarding deep segmentation refinement, our contribution shows similarity to Ravishankar et al.'s work [6] in the architectural aspect, as their construction also yields two Encoder-Decoder modules, which are nevertheless trained separately. Newell et al. [7] propose a similar concept of stacked hourglass modules for human pose estimation. Main differences regarding architecture lie in the arbitrary number of hourglass modules, their use of residual blocks and the. The use of intermediate supervision between modules is comparable to our approach. To this end, we propose a 2D end-to-end double U-Net architecture, that is trained by minimizing a result dependent loss function.

2   Materials and methods

In the following, our proposed deep refinement approach by means of a double U-Net architecture is described. Afterwards, the evaluation details are outlined.

2.1   Deep segmentation refinement

Our proposed network topology is based on Ronneberger et al.'s successful U-Net architecture [5]. As can be seen in Fig. 1, our network is a Fully Convolutional Network, consisting of two U-Net modules. The first U-Net module aims at segmenting the input image, whereas the second module's task is to refine the first module's segmentation output. The segmentation module is only a slight alteration of the original U-Net, as it uses two subsequent Convolutional Layers in

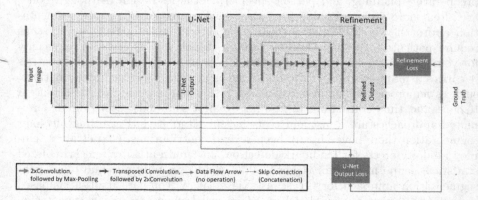

Fig. 1. Our double U-Net architecture consists of a first U-Net module for segmentation and a second U-Net module for refinement, that additionally receives skip connections from the previous module.

each resolution level, and starts with 16 convolutional kernels in the first resolution level instead of 64. Furthermore, we use padded convolutions to receive
segmentation outputs, that are of the same size as the input. We choose a kernel
size of 10×10 for every convolutional layer and 2×2 max-pooling. The second
module is composed in the same way as the segmentation module, except for
the decoding component. By means of additional skip connections from the first
module's encoder, we equip the refinement decoder component with the hierarchical features, extracted from the input image by the segmentation module. We
argue that this extension allows the second module to learn more context-aware
refinements. We use the Dice Similarity Coefficient (DSC) to formulate a loss
function $\mathcal{L}_{\text{unet}}$ for the segmentation output of the first U-Net module and a loss
function $\mathcal{L}_{\text{refine}}$ for the segmentation output of the refinement module. For both
loss functions the respective module outputs O_{unet} and O_{refine} are evaluated by
means of the DSC and the corresponding ground truth (GT). The resulting DSC
is subtracted from 1, leading to loss values in the range $[0, 1]$, i.e

$$\mathcal{L}_{\text{unet/refine}} := 1 - \frac{2 \cdot \sum_p GT(p) \cdot O_{\text{unet/refine}}(p) + \epsilon}{\sum_p GT(p) + \sum_p O_{\text{unet/refine}}(p) + \epsilon} \tag{1}$$

where $\epsilon > 0$ is a small number and p depicts a point in the output/ground truth
image. The two loss functions are combined to an overall loss function

$$\mathcal{L}_{\text{total}} := \alpha \mathcal{L}_{\text{unet}} + (1 - \alpha)\mathcal{L}_{\text{refine}} \tag{2}$$

where $\alpha \in [0, 1]$ is a weighing factor. For a result-dependent learning behavior,
we let α vary during the training process. In the beginning, it is more crucial
to adapt the weights contributing $\mathcal{L}_{\text{unet}}$ whereas optimizing the network weights
contributing to $\mathcal{L}_{\text{refine}}$ becomes relevant, once feasible segmentation results can
be expected from the segmentation module. Instead of relying only on time-
dependency, we introduce a result-dependent weighing scheme, by setting α to
the current loss of the first module $\mathcal{L}_{\text{unet}}$ The better the segmentation of the first
module, the more important becomes minimizing $\mathcal{L}_{\text{refine}}$ i.e. achieving a sufficient
refinement result. When taking the gradient of $\mathcal{L}_{\text{total}}$ during training, the U-Net
within α is not considered in our implementation.

2.2   Evaluation

We evaluated our architecture on the example of hip joint segmentation in T1-
weighted MRI and compared our results to segmentations, achieved by a separately trained U-Net topology. We used eight hip joint MRI data sets, approved
by our institution's ethics committee, comprising six different patients. For two
of these patients, MRI scans were obtained before and after a surgical procedure. The MR images were recorded using a Siemens Magnetom Area 1,5 Tesla
MR tomograph and each volume consists of 40 to 44 axial slices. The respective
ground truths have been validated by clinical experts. We denote the data sets as
P1,...,P6 and label the post operative data sets as P1PO and P2PO. We resized

Table 1. DSC, precision and recall from a standard U-Net compared to the proposed refinement architecture for the segmentation of the proximal femur.

	P1	P1PO	P2	P2PO	P3	P4	P5	∅
DSC [%]								
U-Net	85.09	82.32	87.39	87.71	88.25	90.35	87.45	86.94±1.85
Ref-Net	84.78	78.55	78.74	91.01	90.70	91.90	87.53	86.17±4.70
Precision [%]								
U-Net	79.35	80.23	92.10	91.70	85.69	86.58	89.76	86.49±4.05
Ref-Net	82.88	68.32	95.08	94.11	88.04	90.05	81.27	85.68±7.02
Recall [%]								
U-Net	91.73	84.52	83.13	84.05	90.97	94.45	85.25	87.73±3.99
Ref-Net	86.77	92.38	67.19	88.11	93.52	93.83	94.85	88.09±6.35

the MRI slices to an input size of 128×128 The experiments were conducted in a leave-one-out cross validation manner, in which one data set is kept for testing, and the remaining data sets were used for training. In case of P1, P1PO, P2, and P2PO only those data sets were used for training, which do not correspond to the same patient. P6 was used as arbitrary validation data set to monitor the training process. We increased the number of slices by augmenting the training data by means of rotation and translation. Our architecture is implemented in Tensorflow and we ran our experiments on a NVIDIA GTX 1080 ti GPU. For training we used the Adam optimizer with a learning rate of 10^{-3} and a batch size of 4 slices, and trained our model for 40 epochs. For evaluation we use the Dice similarity coefficient (DSC), Precision, and Recall as quality metrics. These refer to the 3D segmentations, achieved by stacking the 2D outputs of our network. Since our proposed architecture outputs a multi label segmentation, we evaluate the segmentation quality of the proximal femur and the pelvic bones separately.

3 Results

Tab. 1 shows the resulting DSCs, Precision and Recall values for the segmentation of the proximal femur, comparing the standard U-Net approach with the achieved results of our proposed refinement architecture. An average DSC of $86.94 \pm 1.85\,\%$ is achieved by the standard U-Net approach, whereas our refinement architecture results in a slightly lower mean DSC of $86.17 \pm 4.70\%$ The mean precision of the U-Net is $86.49 \pm 4.05\,\%$ and the mean recall 87.73 ± 3.99 while our approach results in a lower average precision of $85.68 \pm 7.02\,\%$ and a slightly higher mean recall of $88.09 \pm 6.35\,\%$ The refinement architecture does not seem to have great impact on the segmentation quality of the femur, as the slightly worse results do not show any major differences to those, achieved by U-Net. Tab. 2 on the other hand allows insight into the cross-validation results for the segmentation of the pelvic bones, also comprising DSC, precision and recall. The average DSC is $77.31 \pm 5.09\,\%$ for the standard U-Net with a mean

Table 2. DSC, precision and recall from a standard U-Net compared to the proposed refinement architecture for the segmentation of the pelvic bones.

	P1	P1PO	P2	P2PO	P3	P4	P5	∅
DSC [%]								
U-Net	73.43	65.53	83.27	83.40	78.19	82.20	75.17	77.31±5.09
Ref-Net	76.86	75.70	83.46	83.87	81.28	87.84	78.19	81.03±3.52
Precision [%]								
U-Net	73.87	63.49	88.61	87.30	72.21	81.81	76.49	77.68±7.05
Ref-Net	76.36	78.93	89.05	88.23	79.42	83.51	71.70	81.03±5.06
Recall [%]								
U-Net	72.98	67.71	78.55	79.83	85.26	82.60	73.89	77.26±4.91
Ref-Net	77.37	72.73	78.52	79.92	83.22	92.63	85.98	81.48±4.97

precision of $77.68 \pm 7.05\,\%$ and a mean recall of $77.26 \pm 4.91\,\%$ Our proposed architecture with its result-depending learning capability yields in a mean DSC of $81.03 \pm 3.52\,\%$, an average precision of $81.03 \pm 5.06\,\%$ and a mean recall of 81.48 ± 4.97 which shows improvement in all three metrics compared to the U-Net results. It is noticeable, that in contrast to the proximal femur segmentations, our approach results in better pelvic bone segmentations for each data set regarding the DSC.

4   Discussion

For the segmentation of the proximal femur, our proposed architecture does not yield any improvements compared to the U-Net, as the U-Net does not seem to have much difficulty to extract the femur from the 2D axial slices. This may be due to the fact, that the femoral components in the axial image slices are mostly of near-spherical nature. Therefore, our refinement architecture fails to achieve further refinement to improve the segmentation. However, regarding pelvic bone segmentation, our proposed network seems to contribute to a better segmentation result, improving mean DSC, precision and recall by approximately $3-4\%$.

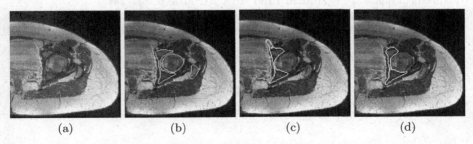

(a)   (b)   (c)   (d)

Fig. 2. (a) Exemplary axial MRI slice, (b) Ground Truth, (c) U-Net segmentation of femur (magenta) and pelvic bone (white), (d) Our segmentation of femur (magenta) and pelvic bone (white).

The pelvic bones show more variance in shape and texture appearance along the longitudinal axis, rendering the segmentation of pelvic bones a more challenging task. Fig. 2 shows exemplary segmentation results from the U-Net and our architecture, respectively, for both femur und pelvic bone. As can be observed, the femur segmentations do not show significant differences. For the pelvic bones, however, the U-Net tends to oversegment, which does not occur to this extend in our refinement architecture. The lower tendency to oversegmentation becomes also apparent in the better precision values in most data sets.

4.1   Conclusion

In this work we present a 2D end-to-end deep learning architecture with a result-dependent loss adaptation scheme. We introduced skip connections from the first segmentation module to the refinement module in our double U-Net architecture for more context-aware refinement and proposed a loss function for adaptive loss weighing. In our evaluation we could not register significant differences to the U-Net results regarding femur segmentation. However, the segmentation performance for more complex pelvic bones shows promising improvements compared to the U-Net with respect to DSC, precision and recall. In the future, we intend to incorporate this result-dependent learning approach to multi task networks for performance adaptive loss weighting of end-to-end architectures.

References

1. Chu C, Chen C, Liu L, et al. FACTS: fully automatic CT segmentation of a hip joint. Ann Biomed Eng. 2015;43(5):1247–1259.
2. Xia Y, Fripp J, Chandra SS, et al. Automated bone segmentation from large field of view 3D MR images of the hip joint. Phys Med Biol. 2013;58(20):7375.
3. Chandra SS, Xia Y, Engstrom C, et al. Focused shape models for hip joint segmentation in 3D magnetic resonance images. Med Image Anal. 2014;18(3):567–578.
4. Klein A, Warszawski J, Hillengaß J, et al. Towards whole-body CT bone segmentation. Proc BVM. 2018; p. 204–209.
5. Ronneberger O, Fischer P, Brox T; Springer. U-net: convolutional networks for biomedical image segmentation. Proc MICCAI. 2015; p. 234–241.
6. Ravishankar H, Venkataramani R, Thiruvenkadam S, et al.; Springer. Learning and incorporating shape models for semantic segmentation. Proc MICCAI. 2017; p. 203–211.
7. Newell A, Yang K, Deng J. Stacked hourglass networks for human pose estimation. Proc ECCV. 2016; p. 483–499.

Abstract: Automatic Estimation of Cochlear Duct Length and Volume Size

Ibraheem Al-Dhamari[1], Sabine Bauer[1], Dietrich Paulus[1], Rania Hilal[2], Friedrich Lissek[3], Roland Jacob[3]

[1]Koblenz and Landau University, Koblenz
[2]Germany Ain Shams University, Cairo, Egypt
[3]Military Hospital, Koblenz, Germany
idhamari@uni-koblenz.de

The exact cochlear length and size are required is an important factor of selecting the suitable cochlear implant. We present a fast cochlear length and volume size estimation method from clinical multi-modal medical images. The method utilizes atlas-model-based segmentation to estimate a transformation from a model to an input volume. The result is used to transform a well-defined segmentation and a points-set of a scala tympani to the input image that segments and estimates the scala tympani length in a few seconds using standard hardware e.g. a laptop. The method is based on automatic cochlea image registration (ACIR) [1]. The error is estimated using the known length of the cochlear implants. A dataset of 71 3D images of 21 patients from various age and gender groups is used. The estimated average scala tympani length was 29.54 mm, with 0.27 mm standard deviation. The average scala tympani volume size was 41.56 mm^3, with 0.19 mm^3 standard deviation (Fig. 1). The method is available as an open source 3D Slicer plug-in. The source code and the data can can be downloaded from a public server as described in [2].

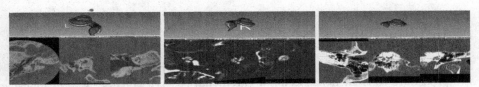

Fig. 1. Samples of segmentation results, left: CBCT, middle: MR and right: CT.

References

1. Al-Dhamari I, Bauer S, Paulus D, et al. ACIR: automatic cochlea image registration. Proc SPIE. 2017;10133(10):1–5.
2. Al-Dhamari I, Bauer S, Paulus D, et al. Automatic cochlear length and volume size estimation. OR 20 Context-Aware Oper Theaters, Comput Assist Rob Endosc. 2018; p. 54–61.

Interactive Neural Network Robot User Investigation for Medical Image Segmentation

Mario Amrehn[1], Maddalena Strumia[2], Markus Kowarschik[2], Andreas Maier[1,3]

[1]Pattern Recognition Lab, Friedrich-Alexander University
Erlangen-Nürnberg (FAU), Germany
[2]Siemens Healthcare GmbH, Forchheim, Germany
[3]Erlangen Graduate School in Advanced Optical Technologies (SAOT), Germany
mario.amrehn@fau.de

Abstract. Interactive image segmentation bears the advantage of correctional updates to the current segmentation mask when compared to fully automated systems. Especially in the field of inter-operative medical image processing of a single patient, where a high accuracy is an uncompromisable necessity, a human operator guiding a system towards an optimal segmentation result is a time-efficient constellation benefiting the patient. There are recent categories of neural networks which can incorporate human-computer interaction (HCI) data as additional input for segmentation. In this work, we simulate this HCI data during training with state-of-the-art user models, also called robot users, which aim to act similar to real users given interactive image segmentation tasks. We analyze the influence of chosen robot users, which mimic different types of users and scribble patterns, on the segmentation quality. We conclude that networks trained with robot users with the most spread out seeding patterns generalize well during inference with other robot users.

1 Introduction

The trans-catheter arterial chemoembolization (TACE) [1] is a minimally invasive procedure to treat hepatocellular carcinoma (HCC). During the treatment, volumetric cone-beam C-arm computed tomography (CBCT) [2] images of the patient's abdomen are generated. The physician maximizes the efficacy of the operation selecting all cancerous cells while reducing the toxicity of the treatment by omitting surrounding healthy tissue during lesion segmentation. Therefore, a crucial step during the intervention is the accurate segmentation of liver lesions in order to precisely isolate the conspicuous tissue's cells from the oxygen supply of the liver.

In recent years, fully-automatic segmentation systems based on convolutional neural networks (CNN) like the U-net [3] outperformed more traditional learning based approaches to medical image segmentation. In 2017, interactive CNNs were published [4, 5] which, to some degree, include guidance from a human user for their final segmentation result. The guidance is provided by post-processing the current segmentation result. In that year, Amrehn et al. [6, 7] and Wang et al. [8]

demonstrated the potential of rule-based seed drawing robot users and feasibility of a combination of interaction input data with traditionally fully-automatic CNN segmentation systems.

All of these systems model the user in a specific way via a set of fixed rules. Kohli et al. [9] described a way to realistically simulate some groups of users. However, most often, the similarity analysis of a simulated user to actual humans interacting with the system is omitted when a new interactive method with its custom interacting robot user are presented. In this work, we quantify the similarity between proposed robot users and illustrate their differences.

2   Materials and methods

The network topology used is a fully convolutional neural network based on U-net [3] with $3.12 \cdot 10^7$ trainable parameters as depicted in Fig. 1. The network utilized 19 convolutional layers. The proposed network utilizes three input channels, with size of 256^2 pixels each, to encode gray-valued image data as well as user provided seed information. Convolution operations are performed utilizing $3 \times 3 \times n$ kernels, where $n \in \{2^6, 2^7, 2^8, 2^9, 2^{10}\}$ depending on the depth of the network. A 2×2 neighborhood is used for pooling. Three input channels encode the gray-valued C-arm CT image data as well as user provided seed information. The seeding channels consist of background respective foreground seeds transformed by the Euclidean distance function. A distance transform as a pre-processing step on the sparse seed images decreases the necessary size of the network's minimum receptive field, which is especially important for its initial layers to capture the seed information as context to the gray-valued input image. Utilizing a distance transform, the seed formation is spread over the whole input channel and seed information is preserved even with small kernel sizes.

The robot user mimics the interaction of a real user. It is assumed, that a human user sets additional seed points during segmentation based on the structures seen on the gray-valued input image, the previously set foreground and background seeds, the current segmentation mask image, as well as a notion of the segmentation ground truth which the physician has from their domain knowledge. These five inputs are also commonly used for a rule-based robot

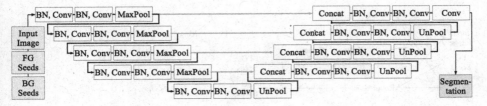

Fig. 1. Schematic representation of a U-net convolutional neural network topology. The input channels include foreground (FG) and background (BG) seed information. Skip-connections are depicted as links in gray. Before each convolution, batch normalization (BN) is applied. The outcome is a dense segmentation mask of size 256^2 pixels (green).

user, as depicted in Fig. 2. In the following analysis, five different robot users are evaluated.

2.1   Random sampling over whole image (rand)

Seeds are placed at random on the seed input channels. Here, a fraction of $r_{rand} = 0.1$ of seeds are drawn with the label inverted i. e. these seeds are misplaced.

2.2   Random sampling from GT (rand_gt)

This robot user samples seed point positions at random and copies labels from the ground truth. Note that *rand_gt* equals rand with $r_{rand} = 0.0$. Here, the number of seeds per interaction is $n_{rand\_gt} \in \{1, 5, 10\}$.

2.3   Robot user by Kohli et al. (kohli12)

Proposed in [9] and selected for user simulation in [5], this robot user utilizes the current segmentation image and the ground truth in order to place one seed point in the center of the largest, wrongly labeled image area.

2.4   Robot user by Xu et al. (xu16)

The robot user proposed in [4] samples $f_{xu16} \in \{1, 5, 10\}$ foreground and $b_{xu16} \in \{1, 5, 10\}$ background seed points at random constrained by a minimum distance to established seeds (such that $2 \le n_{xu16} \le 20$). Possible background seed locations are either sampled inside a 20 pixel wide margin around the GT object's contour line (called *strategy 1* in the original paper), or in the entire background region (strategy 2), depending on parameter $s_{xu16} \in \{1, 2\}$.

2.5   Robot user by Wang et al. (wang17)

In [8, 6] the robot user utilized places seed points at random on wrongly labeled image areas. This behaviour is similar to *kohli12*, but not limited to the center

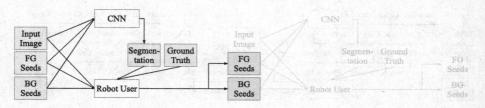

Fig. 2. A robot user bases its seed placement decision process on up to five different inputs (gray): the gray-valued input image, the previous foreground and background seeds, the current segmentation mask, and the ground truth segmentation mask. The outcome of a robot user system is a new set of proposed seed points (green).

of the image areas. Whether a region is ignored during placement of additional seed points is determined by an area size threshold $t_{wang17} \in \{10, 20, 30, 40\}$ in pixels.

When training a new network with robot user interaction input, a classical chicken or the egg causality paradox emerges. A fully trained network would be needed in order to segment the input image. Thereafter, additional correcting seed points may be selected by a robot user, which leads to an updated segmentation result. This interaction data may be used for training the new network. However, a fully trained network would need exactly these steps to be trained first. Therefore, in this work, we initialize the new network with user interaction training data acquired by interaction with a non-learning-based method. Here, robot user interactions are recorded via iterative segmentation utilizing GrowCut [10]. In preliminary experiments, we determined that segmentation methods like GrabCut, which are more robust and therefore more independent of user input patterns do not qualify for the proposed initialization of a new network. The GrowCut method is chosen due to its well known tendency to benefit from careful placement of large quantities of seed points. The figure of merit for segmentation quality is a Dice score, also known as intersection over union (IoU), generated after each GrowCut iteration step, as depicted in Fig. 3.

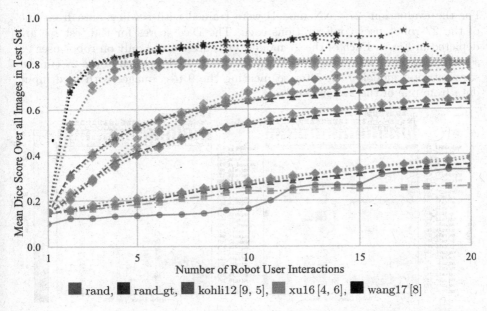

Fig. 3. The mean Dice scores per robot user over all input images and per interaction is depicted. Each robot user provides seeds during interactive segmentation. A segmentation's quality is measured as Dice score after each GrowCut [10] iteration step.

3   Experiments

The data utilized in the experiments are 2-D slices of volumetric CBCT images of liver lesions depicting HCC. The lesions in the volumetric images are fully annotated by medical experts. Subsequently, the image data are cropped to a volume of interest (VOI), with voxel resolutions from $0.46^3\ mm^3$ to $0.68^3\ mm^3$. All annotated lesions are smaller than $117^3\ mm^3$ which allows for a (VOI) of 256^3 voxels depicting the largest lesion outlines. For training and testing, 90 slice images are drawn from the 38 3-D VOI images of 38 individual patients. 90% of images are used for training, 10% for testing.

One network $\mathbb{M}_i$ is trained for every robot user and every parameter configuration tested for a robot user as described in Sec. 2, where $i \in [0, 27)$. The quality of their segmentation outcome is analyzed via the Dice score for the current segmentation mask with the ground truth. It is analyzed, which robot user input patterns during training will generate networks able to generalize to other input patterns during inference.

4   Results

For the evaluation, 27 CNN models were trained with seeding data from one of the 27 robot user configurations each. The Dice scores for the test set are depicted in Fig. 4. Each of the 27 models $m(i)$ are trained only on robot user i's seeding training data. A mean Dice score is computed for each of the 27 trained segmentation models $m(.)$ after segmenting the 9 test images with seed input data from one of the 27 robot users.

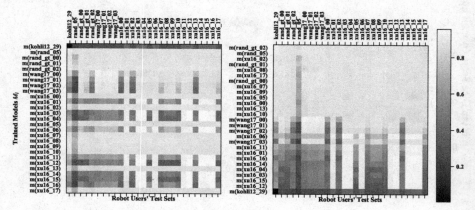

Fig. 4. Each of the 27×27 cells on the left represents the segmentation quality in Dice score given a trained segmentation model $m(.)$ (row) and a robot user's (column) seed input data for the test set. Each model $m(i)$ was trained beforehand only on robot user i's seeding training data. On the right, the rows are sorted by sum of Dice scores per row descending.

5   Discussion and outlook

It becomes apparent from Fig. 4 (right), that (1) CNNs trained with robot users based on rules to place seeds almost at random (rand, rand_gt, xu16) yield similar segmentation results when other user input patterns are utilized during inference. (2) Robot user input with more distinct seeding patterns like wang17 generates trained networks which are better adjusted to their seeding (Fig. 4 wang17, on the left), but not generalizing well to other input patterns.

An interpretation of this result is, that when improving on randomized seeds for training, it is not feasible to train on generalized user input patterns for all use cases, due to (1). Therefore, it is a necessity to train on personalized seeding patterns formalized as individual robot users (2), where a high similarity to the input patterns of the real user operating the system is imperative.

Disclaimer. The concept and software presented in this paper are based on research and are not commercially available. Due to regulatory reasons its future availability cannot be guaranteed.

Acknowledgement. Thanks to PD Dr.-Ing. habil. Stefan Steidl for helpful conversations and feedback during the time of writing.

References

1. Lewandowski RJ, Geschwind JF, Liapi E, et al. Transcatheter intraarterial therapies: rationale and overview. Radiol. 2011;259(3):641–657.
2. Strobel N, Meissner O, Boese J, et al. 3D imaging with flat-detector C-arm systems. Multislice CT. 2009; p. 33–51.
3. Ronneberger O, Fischer P, Brox T. U-net: convolutional networks for biomedical image segmentation. proc MICCAI. 2015; p. 234–241.
4. Xu N, Price B, Cohen S, et al. Deep interactive object selection. Proc CVPR. 2016; p. 373–381.
5. Liew JH, Wei Y, Xiong W, et al. Regional interactive image segmentation networks. Proc ICCV. 2017; p. 2746–2754.
6. Amrehn MP, Gaube S, Unberath M, et al. UI-net: interactive artificial neural networks for iterative image segmentation based on a user model. Proc VCBM. 2017; p. 143–147.
7. Amrehn MP, Steidl S, Kowarschik M, et al. Robust seed mask generation for interactive image segmentation. Proc NSS/MIC. 2017; p. 1–3.
8. Wang G, Zuluaga MA, Li W, et al. DeepIGeoS: a deep interactive geodesic framework for medical image segmentation. Trans Pattern Anal Mach Intell. 2018;.
9. Kohli P, Nickisch H, Rother C, et al. User-centric learning and evaluation of interactive segmentation systems. Proc IJCV. 2012;100(3):261–274.
10. Vezhnevets V, Konouchine V. GrowCut: interactive multi-label ND image segmentation by cellular automata. Comput Graph Appl (Graphicon). 2005; p. 150–156.

Tracing of Nerve Fibers Through Brain Regions of Fiber Crossings in Reconstructed 3D-PLI Volumes

Marius Nolden[1], Nicole Schubert[1], Daniel Schmitz[1], Andreas Müller[2], Markus Axer[1]

[1]Institute of Neuroscience and Medicine (INM-1), Research Centre Jülich
[2]SimLab Neuroscience, Jülich Supercomputing Centre, Research Centre Jülich
m.nolden@fz-juelich.de

Abstract. Three-dimensional (3D) polarized light imaging (PLI) is able to reveal nerve fibers in the human brain at microscopic resolution. While most nerve fiber structures can be accurately visualized with 3D-PLI, the currently used physical model (based on Jones Calculus) is not well suited to distinguish steep fibers from specific fiber crossings. Hence, streamline tractography algorithms tracing fiber pathways get easily misdirected in such brain regions. For the presented study, we implemented and applied two methods to bridge areas of fiber crossings: (i) extrapolation of fiber points with cubic splines and (ii) following the most frequently occurring orientations in a defined neighborhood based on orientation distribution functions gained from 3D-PLI measurements (pliODFs). Applied to fiber crossings within a human hemisphere, reconstructed from 3D-PLI measurements at 64 microns in-pane resolution, both methods were demonstrated to sustain their initial tract direction throughout the crossing region. In comparison, the ODF-method offered a more reliable bridging of the crossings with less gaps.

1 Introduction

The human brain contains about 100 billion nerve cells (neurons), whose long projections intricately connect brain regions with each other [1]. Three-dimensional (3D) polarized light imaging (PLI) utilizes the birefringence of of myelinated axons (here, referred to as fibers) to determine their local orientations in serial unstained histological brain sections. To track fiber tracts within a 3D reconstructed volume of orientations, deterministic tractography algorithms based on Runge-Kutta procedures can be used [2]. However, 3D-PLI cannot easily provide unambiguous fiber orientations in all types of fiber crossings, in particular, in cases of equally distributed perpendicular fibers within a voxel. As a result, simple streamline tractography methods are not able to correctly bridge such areas. Two methods have been implemented to continue tractography within crossing regions. The first method interprets a fiber tract as a space curve and extrapolates the further course using parametric cubic splines. The second method analyzes the neighborhood surrounding the fiber crossing in order to determine most frequently occurring orientations using orientation distribution functions (ODFs). Both methods have been applied to selected fiber crossings within a subsample of a human hemisphere, which was reconstructed from 3D-PLI measurements with a resolution of $64 \times 64 \times 60\,\mu m$.

2   Materials and methods

3D-PLI determines local fiber orientations based on signal changes resulting from the birefringence of myelin sheaths which surround most nerve fibers. The 3D-PLI workflow as developed at the Institute of Neuroscience and Medicine (INM-1) starts with the preparation of the brain. Postmortem brains are formalin-fixated, deep-frozen and cryo-sectioned at 60 μm thickness. During sectioning en-face (blockface) images are taken from above the cryo-block. 3D reconstructed blockface images provide an undistorted reference volume in order to reconstruct PLI images in 3D [3]. Each section is then measured in a customized polarimeter by passing polarized light through the sample [4]. The birefringence of the myelin sheaths changes the light intensity measured by a camera above the section [5]. An analysis of the 3D-PLI signal allows to determine local fiber orientations per voxel [3]. The voxel sizes used for the presented study are $64 \times 64 \times 60\mu m$. Fiber orientation maps, which represent color coded fiber orientations for one section each, can be seen in Fig. 1(a) and (d). By means of the 3D reconstructed blockface volume, the 3D-reconstruction process results in a 3D vector field of fiber orientations.

Various methods to interpret orientations fields in terms of connectivity are already well established in Diffusion Magnetic Resonance Imaging and are referred to as tractography apporaches [6]. Depending on the acquired data types and the study aims, tractography algorithms can be broadly classified into streamline, probabilistic and global methods [7, 8]. In our study, a streamline-based approach was selected.

To realize streamline tractography for 3D-PLI data, Runge-Kutta methods were used. Similar to tracking the main directions of diffusion tensors for DTI data, the tracking directions 3D-PLI data were determined by trilinear interpolation in the 3D volume of fiber orientations. Runge-Kutta methods of first (Euler method), second and fourth order (classic Runge-Kutta) were implemented. While these streamline techniques provided plausible results in areas with homogeneous fiber structures, they were not able to correctly represent fibers in crossing regions due to the interpolation of ambiguous fiber orientations.

Therefore, additional crossing algorithms have been developed which temporarily interrupt the standard tractography and continue the fiber tracts in a different way. The first algorithm interprets the previously followed fiber path as a space curve, which is artificially continued until leaving the crossing region. For this purpose, parametric cubic splines are applied, which interpolate the last fiber points passed through by the current fiber tract. The continuation of the generated function is done by extrapolating the last spline function, whereby the distance of the extrapolated fiber point to the last fiber point corresponds to the average distance of the support points used for the splines.

This raises the question of how crossing areas can be identified. Two methods have been tested: (i) Consider angles between successively traced directions. When a previously defined threshold value is exceeded, a fiber crossing is assumed. (ii) Crossing areas are labeled manually based on the fiber orientation maps. The dashed rectangles in Fig. 1(b) and (c) represent the selected areas for one section, respectively.

The second implemented crossing algorithm calculates most frequently occurring fiber orientations by ODFs. To determine most frequently occurring orientations for a given voxel, the surrounding neighborhood is analyzed. Therefore, a supervoxel is defined, which can be described as a cube with edge length n that contains a set of $n \times n \times n$ voxels. If the crossing is labeled, only voxels outside of the labeled area are used for the calculation. The orientation histogram is approximated by spherical harmonics, representing the pliODF [9]. The maxima of the pliODF are interpreted as the most frequently occurring orientations. For their estimation, a discrete sample of direction vectors in the unit circle is tested. In order to preferably follow different nerve fibers and not assign multiple fiber tracts to the same fiber, the minimum angle between most frequently occurring directions is defined. Like the first algorithm, it can work with or without a labeling of the crossing region. An adequate labeling prevents ambiguous fiber orientations from being taken into account to calculate ODFs.

3 Results

The tractography algorithms have been applied to different fiber crossings in a human hemisphere. The entire dataset includes 228 sections, each containing 1350×1950 voxels. To apply the algorithms, sub-volumes of $55 \times 57 \times 31$ and $66 \times 66 \times 30$ voxels were selected. For all implemented Runge-Kutta methods a standard streamline approach just following local fiber orientations was not able to correctly reconstruct the transitions into and out of the crossing regions. As can be seen in Fig. 1(e) and (j), the fiber tracts did not bridge the investigated regions.

For extrapolation with cubic splines, in case of crossing detection via angle determination, ambigous signals from within the crossing region influenced the extrapolation curve. This can be noticed by the gaps in the crossing areas of the tractography results (Fig. 1(f) and (k)). With an adequate labeling, the extrapolation with splines led to smooth transitions into and out of the crossing regions and a lot of fiber tracts were able to cross them. The applied masks for one section are illustrated in Fig. 1(b) and (c) by the dashed rectangles. Using them for crossing detection, the number and size of gaps were smaller. This difference was noticeable especially by the tractography results depicted in Fig. 1(l).

For tracing the most frequently occurring orientations with ODFs, the fiber tracts were able to bridge crossing regions, independently of whether the crossing

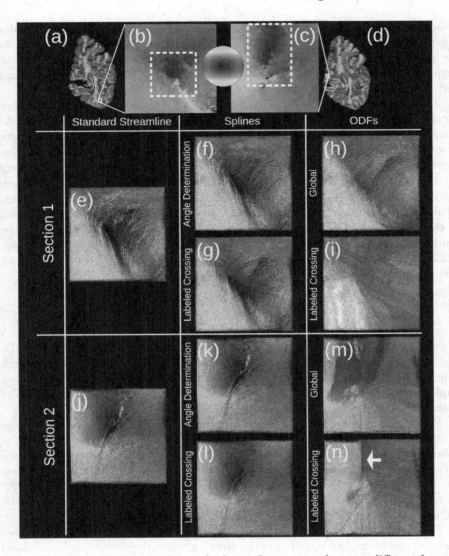

Fig. 1. The different tractography methods are demonstrated at two different human hemispheric sections (a,d) at two selected crossing regions (b,c). The results of the standard streamline tractography show that the tracking algorithm stops shortly after entering the crossing area (e,j). Extrapolating fiber points with cubic splines has been done with crossing detection via angle determination between successive directions (f,k), which results in abrupt transitions around the crossing area. The method has also been applied with a manual labeling of the crossing region, illustrated by the dashed rectangles (b,c), resulting in smoother transitions (g,l). Following the most probable directions calculated by ODFs has been done globally, taking every voxel of the examined volumes into account, providing a gap-free tractography result throughout the volumes (h,m). Adequate labelings improve this results because highly inclined fiber orientations are not taken into account (i,n), but sharp borders can arise (n).

areas had been labeled or not. Furthermore, in comparison with the results regarding the extrapolation with splines, there were no more gaps visible in the crossing region because every fiber orientation that was one of the most frequently occurring directions, according to the ODF, was traced. Fig. 1(h) and (m) illustrate the corresponding tractography results.

The orientations inside of manually labeled areas were not taken into account for the calculation of pliODFs. Thus, adequate labelings led to the fact that the fiber tracts sustained their initial direction throughout the region. They were able to bridge the labeled crossings, given the supervoxels were large enough. The corresponding results can be seen in Fig. 1(i) and (n). However, in some cases there were sharp borders within the tractography results. They arised because the main directions followed on the two sides of this borders were very different. This effect is also illustrated in Fig. 1(n), where the border is visible at the top of the volume, marked by the white arrow. In this case, on the left side of the border an approximately vertical main orientation is most strongly represented, while on the right side only a nearly orthogonal orientation is considered most frequently occurring.

4   Discussion

A validation of the tractography results inside crossing regions based on 3D-PLI data requires the ground truth in form of the local nerve fiber architecture, which is not available. Therefore, the results were compared visually. The two implemented crossing tractography methods enabled fiber tracts to cross the examined fiber crossings.

For the extrapolation with splines, an adequate labeling of the crossing helps to smooth out transitions into and out of the crossing region. Without such a labeling, ambiguous 3D-PLI orientations can lead to undesired effects to the space curve. The major problem is that the orientations in specific crossing regions are often misinterpreted as highly inclined fiber structures. That means that the z-component is unusually large in comparison to the x- and y-components. Thus, the space curve is deflected vertically out of the volume.

Following the most likely orientations calculated by ODFs always provided smooth transitions, but labelings of the crossing regions prevented highly inclined fiber orientations from getting taken into account for the calculation. Therefore, Fig. 1(i) and (n) show the tractography results with the smallest number of highly inclined fiber tracts. However, labeling crossing areas for ODFs can result in sharp borders, as can be seen in Fig. 1(n). On one side of the line, a lot of fiber tracts were traced in one main orientation and the other orientations were considered to be irrelevant, while on the other side fiber tracts with a different orientation were more dominant and the previous orientation was not relevant enough anymore to be traced. The best overall results from a visual point of view were achieved by following most frequently occurring directions calculated by ODFs, where a labeling of the crossing regions had been done beforehand.

However, a detailed validation with help of neuroanatomical experts and simulations of the fiber architecture will be performed in near future. Furthermore, for an automatic detection of fiber crossings confidence levels will be used, which can be evaluated duringthe 3D-PLI signal analysis [10]. Classification of crossing-and non-crossing voxels is then done by defining a threshold regarding the local confidence level. Alternatively, instead of dividing voxels into this two classes, they could all get taken into account when calculating ODFs, but weighted by their individual confidence level. Evaluating the effectiveness of using confidence levels requires further investigations.

Acknowledgement. This project has received funding from the European Union's Horizon 2020 Research and Innovation Programme under Grant Agreement No. 785907 (HBP SGA2). The authors gratefully acknowledge the computing time granted through JARA-HPC on the supercomputer JURECA at Forschungszentrum Jülich.

References

1. Herculano-Houzel S. The human brain in numbers: a linearly scaled-up primate brain. Front Hum Neurosci. 2009;3:31.
2. Mori S, van Zijl PCM. Fiber tracking: principles and strategies: a technical review. NMR Biomed. 2002;15(78):468–480.
3. Schober M, Schlömer P, Cremer M, et al. Reference volume generation for subsequent 3D reconstruction of histological sections. Proc BVM. 2015; p. 143–148.
4. Axer M, Amunts K, Grässel D, et al. A novel approach to the human connectome: ultra-high resolution mapping of fiber tracts in the brain. Neuroimage. 2011;54(2):1091 – 1101.
5. Schmitt FO, Bear RS. The optical properties of vertebrate nerve axons as related to fiber size. J Cell Comp Physiol. 1937;9(2):261–273.
6. Basser JP, Pajevicand S, Pierpaoli C, et al. In vivo fiber tractography using DT-MRI data. Magn Reson Med. 2000;44(4):625–632.
7. Mori S, Zhang J. Principles of diffusion tensor imaging and its applications to basic neuroscience research. Neuron. 2006;51(5):527 – 539.
8. Maxime D. Wiley encyclopedia of electrical and electronics engineering. HARDI. 2015; p. 1–25.
9. Axer M, Strohmer S, Gräßel D, et al. Estimating fiber orientation distribution functions in 3D-Polarized light imaging. Front Neuroanat. 2016;10:40.
10. Schmitz D, Amunts K, Lippert T, et al. A least squares approach for the reconstruction of nerve fiber orientations from tiltable specimen experiments in 3D-PLI. Proc IEEE Int Symp Biomed Imaging. 2018; p. 132–135.

Dilated Deeply Supervised Networks for Hippocampus Segmentation in MRI

Lukas Folle, Sulaiman Vesal, Nishant Ravikumar, Andreas Maier

Pattern Recognition Lab, Friedrich-Alexander-Universität Erlangen-Nürnberg,
Germany
lukas.folle@fau.de

Abstract. Tissue loss in the hippocampi has been heavily correlated with the progression of Alzheimer's Disease (AD). The shape and structure of the hippocampus are important factors in terms of early AD diagnosis and prognosis by clinicians. However, manual segmentation of such subcortical structures in MR studies is a challenging and subjective task. In this paper, we investigate variants of the well known 3D U-Net, a type of convolution neural network (CNN) for semantic segmentation tasks. We propose an alternative form of the 3D U-Net, which uses dilated convolutions and deep supervision to incorporate multi-scale information into the model. The proposed method is evaluated on the task of hippocampus head and body segmentation in an MRI dataset, provided as part of the MICCAI 2018 segmentation decathlon challenge. The experimental results show that our approach outperforms other conventional methods in terms of different segmentation accuracy metrics.

1 Introduction

Neurodegenerative brain disorders are a major cause of disability, and early mortality, in many developed and developing countries worldwide. Alzheimer's disease is a type of dementia that affects 20 % of the population over 80 years of age, worldwide [1]. Currently, AD is typically only diagnosed in patients presenting with symptoms of cognitive impairment, and behavioural changes [2]. With high-resolution MRI structural changes in the brain which accompany the onset of AD, can be recognized in vivo [3]. Early disease stages classified as mild cognitive impairment that occur prior to AD, can also be identified in some cases, and the associated structural changes within the brain can subsequently be used as biomarkers to predict the risk of conversion to AD. Additionally, the rate of tissue atrophy of the hippocampus can be used as a temporal marker to monitor the progression of AD. The current clinical protocol to detect volumetric changes in the hippocampus is manual segmentation, which is time-consuming, observer-dependent and challenging [2]. Consequently, an automated approach to hippocampus segmentation is imperative to improve the efficiency and accuracy of the diagnostic workflow. Several automatic and semi-automatic segmentation approaches have been proposed, which utilize T1-weighted structural MRIs, to segment the hippocampus. A multi-atlas segmentation approach was proposed in [4], to jointly localize and segment the hippocampi using the average of all registered atlases. In [5], robust segmentation approach was proposed, using subject-specific 3D optimal local maps, with a hybrid active contour model to automatically segment hippocampus.

In recent years, convolution neural networks (CNNs) have achieved state-of-the-art performance in a variety of medical image segmentation tasks. Specifically, the U-Net [6], an encoder-decoder network, has received tremendous attention within the medical imaging community. Expanding the U-Net to process 3D volumes rather than 2D slices was proposed in [7] using 3D convolutions (3D U-Net). This was modified in [8] by increasing the channels in the center part of the network (V-Net). In this paper, we propose a CNN for automatic segmentation of the hippocampus. Our network is based on the 3D U-Net, with dilated convolutions in the lowest layer between the encoder and decoder paths [9], residual connections between the convolution blocks in the encoder path, and residual connections between the convolution blocks and the final layer of the decoder path. A schematic of the network is presented in Fig. 2. The main contribution of this paper is the combination of dilated convolutions in the lowest part of the network with the ensemble of the decoder outputs for the final prediction, providing a mechanism for "deep supervision". We evaluated the performance of the network using the hippocampus dataset provided as part of the Medical Segmentation Decathlon challenge[1] hosted at MICCAI 2018, and compared it to different 3D U-net based architectures.

---

[1] http://medicaldecathlon.com/

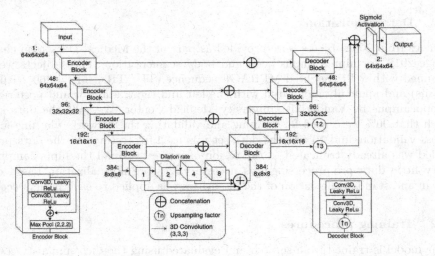

Fig. 1. Network Architecture with residual connections in the encoder path, dilated convolutions at the lowest layer and residual connections between the decoder stages and the final layer.

2   Methodology

Segmentation tasks often require integration of local and global context, in addition to learning multi-scale features. However, training segmentation networks that incorporate these properties and act directly on volumetric data, is computationally intensive. We address this by including dilated convolutions within the network to imbue greater global context during feature extraction and combine the output of the decoder layers for the final mask prediction, thereby encouraging the learning of multi-scale features, while providing a means for efficient backpropagation of gradients through the network. Beyond that, this modification yields the benefit of residual connections to the decoding part while retaining the same number of model parameters.

The proposed network consists of four encoder and decoder blocks, each containing two 3D convolution layers with kernel size of 3x3x3, batch normalization and leaky rectified linear units (leaky RELU) as activation functions. The encoder blocks additionally use residual connections and 3D max-pooling operations, as illustrated in Fig. 2. The decoder blocks use 3D up-sampling with a factor of two. The four dilated convolution layers employed in the bottleneck of the network are configured such that the first layer uses a dilation rate of one, and each subsequent layer increases the dilation rate by a multiple of two, as proposed in [9]. The output of each decoder block is up-sampled to match the dimensions of the final mask predicted by the network, following which, they are all concatenated.

2.1   Data acquisition

Images from 263 subjects were provided as part of the Medical Decathlon challenge 2018, for hippocampus head and body segmentation. The subjects were scanned with a T1-weighted MPRAGE sequence (TI / TR / TE = 860 / 8.0 / 3.7ms) and manually annotated with the left and right, anterior and posterior, hippocampus by Vanderbilt University Medical Center. We split the data set such that 90% were used for training and validating the network, via nine-fold cross-validation, and 10% of the data-set was used for testing. As the data provided was already truncated to the region of interest around the hippocampus, very little data pre-processing was necessary. Z-score normalization based on mean and standard deviation of the intensities was applied to each patient scan.

2.2   Training procedures

Our model is trained from scratch and evaluated using the dice similarity coefficient (DSC), Jaccard index (JI) and normalized surface distance (NSD). DSC and JI measure the overlap of the ground-truth and model-predicted segmentations, while NSD is computed between the reconstructed surfaces. These were the official metrics used to assess segmentation accuracy in the decathlon challenge as well. The dice coefficient loss is widely used for training segmentation

Table 1. Segmentation accuracy evaluated in terms of DSC, JI and NSD for the V-Net, 3D U-Net, dilated 3D U-Net and the proposed method.

	Training	Validation	Testing		
Methods	DSC	DSC	DSC	JI	NSD
V-Net	0.968	0.872	0.848	0.736	0.954
3D U-Net	0.965	0.858	0.865	0.740	0.960
3D U-Net + Dilation	0.977	0.878	0.879	0.785	0.960
Proposed method	0.984	0.882	0.882	0.790	0.962

networks [8]. We used a combination of binary cross entropy and DSC loss functions to train all networks investigated in this study, as proposed in [9]. This combined loss (Eq.1) is less sensitive to class imbalance and leverages the advantages of both loss functions. Our experiments demonstrated better segmentation accuracy when using the combined loss in comparison to employing either individually

$$\zeta(y, \hat{y}) = \zeta_{dc}(y, \hat{y}) + \zeta_{bce}(y, \hat{y}) \tag{1}$$

In Eq.1 $\hat{y}$ denotes the output of the model and the ground truth labels are denoted by y. We use the two-class version of the DSC loss $\zeta_{dc}(y, \hat{y})$ proposed in [8, 9], the Adam optimizer with a learning rate of 0.0005, and trained the network for 500 epochs. Additionally, the learning-rate was reduced gradually (using a factor of 0.1), if the validation loss did not improve after 10 epochs. To prevent overfitting and improve the robustness of our approach to varied hippocampal shapes, we augmented the dataset with random rotations and flipping. Based on our experiments, we found that augmenting with large rotation angles produced worse segmentation masks, consequently, we reduced the rotation angles to be in the range of ±10 degrees.

3   Results and discussion

In order to assess the performance of different networks, we used the Dice Coefficient Score (DSC), Jaccard index and Normalised Surface Distance (NSD) with 4mm tolerance. The segmentation performance of our model, V-Net, 3D U-Net and 3D U-Net with dilated convolutions are compared in Table 1. The V-Net achieved mean DSC scores of 96.8%, 87.2% and 84.8%, for the training, validation and test sets, respectively. The performance of the 3D U-Net is close to the V-Net performance with mean DSC scores of 96.5%, 85.5% and 86.5% respectively. 3D U-Net with dilated convolutions was able to improve the scores to 97.7%, 87.8% and 87.9%, respectively. However, the proposed approach outperformed the others with scores of 98.4%, 88.2% and 88.2% for the training, validation, and test sets, respectively. Additionally, our approach consistently outperformed the other state-of-the-art networks, in terms of the JI and NSD metrics as well, as highlighted in Table 1.

In Fig. 2 the segmentation quality of the proposed method is visually compared with V-Net, 3D U-Net, and 3D U-Net with dilated convolutions. Here, red represents the ground-truth, yellow, green and cyan represent the predictions of V-Net, dilated 3D U-Net and the proposed method, respectively. In the second column, the advantage of dilated convolutions is highlighted, in comparison to the V-Net, which failed to segment the small disjoint parts of the mask in the top right. However, the dilated 3D U-Net and the proposed method were able to capture those areas due to the increased global context imbued in the learned features. Fig. 3 depicts 3D surface meshes of two different patients. Columns two and three illustrate the outputs of V-Net and our method, respectively. The lower boundary of the red part (body) of the hippocampus in the ground-truth surfaces, contains ridge-like structures which are typical of hippocampal structure. While the V-Net predicted surfaces are relatively smooth in this region, the proposed approach is more successful in capturing these subtle shape variations.

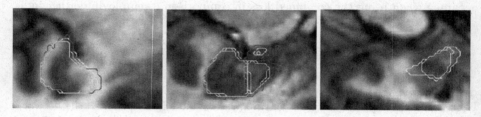

Fig. 2. Each image represents a different MRI slice from a different patient. The corresponding segmentations are overlaid: Red contour represents ground-truth, yellow V-Net, green 3D U-Net with dilated convolutions and cyan our proposed method.

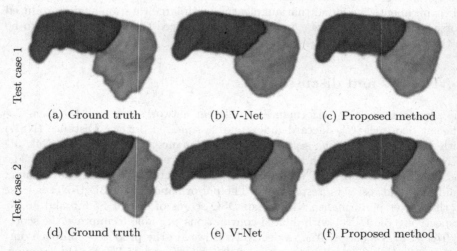

Fig. 3. Rows represent 3D surface visualizations for two different patients. Columns from left to right are the ground truth surfaces, and those predicted by the V-Net and our approach, respectively. Hippocampus head is visualized in green and body in red.

4   Conclusion

We proposed a 3D U-Net based segmentation framework with dilated convolutions in the deepest part of the network and deep supervision in the decoder part of the network. The dilated convolutions capture global context due to their larger receptive fields. Deep supervision helped further improve segmentation accuracy, by incorporating multi-scale information more efficiently during the training process. We showed that our network consistently outperforms the V-Net, 3D U-Net, and 3D U-Net with dilated convolutions, in terms of all metrics evaluated. Future work will aim to use the proposed framework for segmentation in whole brain MRI volumes, and on different segmentation tasks in medical imaging.

Acknowledgement. This work was supported by the EFI Project: BIG-THERA.

References

1. Ferri C, Prince M, Brayne C, et al. Global prevalence of dementia: a delphi consensus study. Lancet. 2005;366(9503):2112–2117.
2. Hampel H, Teipel SJ, Buerger K. Neurobiologische Frühdiagnostik der Alzheimer-Krankheit. Nervenarzt. 2007;78:1310–1318.
3. Schuff N, Woerner N, Boreta L, et al. MRI of hippocampal volume loss in early alzheimer's disease in relation to ApoE genotype and biomarkers. Brain. 2009;132(4):1067–1077.
4. Plassard AJ, McHugo M, Heckers S, et al.; International Society for Optics; Photonics. Multi-scale hippocampal parcellation improves atlas-based segmentation accuracy. Proc SPIE. 2017;10133:101332D.
5. Zarpalas D, Gkontra P, Daras P, et al. Accurate and fully automatic hippocampus segmentation using subject-specific 3D optimal local maps into a hybrid active contour model. IEEE J Trans Eng Health Med. 2014;2:1–16.
6. Ronneberger O, Fischer P, Brox T; Springer. U-net: convolutional networks for biomedical image segmentation. Proc MICCAI. 2015; p. 234–241.
7. Çiçek Ö, Abdulkadir A, Lienkamp S, et al. 3D U-net: learning dense volumetric segmentation from sparse annotation. Proc MICCAI. 2016;9901:424–432.
8. Milletari F, Navab N, Ahmadi SA. V-net: fully convolutional neural networks for volumetric medical image segmentation. Proc 3DV. 2016; p. 565–571.
9. Vesal S, Ravikumar N, Maier A. Dilated convolutions in neural networks for left atrial segmentation in 3D gadolinium enhanced-MRI. arXiv:180801673. 2018;.

Automatic Detection and Segmentation of the Acute Vessel Thrombus in Cerebral CT

Christian Lucas[1], Jonas J. Schöttler[1], André Kemmling[2], Linda F. Aulmann[3], Mattias P. Heinrich[1]

[1]Institute of Medical Informatics, University of Lübeck, Lübeck
[2]Department of Clinical Radiology, University Hospital Münster, Münster
[3]Institute of Neuroradiology, University Medical Center Schleswig-Holstein, Lübeck
lucas@imi.uni-luebeck.de

Abstract. Intervention time plays a very important role for stroke outcome and affects different therapy paths. Automatic detection of an ischemic condition during emergency imaging could draw the attention of a radiologist directly to the thrombotic clot. Considering an appropriate early treatment, the immediate automatic detection of a clot could lead to a better patient outcome by reducing time-to-treatment. We present a two-stage neural network to automatically segment and classify clots in the MCA+ICA region for a fast pre-selection of positive cases to support patient triage and treatment planning. Our automatic method achieves an area under the receiver operating curve (AUROC) of 0.99 for the correct positive/negative classification on unseen test data.

1 Introduction

Stroke is a cerebrovascular disease, which is among the leading causes of deaths in the industrialized world [1]. Ischemic stroke is a condition where a blood clot blocks the blood flow that provides brain cells with oxygen. The underperfusion can lead to a necrosis of irreversibly damaged brain tissue if not treated within hours of onset. In fact, time is one of the most important factors on the outcome of a stroke [2], making the immediate detection of the clot a vital precondition to successful tissue and patient salvation.

Thrombi can be detected through hyperdensities in fast native CT imaging, but there might be several other causes for bright signals in the standard CT such as normal hyper-dense structures of the brain (or head) and calcification outside the brain arteries. While other parameters such as perfusion have been investigated widely to predict clinical and tissue outcomes [3], these methods assume that a subject has been already selected to be in a potentially critical clinical situation.

The patients arriving at the emergency room can have various indications and multiple diseases. If an ischemic stroke condition was automatically detected after imaging, the attention of the physician could directly be drawn to the time-critical treatment of such by marking positive cases with "red flags". This enables the doctor to choose the best therapy option through an early examination, e.g. to decide for thrombolysis against mechanical thrombectomy.

1.1 Related work

The computer-aided detection (CAD) of ischemic stroke depends on high-quality brain CT acquisition, enhancing and detecting specific stroke signs, as well as the appropriate analysis of these for automated detection of e.g. the common middle cerebral artery (MCA) or internal carotid artery (ICA) occlusion. Traditional methods have steadily improved the CAD pipeline, such as Inoue et al. [4] who increased the contrast of standard CT using a specific reconstruction method (IMR) with less noise to better diagnose acute MCA strokes.

The diagnosis itself can be based on several stroke signs. In this work we focus on the hyperattenuating MCA sign of the thromboembolus in standard CT. One existing method automatically detects the MCA dot sign using a multi-step approach [5] and without deep learning. Hand-crafted features are computed on candidate regions as a basis to eliminate false-positives and also anatomically implausible outliers before a Support-Vector Machine eventually classifies the remaining candidates.

Lisowska et al. [6] recently proposed a segmentation of vessel and ischemia as a stroke sign detection by incorporating contextual information in the form of atlas coordinates and bilateral comparison that enables the network to properly detect the dense vessel (in which the thrombus can only occur) and ischemia as a sign of stroke. However, there exists no combined approach for detection of clots and their segmentation.

Ischemic clots lead to increased attenuation and intensity values in CT along with other calcifications or hyper-dense brain structures. They can often be observed as small dot- or tube-like structures within the MCA. This makes the detection of such clots – to some degree – comparable with the task of lung nodule detection in 3D volumes: The (variance in the) general appearance of lung nodules is certainly different to the appearance of ischemic clots in the MCA, but the problem remains to distinguish the small targets from similarly appearing structures in the proximity.

Deep learning can help to recognize those subtle differences for e.g. the detection of lung nodules, as proposed by Setio et al. [7] using a false-positive reduction approach for their CAD system that employs a 2.5D neural network. The detection by Sakamoto et al. [8] inputs only three consecutive 2D slices for another false-positive reduction approach using a multi-stage neural network. These methods perform detection without segmentation.

In this work, our contributions are the presentation of a novel approach employing a cascaded convolutional neural network (CNN) for the fully automated detection of ischemic stroke clots (limited to the MCA+ICA region for which we have ground truth data). The algorithm directly outputs the binary result (stroke clot: yes/no) including the hemispheric side of the stroke and the clot (candidates) segmentation in the case of a positive test result.

2   Methods

We propose a cascaded neural network that consists of two sub-networks (Fig. 1), each trained on a specific sub-task. The first network learns to segment potential clots in the MCA+ICA region of interest (ROI), while the second network learns to correctly classify those candidates as clot or not. Designing a cascaded network follows the false-positive reduction principle (as described in several of the related works above) in order to optimally use all available training data, in particular for small clots. The training of the two networks is conducted sequentially, first the segmentation network, and afterwards the classification network, each following a different objective.

2.1   Clot candidates segmentation

The segmentation network aims to detect any potential clot in the MCA or ICA, so that a true thrombus is among those candidates. The network learns a high variety of thrombotic clots by training on the ROI (MCA+ICA area) of positive training samples only. This should result in the true clot segmentation among other false-positive candidates. A U-Net [9] architecture was employed for this task with three resolution levels (two 2×2 max-pooling and max-unpooling layers) and 13 convolution layers (each with 3×3 kernels), where the channel numbers range from 32 to 256.

In the first layer, a dilation size of 3 is used to cover a larger receptive field, which we empirically found to be useful. Further, the next resolutions levels contain three instead of two consecutive convolutions as in the original paper. The network expects the entire ROI image as input. A cross-entropy loss is computed on the output layer and back-propagated to optimize the network weights with AdaDelta.

2.2   Clot classification

The second network is trained with both positive and negative cases to learn the decision boundary between *clot* and *no clot* and aims to reduce the potential clot candidates to a final binary decision for the target being present among these candidates or not. Again, we use a CNN architecture, but this time use the

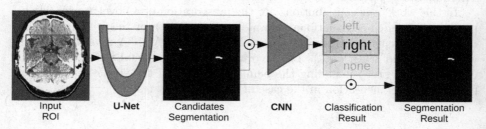

Fig. 1. The proposed cascaded network design for clot detection and segmentation.

element-wise product of the native CT and the estimated clot candidates from the first network as input. This provides the second network with location, shape, density and volume of potential clots to decide if a clot is present. Instead of using a U-Net architecture, three 3×3 convolutional layers are now interspersed with two max-pooling layers, followed by an adaptive pooling layer that reduces resolution of the intermediate feature map from $27 \times 24 \times 24$ to $2 \times 2 \times 2$ before two linear layers predict the probabilities of the three output classes.

The overall design of our algorithm is split into two sub-tasks to ease the learning of the clot classification by first learning to segment potential candidates and to classify those in a separate step: The algorithm is guided to learn the relationship between the clot label and the relevant hyper-dense regions in the MCA+ICA area. Similarly, we simplified the classification task itself and made the clot label more informative by learning a ternary classification: Distinguishing between *no clot*, *left clot*, and *right clot* potentially enables the algorithm to relate a positive label only to candidates in a single hemisphere during training. The classification result can later be used at test time to remove false-positive segmentation candidates from the opposite hemisphere.

3 Experiments

We run an evaluation on a single split with 60% of the data used for training, 30% for validation during training, and 10% for testing (running a full 10-fold is very time demanding and was left for future work). The prototype was implemented in PyTorch 0.3 (Python) and trained on a GeForce GTX 1080. Inference of the cascaded network for a full image takes about 25 seconds on CPU (Intel Xeon).

3.1 Data

The images must be co-registered in a common space, so that the algorithm works within a valid ROI. There is consequently no need to skull-strip the image, because the ROI for the MCA is directly extracted from the CT image. The ROI has been computed on the training data as the minimum bounding box of all MCA and ICA clot segmentations with an additional margin of 5 voxels in each direction and is of size $118 \times 98 \times 98$ voxels. FSL-FLIRT with a mutual information cost function was used for the registration of the images onto a mean atlas image provided with the dataset.

Our retrospectively collected non-contrast cerebral CT dataset consists of 108 positive cases with clot segmentation masks in the ICA or MCA and 108 negative cases. During training each case is laterally flipped to avoid preference for either hemisphere side, leading to a total of 432 samples (the segmentation network is trained only on the 216 positive cases).

3.2 Results

Our fully-automatic pipeline achieves a sensitivity of 0.86 at a specificity of 1 (Fig. 2, ROC). If a threshold of 0.13 or lower (instead of 0.5) was chosen to be exceeded by the combined clot probabilities (left + right), the method could detect all positive cases at a very reasonable false-positive rate of less than 5%. False-positives are more tolerable, because the algorithm is supposed to serve as a pre-selection of urgent cases that have to be diagnosed in-depth by a physician. Moreover, the hemisphere location is correctly detected for all true-positives.

The first network achieves a Dice overlap of 0.5 with the expert rater segmentations (Fig. 2, DSC) when evaluated on the unseen test scans of our dataset. Given that the network was trained on positive cases only and that the targets are very small – which makes the partial volume effect a prominent factor for ambiguities – this result is very promising (Fig. 3). The accuracy can be improved by using the classification result of the second network to remove candidates from the "wrong" hemisphere, which leads to a drastic reduction in outliers. The median number of candidates is reduced from 6.5 to 3.5, while the Hausdorff distance median decreases even more from 49 mm down to 14 mm (Fig. 2, HD).

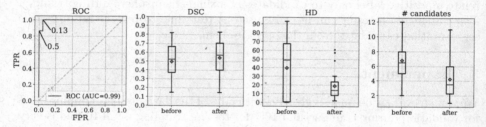

Fig. 2. Results on balanced test data (22 positive, 22 negative) from left to right: Final clot/non-clot classification ROC curve with clot thresholds; Segmentation Dice (DSC), Hausdorff distance in mm (HD), and number of candidates before and after removing them from the opposite hemisphere. (Blue: Median, Green: Arithmetic mean).

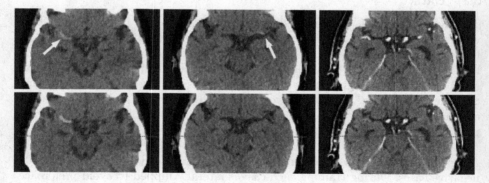

Fig. 3. Example results on test data (top: CT image; bottom: segmentation overlays). Left: True-positive with segmentation candidate (green) overlapping the true clot. Center: False-negative, where clot (red) is segmented among the candidates. Right: True-negative, where no clot was classified being present among the candidates (red).

4 Discussion

In this work we could show that a deep-learning based highly sensitive segmentation of clot candidates is suitable to classify patients as *urgent-to-be-diagnosed* with respect to the occurence of hyper-dense acute ischemic stroke signs. If integrated into a radiology information system, the algorithm could automatically pre-select highly probable acute stroke patients and mark them with a "red flag". Although the segmentation usually consists of multiple object instances (candidates), these enable the physician to be pointed directly to the clot suspects in a CT scan (around four candidates per patient) to verify the acute stroke.

In contrast to state-of-the-art lung nodule detection algorithms, which directly classify nodule ROI candidates as in [8], our approach performs localized detection that implicitly outputs a corresponding segmentation mask for the entire MCA+ICA area. Reducing the memory and computational demand of the first network should be investigated more closely. It could be worthwhile to evaluate simpler and more efficient approaches (without expensive CNN networks) for the candidate proposal in the first stage, so that more resources can be reserved for the second network to be more sensitive. If also the training data was augmented with affine transformations, the preprocessing the images with linear registration could possibly omitted.

References

1. Mackay J, Mensah G, eds. The atlas of heart disease and stroke. WHO. 2004; p. 18–19.
2. Kemmling A, Flottmann F, Forkert ND, et al. Multivariate dynamic prediction of ischemic infarction and tissue salvage as a function of time and degree of recanalization. J Cereb Blood Flow Metab. 2015;35(9):1397–1405.
3. Winzeck S, Hakim A, McKinley R, et al. ISLES 2016 and 2017-benchmarking ischemic stroke lesion outcome prediction based on multispectral MRI. Front Neurol. 2018;9:679.
4. Inoue T, Nakaura T, Yoshida M, et al. Brain computed tomography using iterative reconstruction to diagnose acute middle cerebral artery stroke: usefulness in combination of narrow window setting and thin slice reconstruction. Neuroradiol. 2018;60(4):373–379.
5. Takahashi N, Lee Y, Tsai DY, et al. An automated detection method for the MCA dot sign of acute stroke in unenhanced CT. Radiol Phys Technol. 2014;7(1):79–88.
6. Lisowska A, O'Neil A, Dilys V, et al. Context-aware convolutional neural networks for stroke sign detection in non-contrast CT scans. Med Image Underst Anal. 2017; p. 494–505.
7. Setio AAA, Ciompi F, Litjens G, et al. Pulmonary nodule detection in CT images: false positive reduction using multi-view convolutional networks. IEEE Trans Med Imaging. 2016;35(5):1160–1169.
8. Sakamoto M, Nakano H, Zhao K, et al. Multi-stage neural networks with single-sided classifiers for false positive reduction and its evaluation using lung X-ray CT images. Proc ICIAP. 2017; p. 370–379.
9. Ronneberger O, Fischer P, Brox T. U-net: convolutional networks for biomedical image segmentation. Proc MICCAI. 2015; p. 234–241.

Sparsely Connected Convolutional Layers in CNNs for Liver Segmentation in CT

Alena-Kathrin Schnurr[1], Lothar R. Schad[1], Frank G. Zöllner[1]

[1]Computer Assisted Clinical Medicine, Medical Faculty Mannheim, Heidelberg University
alena-kathrin.schnurr@medma.uni-heidelberg.de

Abstract. Convolutional neural networks are currently the best work-ing solution for automatic liver segmentation. Generally, each convolu-tional layer processes all feature maps from the previous layer. We show that the introduction of sparsely connected convolutional layers into the U-Net architecture can benefit the quality of liver segmentation and re-sults in the increase of the dice coefficient by 0.32% and a reduction of the mean surface distance by 3.84 mm on the LiTS data. Evaluation on the IRCAD data set with the application of post-processing showed a 0.70% higher Dice coefficient and a 0.26 mm lower mean surface distance.

1   Introduction

Exact delineation of the liver contour is an important step in computer-assisted surgery and radiotherapy planning. It can also be used as a preprocessing step in the tumor localization and is needed for volume measurements. Manual annota-tion of Ct scans is time consuming and unfeasible with the increasing number of scans produced in medical facilities. Therefore, the fast and reliable automatic annotation of the organ contour becomes a more important topic.

In recent years, liver and liver lesion segmentation has been a subject of in-tense research in the medical image processing community due to the availability of the Liver Tumor Segmentation (LiTS) challenge [1] data set. All top scoring automatic segmentation methods in the LiTS challenge used CNNs. The first round of the LiTS challenge was won by Han [2]. This solution consists of two cascading U-Net-like networks [3], of which the first extracted a coarse liver seg-mentation. The second network refined the liver boundary and also delineated the tumors. Han extended the U-Net with short range residuual connections.

Convolutions in CNNs are usually fully connected channel-wise, meaning that each convolution kernel will always process all feature maps resulting from the previous convolution. However, Changpinyo et al. showed that sparsely con-nected convolutions can increase the network performance in classification tasks, while simultaneously reducing the number of weights [4]. They theorized that the sparse connection pattern leads to more diverse features. Another way to interpret the change might be the introduction of parallel information pathways which can also be found in Google's inception modules [5].

We suggest sparsely connected convolutions as a possible building block in U-Net architectures. To show how the can benefit the segmentation, we compare three networks: a dense version and two sparse versions with the proposed modifications.

2 Materials and methods

2.1 Network

We base our networks on the architecture presented by Han. The architecture of our networks is shown in 1. Each stage consists of n convolutional layers, which are composed of a 3×3-convolution, batch normalization and rectified linear units. The result of the first convolutional layer is added to the result of the last forming a residual connection. At the end of each encoding stage the feature maps are scaled down using 2×2 max-pooling. The first two stages have $n = 2$, the third has $n = 3$. Similarly, the bottom stage consists of three convolutional layers. This stage is then followed by the decoding stages. In each decoding stage the first operation is an upscaling via transposed convolution. The resulting feature maps are then concatenated with the feature maps from the according encoding stage, forming a skip connection. The first decoding stage has $n = 3$, the following $n = 2$. The first stage has 32 channels, this number is doubled with every encoding stage and the bottom stage. Each decoding stage halves the number of channels. A final 1×1 convolutional layer is appended to the final stage to produce the logits.

In the dense version of the network all convolutions are connected to all feature maps from the previous layer. For the two sparse versions of the network, we restrict the connection pattern between convolutional layers. In the dense network the number of weights $|w|$ in a convolutional layer is defined as the product of the number of input channels c_{in}, the spatial kernel dimensions x and y, as well as the number of output channels c_{out}

$$|w| = c_{\text{in}} \cdot x \cdot y \cdot c_{\text{out}} \tag{1}$$

We introduce a cardinality parameter C, which controls the number of sub-operations into which the convolution is split. The input channels are divided into an according number of sets and for each set a convolution with c_{out}/C output channels is performed. The resulting feature maps from all sub-operations are then concatenated. This way the operation produces the same number of output channels while the number of weights is reduced in comparison to the dense version

$$|w| = \frac{c_{\text{in}}}{C} \cdot x \cdot y \cdot \frac{c_{\text{out}}}{C} = \frac{c_{\text{in}} \cdot x \cdot y \cdot c_{\text{out}}}{C^2} \tag{2}$$

To evade the problem of checking for dead information pathways, which have no connection to output or input, we only use sparsely connected convolutions in every second convolutional layer. We refrain from using randomized channel splitting as this would require several more slicing and concatenation operations, which we deem too time consuming. For a proof of principle we test $C \in [2, 4]$. Higher cardinalities would lead to a too small number of channels in the sub-operations of the first stage.

2.2   Data

The LiTS [1] data set consists of 131 contrast-enhanced abdominal CT scans from different clinical sites. The challenge provides reference annotations for the liver contours as well as for liver lesions. The scans vary in in-plane resolution and slice thickness. We aligned the directions of all images, but kept the different resolutions, so that the networks are able to process a range of resolutions and the results can be compared to the original labels.

For evaluation we additionally use the IRCAD data set [6]. It is composed of CT-scans of 10 women and 10 men. As this data set is aimed at liver segmentation the annotations have a higher quality than the LiTS.

2.3   Training

For the training we use patches of 256×256 voxels with a batch size of 16. To counteract the class imbalance, we differentiate the slices from each scan into one of two classes:

1. Liver: slice contains liver annotations.
2. Background: slice does not contain any annotations.

All liver slices are used for sample extraction. We select two patches from each liver slice. The possible patch centers are constrained to $\mu + 3\sigma$ of the position of the liver annotations along each axis. We use equal quantities of liver and background patches, but from each background slice we only sample a single patch to get a diverse representation of non-liver structures. The ratio we apply for sampling was also used in the batches. We perform data augmentation in the

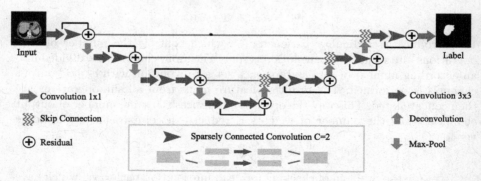

Fig. 1. Architecture: The U-Net is extended with sparsely connected convolutions. Using $C = 2$, the feature maps are divided into two subsets and a kernel is learned for each subset. The resulting feature maps are then concatenated.

form of a rotation r around the cranial-caudal axis with $r \in [-9\,°, 9\,°]$ to mimic possible patient positions.

Training is performed with the Adam optimizer, applying a learning rate of $lr = 10^{-3}$. We use L2-regularization and minimize the Tversky loss function between probabilities P and labels Y. Where P_l denotes the liver probability and P_b the background probability, accordingly in Y_l the liver is denoted by 1 and in Y_b the background is 1. The weights are set to $\alpha = 0.3$ and $\beta = 0.7$ as suggested by Salehi et al. [7]

$$T_{\alpha,\beta}(P,Y) = \frac{\sum_{i=0}^{|Y|} p_{l,i} y_{l,i}}{\sum_{i=0}^{|Y|} p_{l,i} y_{l,i} + \alpha \sum_{i=0}^{|Y|} p_{l,i} y_{b,i} + \beta \sum_{i=0}^{|Y|} p_{b,i} y_{l,i}} \tag{3}$$

2.4 Experimental design and evaluation metrics

The described networks were implemented using Tensorflow 1.10 [1] and Python 3.5. We performed three-fold-cross-validation on the LiTS data. Each network was trained for 25 epochs, which equaled 52500 iterations. Training and testing were performed on an NVIDIA Quadro P5000 graphics card. We used two metrics to compare the network predictions $\hat{Y}$ to the labels Y. Firstly, the dice coefficient to assess the overlap

$$D\left(\hat{Y}, Y\right) = \frac{2\,|\hat{Y} \cap Y|}{|\hat{Y}| + |Y|} \tag{4}$$

Secondly, the mean surface distance (MSD) which is more sensitive to shape and alignment

$$\text{MSD}\left(\hat{\text{Y}}, \text{Y}\right) = \frac{1}{|\hat{\text{Y}}|} \sum_{i=0}^{|\hat{\text{Y}}|} \min(\text{d}(\hat{y}_i, \text{Y})) \tag{5}$$

We used the SimpleITK [2] implementations. No postprocessing was performed for the evaluation on the LiTS data set, therefore, the performance of the networks can be directly compared. For the IRCAD data we performed a connected component analysis on the network predictions to verify the performance without the presence of outliers.

3 Results

3.1 LiTS

The dense network achieved an average D=0.940 and a MSD=22.738 mm. Our network with sparsely connected convolutions and $C = 2$ accomplished a D=0.9411 and MSD=22.738 mm. Using $C = 4$ resulted in a D=0.944 and

---

[1] https://www.tensorflow.org/
[2] http://www.simpleitk.org/

MSD=19.893 mm. A visualization of the results across all test cases can be seen in Fig. 4. As stated before, the splitting and concatenating operations are computationally expensive, which leads to a slight increase in prediction time per slice from 0.036 seconds to 0.039 seconds for $C = 2$ and to 0.043 seconds for $C = 4$.

3.2   IRCAD

All networks trained on the LiTS data were applied to the IRCAD data set. The densely connected U-Nets achieved an average D=0.953 and a MSD=1.820 mm. The $C = 2$ sparse networks accomplished a D=0.956 and MSD=1.820 mm. Using $C = 4$ resulted in a D=0.960 and MSD=1.560 mm. Slices from an exemplary case with labels and predictions are shown in Fig. 3.

4   Discussion

Our experiments have shown that sparsely connected convolutions can be a beneficial building block in segmentation networks. Our network benefits from parallel information pathways, while maintaining a U-Net structure and using less weights. The difference in quality low in the the Dice coefficient, but more prominent for the MSD. $C = 2$ performed only slightly better than the dense - Unet. However, on the IRCAD data the Dice coefficient achieved by our network with cardinality $C = 4$ was 0.7% higher in comparison to a densely connected U-Net. While the MSD was decreased by 14.2% mm. The sparse versions had a slightly higher prediction time per slice. However, due to the enhanced quality we deem this justifiable and recommend sparsely connected convolutions with $C = 4$ for segmentation tasks.

Acknowledgement. The authors declare that they have no conflict of interest. This research project is part of the Research Campus M^2OLIE and funded by the German Federal Ministry of Education and Research (BMBF) within the framework "Forschungscampus: public-private partnership for innovations"

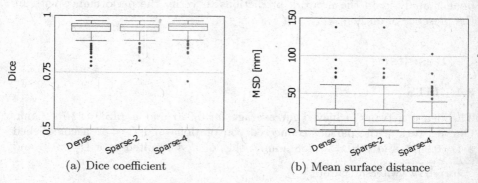

(a) Dice coefficient   (b) Mean surface distance

Fig. 2. Comparison of the LiTS segmentation quality across all three cardinalities.

Fig. 3. IRCAD example case: The annotated ground truth is shown in green. Dense U-Net prediction is shown in blue. Results from the sparsely connected U-Nets are shown in red ($C = 2$) and magenta ($C = 4$).

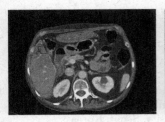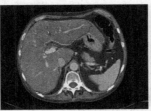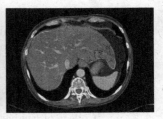

under the funding code 13GW0092D. We gratefully acknowledge the support of NVIDIA Corporation with the donation of the NVIDIA Quadro P5000 used for this research.

References

1. Christ P, Ettlinger F, Lipkova J, et al.. LiTS: liver tumor segmentation challenge; 2017. Available from: http://www.lits-challenge.com/.
2. Han X. Automatic liver lesion segmentation using a deep convolutional neural network method. CoRR. 2017;abs/1704.07239.
3. Ronneberger O, Fischer P, Brox T. U-Net: convolutional networks for biomedical image segmentation. Proc MICCAI. 2015; p. 234–241.
4. Changpinyo S, Sandler M, Zhmoginov A. The power of sparsity in convolutional neural networks. CoRR. 2017;abs/1702.06257.
5. Szegedy C, Liu W, Jia Y, et al. Going deeper with convolutions. Proc CVPR. 2015; p. 1–9.
6. 3D-IRCADb-01; 2018. Available from: https://www.ircad.fr/research/3d-ircadb-01/.
7. Salehi SSM, Erdogmus D, Gholipour A. Tversky loss function for image segmentation using 3D fully convolutional deep networks. Mach Learn Med Imaging. 2017; p. 379–387.

Smooth Ride: Low-Pass Filtering of Manual Segmentations Improves Consensus

Jennifer Maier[1], Marianne Black[2], Mary Hall[2], Jang-Hwan Choi[3],
Marc Levenston[2], Garry Gold[2], Rebecca Fahrig[4], Bjoern Eskofier[1],
Andreas Maier[1]

[1]Pattern Recognition Lab, Friedrich-Alexander-Universität Erlangen-Nürnberg
[2]Stanford University, Stanford, California, USA
[3]College of Engineering, Ewha Womans University, Seoul, Korea
[4]Siemens Healthcare GmbH, Erlangen, Germany
jennifer.maier@fau.de

Abstract. In this paper, we investigate slice-wise manual segmentation of knee anatomy. Due to high inter-rater variability between annotators, often a high number of raters is required to obtain a reliable ground truth consensus. We conducted an extensive study in which cartilage surface was segmented manually by six annotators on three scans of the knee. The slice-wise annotation results in high-frequency artifact that can be reduced by averaging over the segmentations of the annotators. A similar effect can also be obtained by smoothing the surface using low-pass filtering. In our results, we demonstrate that such filtering increases the consistency of the annotation of all raters. Furthermore, due to the smoothness of the cartilage surface, strong filtering produces surfaces that show differences to the ground truth that are in the same order of magnitude as the inter-rater variation. The remaining root mean squared error lies in the range of 0.11 to 0.14 mm. These findings show that appropriate pre-processing techniques result in segmentations close to the consensus of multiple raters, suggesting that in the future fewer annotators are required to achieve a reliable segmentation.

1 Introduction

The validity of medical image-based analyses often heavily depends on the accuracy of a segmentation of the underlying data. A medical application demanding accurate segmentation is the analysis of articular knee cartilage of patients suffering from Osteoarthritis. Particularly, imaging under natural weight-bearing conditions is of interest, because it may further the understanding of this disease and may lead to an improved early diagnosis. Scanning a person in a standing position is enabled by the usage of flexible cone-beam C-arm CT (CBCT) systems. Contrast agent injected into the knee joint makes the contact surface between femoral and tibial cartilage visible in the 3D reconstructions and enables its segmentation. At the same time, the contrast agent poses additional challenges to the segmentation problem, since it fills a whole region instead of marking a clear cartilage border line, and over time diffuses into the spongy cartilage tissue.

Segmentation of structures in medical images is often performed automatically, since the advantages of automatic segmentations are manifold: On average, they can be performed faster than manual segmentations, they are repeatable and they follow predefined objective rules [1]. There exists a variety of automatic segmentation algorithms, based on thresholds, edges or regions, and also more complex methods like shape modeling [1]. More recent studies investigate deep neural networks for segmentation tasks with promising results [2, 3].

In comparison, manual segmentations are time-consuming and subjective with often high inter-rater variability. Still, many studies rely on this process. Especially if the segmentation requires human assessment, or if the underlying data shows quality differences that interfere with automated methods, manual segmentation is often preferred. Both are the case when aiming at segmenting cartilage surfaces in the presented case.

To obtain a stable consensus from manual segmentations of multiple raters, many annotators are needed due to the high inter-rater variability. It is assumed that on average, they are able to segment the true borders. Alternatively to averaging over multiple raters, the issue of inter-rater differences can be tackled by low-pass filtering. In this work, we evaluate the effect of low-pass filtering of segmentations on datasets manually segmented by six experienced raters. Isotropic and anisotropic smoothing kernels of varying size are applied. The unfiltered and filtered segmentations of each rater are evaluated against a consensus computed from an increasing number of other raters.

2   Materials and methods

In the following, the data acquisition and the segmentation process are described. Afterwards, the smoothing process and comparison between raters are explained.

2.1   Data acquisition and segmentation

X-ray images were acquired according to an IRB-approved protocol using a clinical C-Arm CT system (Artis Zeego, Siemens Healthcare GmbH, Erlangen, Germany) with a flat panel detector. The knees of one healthy subject (male, 52 years) were scanned three times. Motion compensated filtered backprojection [4, 5] resulted in 3D images of 512^3 voxels with an isotropic voxel spacing of 0.2 mm. The reconstructed volumes contained only the right knee.

The tibial bone and the contrast agent lines marking the border of tibial cartilage on the lateral and medial side were segmented by 6 experienced raters using AMIRA software (AMIRA, Mercury Computer Systems, Berlin, Germany). Segmentations were performed slice by slice on 2D images in the sagittal plane. For further processing, only the part of the tibial surface below the segmented cartilage surfaces was stored, see gray surface in Fig. 1(c). In total, this resulted in 3 (scans) * 4 (medial/lateral tibia/cartilage) = 12 segmentations per rater. For the comparison of the segmentations, only one z-value per (x,y)-combination was segmented. If a rater marked multiple values per (x,y)-coordinate, only the upper value was stored. Fig. 1(a) shows an example grayscale image and one rater's segmentation as overlay, Fig. 1(b) depicts a magnified region. In Fig. 1(c) surfaces reconstructed from the medial part of the segmentations are shown. The three colors blue, green and pink mark segmentations of three raters, showing high similarity with small fluctuations of their labeling.

2.2   Data processing

The X-ray images were acquired in-vivo, thus there was no possibility to measure a ground truth for segmentation. For this reason, the agreement between raters was evaluated in this work.

Smoothing. Since the raters all were instructed to segment the tibial surface and cartilage surface, their resulting segmentations are similar. However, there are small high-frequency differences in the extent of the surfaces and in the segmented z-values. To tackle the former, only those (x,y)-coordinates in which all six raters segmented a voxel were considered in the comparison of the raters. By smoothing the segmentations in z-direction, the small variations in z-value can be reduced and the segmentations are expected to be more similar afterwards. The segmentations were smoothed with an isotropic mean and median filter of size 3. Since the single lines caused by slice-wise segmentation are clearly visible in the unfiltered segmentations, (Fig. 1(c)) it makes sense to average over a larger extent in the direction perpendicular to the lines to reduce this unevenness. For this reason, anisotropic mean filters of size 7x3 and 11x9 were applied to the segmentations. Furthermore, larger isotropic kernels of size 11, 15 and 21 were used to heavily smooth the segmentations. Finally, isotropic and anisotropic

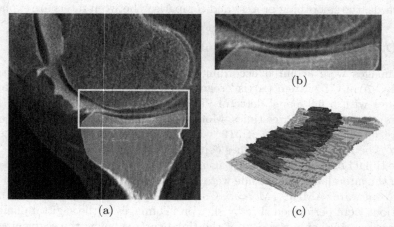

(b)

(a)   (c)

Fig. 1. (a) Grayscale CBCT slice in sagittal plane, segmentations of one rater marked in red. (b) The region in the yellow rectangle is magnified. (c) 3D surfaces created from three raters' segmentations (medial part) marked in blue, green and pink. The segmentation direction is visible, here from the upper left to the lower right.

Gaussian filter kernels with σ between 1 and 3 were evaluated, since they assign larger weights to voxels closer to the kernel center, which may have a higher influence on the considered voxel.

Evaluation. The original and smoothed segmentations of each rater were compared to combinations of a growing number of segmentations of the other five raters, that were formed by averaging the z-values of their original segmentations. Combining the segmentations of k raters, $k \in [1; 5]$, from a total of $N = 5$ raters resulted in $\binom{N}{k}$ combinations for comparison to the remaining rater.

The metric to describe the agreement between a rater and those combinations was the root mean squared error (RMSE) of the point-wise z-value difference. For each of the 12 segmentations of a rater, the RMSE to all combinations of the other 5 raters was computed. As next step, the average RMSE over the 12 surfaces was computed, resulting in $\binom{N}{k}$ mean RMSE values per rater. Lastly, the mean with standard deviation of these $\binom{N}{k}$ values is computed and is interpreted as the overall mean RMSE between one rater and the others.

3   Results

A visual comparison of a segmentation of one rater smoothed with different kernels is shown in Fig. 2. The data was processed in a point-wise manner, but for better visualization, surfaces were generated from the point clouds.

The results show that mean and Gaussian filtering create smoother surfaces compared to median filtering, since they allow for sub-voxel placement of points on the smoothed surface. Furthermore, as expected, larger kernels create smoother outputs. In contrast to the isotropic filters, the anisotropic kernels reduced the visible segmentation direction.

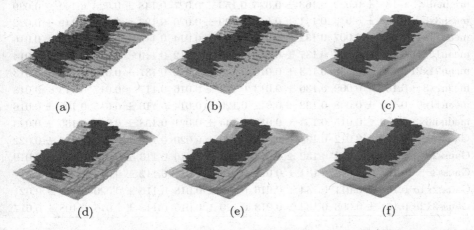

Fig. 2. Surfaces reconstructed from segmentations of one rater (medial tibial and cartilage surface). (a) original segmentation, (b) 3x3 median filtered, (c) 3-σ Gauss filtered, (d) 3x3 mean filtered, (e) 7x3 mean filtered, (f) 11x9 mean filtered.

Table 1. RMSE (mean ± standard deviation) between one rater's original segmentations, and combinations of segmentations of an increasing number of reference raters. Since there is only one possibility to combine five raters, only a mean and no standard deviation is given in the last column.

	1 rater	2 raters	3 raters	4 raters	5 raters
rater 1	0.184 ± 0.028	0.159 ± 0.011	0.149 ± 0.006	0.144 ± 0.003	0.141
rater 2	0.167 ± 0.029	0.137 ± 0.012	0.124 ± 0.006	0.117 ± 0.004	0.113
rater 3	0.199 ± 0.022	0.176 ± 0.007	0.168 ± 0.003	0.164 ± 0.002	0.161
rater 4	0.183 ± 0.029	0.157 ± 0.011	0.147 ± 0.005	0.141 ± 0.003	0.137
rater 5	0.172 ± 0.030	0.144 ± 0.012	0.132 ± 0.007	0.126 ± 0.004	0.122
rater 6	0.222 ± 0.011	0.204 ± 0.004	0.198 ± 0.002	0.195 ± 0.001	0.193

The results of the quantitative evaluation are shown in Tab. 1 and 3. Tab. 1 shows for the original segmentation of each rater the mean RMSEs to all combinations of other raters. For the original and smoothed surfaces, in Tab. 3 the mean RMSEs over all raters are given.

4 Discussion

Manual segmentations are always subjective because every human rater makes decisions based on his experience and intuition. However, a consensus can be computed by averaging over multiple raters. The presented work shows that a consensus that is based on a higher number of raters has a lower mean RMSE to each single rater (Tab. 1). A possible interpretation of this finding is that the

	1 rater	2 raters	3 raters	4 raters	5 raters
original	0.188 ± 0.020	0.163 ± 0.025	0.153 ± 0.027	0.148 ± 0.028	0.144 ± 0.029
mean3x3	0.168 ± 0.013	0.141 ± 0.017	0.129 ± 0.020	0.123 ± 0.021	0.119 ± 0.022
mean11x11	0.162 ± 0.007	0.132 ± 0.012	0.120 ± 0.014	0.113 ± 0.015	0.109 ± 0.016
mean15x15	0.166 ± 0.007	0.137 ± 0.010	0.126 ± 0.012	0.119 ± 0.013	0.115 ± 0.014
mean21x21	0.180 ± 0.008	0.153 ± 0.010	0.143 ± 0.012	0.137 ± 0.012	0.134 ± 0.013
mean7x3	0.164 ± 0.009	0.136 ± 0.013	0.124 ± 0.016	0.117 ± 0.017	0.113 ± 0.018
mean11x9	0.162 ± 0.008	0.132 ± 0.012	0.120 ± 0.014	0.113 ± 0.015	0.109 ± 0.016
median3x3	0.180 ± 0.015	0.154 ± 0.019	0.144 ± 0.021	0.138 ± 0.022	0.135 ± 0.023
Gauss1σ	0.166 ± 0.012	0.138 ± 0.017	0.126 ± 0.020	0.120 ± 0.021	0.116 ± 0.022
Gauss2σ	0.161 ± 0.009	0.132 ± 0.014	0.120 ± 0.016	0.113 ± 0.018	0.109 ± 0.019
Gauss3σ	0.161 ± 0.008	0.131 ± 0.012	0.119 ± 0.014	0.112 ± 0.016	0.108 ± 0.017
Gauss2x1σ	0.163 ± 0.011	0.134 ± 0.016	0.122 ± 0.018	0.116 ± 0.020	0.111 ± 0.021
Gauss3x2σ	0.161 ± 0.008	0.132 ± 0.013	0.120 ± 0.015	0.113 ± 0.016	0.108 ± 0.017

Table 2. Mean RMSE and standard deviation over all raters for the comparison of the original respectively smoothed segmentations with one to five raters.

consensus of a larger number of raters lies closer to the correct segmentation than all individual raters alone.

The second part of the evaluation showed that low-pass filtering the annotations of a rater results in a segmentation that is closer to the consensus compared to the unfiltered segmentation, as shown in Tab. 3. The mean and Gaussian filters outperformed the median, an explanation for this is that the creation of reference combinations was also based on a mean computation. For the smaller filter sizes, anisotropic filtering produced slightly better results than isotropic filtering. More importantly, it considerably reduced the visibility of the segmentation direction, yielding qualitatively better results compared to the unfiltered and isotropically filtered segmentations. Since cartilage is a smooth surface, this filtering step will therefore produce more natural looking results. The smallest mean RMSE values were achieved for the 3σ Gaussian filtered segmentation, but 11x9 and 11x11 mean achieved similar results. If it is assumed that the average rating of the other raters corresponds most closely to the gold standard segmentation, this minimum indicates that a 3σ Gaussian or 11x11 resp. 11x9 mean filter should be considered as filtering method of choice. Note that 15x15 and 21x21 filtering already started to increase the distance to the consensus of the other raters.

The current work shows that smoothing can be used to decrease the variability between raters and suggests the Gaussian filter as best filtering method. The best kernel size is highly problem dependent and is still to be evaluated in a larger study. This study implies that low-pass filtering of manual segmentations yields results similar to the consensus of multiple raters, suggesting that fewer raters are needed to create a reliable consensus.

References

1. Pham DL, Xu C, Prince JL. Current methods in medical image segmentation. Annu Rev Biomed Eng. 2000;2(1):315–337.
2. Ronneberger O, Fischer P, Brox T. U-net: convolutional networks for biomedical image segmentation. In: Proc MICCAI. vol. 9351. Springer; 2015. p. 234–241.
3. Milletari F, Navab N, Ahmadi SA. V-Net: fully convolutional neural networks for volumetric medical image segmentation. In: Proc 3DV. IEEE; 2016. p. 565–571.
4. Choi JH, Fahrig R, Keil A, et al. Fiducial marker-based correction for involuntary motion in weight-bearing C-arm CT scanning of knees: part 1: numerical model-based optimization. Med Phys. 2013;40(9):091905–1–12.
5. Choi JH, Maier A, Keil A, et al. Fiducial marker-based correction for involuntary motion in weight-bearing C-arm CT scanning of knees: part 2: experiment. Med Phys. 2014;41(6):061902–16.

User Loss

A Forced-Choice-Inspired Approach to Train Neural Networks Directly by User Interaction

Shahab Zarei, Bernhard Stimpel, Christopher Syben, Andreas Maier

Pattern Recognition Lab, Department of Computer Science,
Friedrich-Alexander-Universität Erlangen-Nürnberg, Germany
andreas.maier@fau.de

Abstract. In this paper, we investigate whether is it possible to train a neural network directly from user inputs. We consider this approach to be highly relevant for applications in which the point of optimality is not well-defined and user-dependent. Our application is medical image denoising which is essential in fluoroscopy imaging. In this field every user, i.e. physician, has a different flavor and image quality needs to be tailored towards each individual. To address this important problem, we propose to construct a loss function derived from a forced-choice experiment. In order to make the learning problem feasible, we operate in the domain of precision learning, i.e., we inspire the network architecture by traditional signal processing methods in order to reduce the number of trainable parameters. The algorithm that was used for this is a Laplacian pyramid with only six trainable parameters. In the experimental results, we demonstrate that two image experts who prefer different filter characteristics between sharpness and de-noising can be created using our approach. Also models trained for a specific user perform best on this users test data. This approach opens the way towards implementation of direct user feedback in deep learning and is applicable for a wide range of application.

1 Introduction

Deep learning is a technology that has been shown to tackle many important problems in image processing and computer vision [1]. However, all training needs a clear reference in order to apply neural network-based techniques. Such a reference can either be a set of classes or a specific desired output in regression problems. However, there are also problems in which no clear reference can be given. An example for this are user preferences in forced-choice experiments. Here, a user can only select the image he likes best, but he cannot describe or generate an optimal image. In this paper, we tackle exactly this problem by introduction of a user loss that can be generated specifically for one user of such a system.

In order to investigate our new concept, we explore its use on image enhancement of interventional X-ray images. Here, the problem arises that different physicians prefer different image characteristics during their interventions.

Some users are distracted by noise and prefer strong de-noising while others prefer crisp and sharp images. Another requirement for our user loss is that we want to spend only few clicks for training. As such we have to deal with the problem of having only few training samples, as we cannot ask your users to click more than 50 to 100 times. In order to still work in the regime of deep learning, we employ a framework coined *precision learning* that is able to map known operators and algorithms onto deep learning architectures [2]. In literature this approach is known to be able to reduce maximal error bounds of the learning problem and to reduce the number of required training samples [3]. Fu et al. even demonstrated that they are able to map complex algorithms such as the vesselness filter onto a deep network using this technique [4].

2 Methods

We chose an Laplacian pyramid de-noising algorithm as basis [5]. In this section first image denoising using the Laplacial pyramid is described. Then, we follow the idea of precision learning to derive the network topolgy based on the known approach followed by an detailed description of the loss function.

2.1 Subband decomposition

Image densoising using a Laplacian pyramid is carried out in two steps. First the image is decomposed into subbands followed by an soft threshold to reduce the noise. The Laplacian pyramid [5] is an extension of the Gaussian pyramid using differences of Gaussians (DoG). To construct a layer of the Laplacian pyramid the input has to be blurred using a Gaussian kernel with a defined standard deviation σ and mean $\mu = 0$ with a subsequent subtraction from the unblurred input itself.

2.2 Soft-thresholding

After sub-band decomposition, we assume that small coefficients are caused by noise in each band $I_{\mathrm{bp},n}$. We employ soft-thresholding to suppress this noise with magnitudes smaller than ϵ. Note that for both, the Gaussian that is used for the sub-band decomposition, as well as for the soft thresholding function sub-gradients [6] can be computed with respect to their parameters. As such both are suited for use in neural networks [2].

2.3 Neural network

Following the *precision learning* paradigm, we construct a three layer Laplacian pyramid filter as a neural network. A flowchart of the network is depicted in Fig. 1. The low-pass filters are implemented as convolutional layers, in which the actual kernel only has a single free parameter σ. Using point-wise subtraction, these low-pass filters are used to construct the band-pass filters. On each of those filters, soft-thresholding with parameter ϵ is applies. In a final layer, the soft-thresholded band-pass filters are recombined to form the final image. As such we end up with a network architecture with nine layers that only has six trainable parameters $\sigma_1, \sigma_2, \sigma_3, \epsilon_1, \epsilon_2, \epsilon_3$. In the following, we summarize these parameters as a single vector ϕ that can be trained using the back-propagation algorithm [7].

2.4   User loss

Let I_{pref} be the user preferred image, I_{NN} the denoised image produced by our net. Below equation would be the main objective of our net

$$\text{argmin}_\phi \, ||I_{\text{pref}} - I_{\text{NN}}||_2^2 \tag{1}$$

The main problem with this equation is that the user is not able to produce I_{pref}. To resolve this problem, we introduce errors to the optimal image that cannot be observed directly

$$e = ||I_{\text{pref}} - I||_2^2$$

However, if we provide a forced-choice experiment using four images $I_0 \ldots I_3$, we can determine which of the four errors $e_0 \ldots e_3$ is the smallest. This gives us a set of constraints that need to be fulfilled by our neural network. For the training of the network, we define our error in the following way

$$e_q = ||I_{\text{NN}} - I_q||_2^2$$

Let s be the total number of frames, $e_{s,q}$ denote the quality q dedicated to frame s_r and Q denote the number of choices. Assuming $e_{s,*}$ is selected by the user, the following expected relationships between the errors emerge

$$e_{s,*} \leq e_{s,q} \qquad \forall q \in \{0, \ldots, Q-1\} \tag{2}$$

For user selection is $* = 2$, the constraint below are used to set up our loss function. Similar to implementation of support vector machines in deep networks, we map the inequality constraints to the hinge loss using the max operator [8]

$$
\begin{aligned}
e_{s,2} < e_{s,0} &\quad \rightarrow \quad e_{s,2} - e_{s,0} < 0 &\quad \rightarrow \quad \max(e_{s,2} - e_{s,0}, 0) \\
e_{s,2} < e_{s,1} &\quad \rightarrow \quad e_{s,2} - e_{s,1} < 0 &\quad \rightarrow \quad \max(e_{s,2} - e_{s,1}, 0) \\
e_{s,2} < e_{s,3} &\quad \rightarrow \quad e_{s,2} - e_{s,3} < 0 &\quad \rightarrow \quad \max(e_{s,2} - e_{s,3}, 0)
\end{aligned} \tag{3}
$$

Fig. 1. Schematic of the neural network design used in this work. The architecture mimics a Laplacian pyramid filter with soft-thresholding.

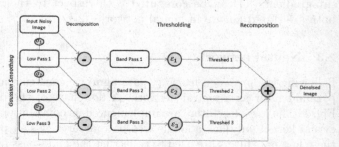

This gives rise to three different variants of the user loss that are used in this work:

1. Best-Match: Only the user selected image is used to guide the loss function

$$\text{argmin}_\phi \sum_{s=1}^{S} e_{s,*} \tag{4}$$

2. Forced-Choice: The user loss seeks to fulfill all criteria imposed by the user selection

$$\text{argmin}_\phi \sum_{s=1}^{S} \sum_{q=0}^{Q-1} \max(e_{s,*} - e_{s,q}, 0) \tag{5}$$

3. Hybrid: The user selected image drives the parameter optimization while all constraints implied by the forced-choice are sought to be fulfilled

$$\text{argmin}_\phi \sum_{s=1}^{S} e_{s,*} + \sum_{q=0}^{Q-1} \max(e_{s,*} - e_{s,q}, 0) \tag{6}$$

Note that the hybrid user loss is mathematically very close to the soft-margin support vector machine, where $e_{s,*}$ takes the role of the normal vector length and $\sum_{q=0}^{Q-1} \max(e_{s,*} - e_{s,q}, 0)$ the role of the additional constraints.

3   Experiments and results

For generating different scenarios, in the first step the Laplacian pyramid is initialized for each input image. Considering the center values of our parameter sets ϕ, the four different scenes are generated using random parameters. The resulting scenes for each frame are then imported to a GUI in order to take the user preferences (Fig. 2). The network is implemented in Python using Tensorflow framework. ADAM algorithm is used as optimizer iterating over 5000 epochs with learning rate of $\mu = 10^{-2}$ and the batchsize is set to 50. The datasets which are used in this work are 2D angiography fluoroscopy image data. The dataset contains 50 images of size 1440×1440 with different dose levels. We created 200 scenarios via randomly initializing the Laplacian pyramid parameters.Our dataset is divided such that 60 % of the dataset for training data, 20 % for validation and 20 % for test set. In this work *stratified K-Fold Cross-Validation* is used for data set splitting.

3.1   Qualitative results

Qualitative results of our approach are presented in Fig. 3 for the first user. These indicate an influence of different loss functions on the parameter tuning of one user's preferences. The *Best Match* loss shows better noise reduction, however reduces the sharpness more than the other losses. In contrast to Best Match, *Forced Choice* loss shows better sharpness and higher noise level. In order to favor both targets the *Hybrid Loss* eliminates noise and preserve sharpness of image data as well.

Table 1. Quantitative comparison of loss functions: Best-Match (BM), Forced-Choice (FC), Hybrid(HY).

Low dose data		User 1			User 2		
		BM	FC	HY	BM	FC	HY
Model Nr. 1	BM	1431.1	—	—	2436.7	—	—
	FC	—	248.8	—	—	253.1	—
	HY	—	—	**1771.1**	—	—	2675.9
Model Nr. 2	BM	1381.5	—	—	2391.5	—	—
	FC	—	249.5	—	—	964.9	—
	HY	—	—	1781.1	—	—	**2359.1**

3.2 Quantitative evaluation

In this section, we evaluate the three loss functions for both of our users against each other. Tab. 1 displays the models created with the respective loss functions versus the test sets of both users. To set fair conditions for the comparision, we only evaluated models with the respective loss functions that were used in their training. The results indicate that Best-Match and Forced-Choice only are not able to result in the lowest loss for their respective user. The Hybrid loss models, however, are minimal on the test data of their respective user. Hence, the Hybrid loss seems to be a good choice to create user-dependent de-noising models.

Fig. 2. Graphical user interface designed for proposed network training.

Fig. 3. Comparison of original low-dose image and its corresponding results obtained from different user losses for the first user. For better visualization windowing is applied on the second row.

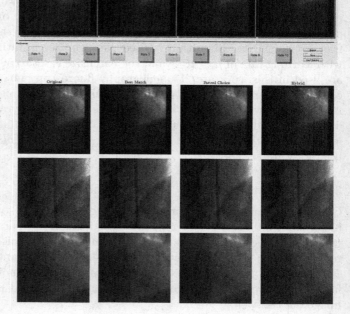

4   Conclusion and discussion

We propose a novel user loss for neural network training in this work. It can be applied to any image grading problem in which users have difficulties in finding exact answers. As a first experiment for the user loss, we demonstrate that it can be used to train a de-noising algorithm towards a specific user. In our work 200 decisions using 50 clicks were sufficient to achieve proper parameter tuning. In order to be able to apply this for training, we used the *precision learning* paradigm to create a suitable network with only few trainable parameters.

Obviously also other algorithms would be suited for the same approach [9, 10, 11, 12, 5]. However, as the scope of the paper is the introduction of the user loss, we omitted these experiments in the present work. Further investigations on which filter requires how many clicks for convergence is still an open question and subject of future work.

We believe that this paper introduces a powerful new concept that is applicable for many applications in image processing such as image fusion, segmentation, registration, reconstruction, and many other traditional image processing tasks.

References

1. LeCun Y, Bengio Y, Hinton G. Deep learning. Nat. 2015;521(7553):436.
2. Maier AK, Schebesch F, Syben C, et al. Precision learning: towards use of known operators in neural networks. CoRR. 2017;abs/1712.00374. Available from: http://arxiv.org/abs/1712.00374.
3. Syben C, Stimpel B, Breininger K, et al. Precision learning: reconstruction filter kernel discretization. Procs Fifth Int Conf Image Form X-Ray Comput Tomogr. 2018; p. 386–390.
4. Fu W, Breininger K, Schaffert R, et al. Frangi-net: a neural network approach to vessel segmentation. BVM 2018. 2018; p. 341–346.
5. Rajashekar U, Simoncelli EP. Multiscale denoising of photographic images. Essent Guide Image Process. 2009; p. 241–261.
6. Rockafellar RT. Convex Analysis. Princeton landmarks in mathematics and physics. Princeton University Press; 1970. Available from: https://books.google.de/books?id=1TiOka9bx3sC.
7. Rumelhart DE, Hinton GE, Williams RJ. Learning representations by back-propagating errors. Nat. 1986;323(6088):533.
8. Bishop CM. Pattern Recognition and Machine Learning (Information Science and Statistics). Berlin, Heidelberg: Springer-Verlag; 2006.
9. Tomasi C, Manduchi R; IEEE. Bilateral filtering for gray and color images. Proc ICCV. 1998; p. 839–846.
10. Petschnigg G, Szeliski R, Agrawala M, et al.; ACM. Digital photography with flash and no-flash image pairs. ACM Trans graph (TOG). 2004;23(3):664–672.
11. Luisier F, Blu T, Unser M. A new SURE approach to image denoising: interscale orthonormal wavelet thresholding. IEEE Trans Image Process. 2007;16(3):593–606.
12. Motwani MC, Gadiya MC, Motwani RC, et al. Survey of image denoising techniques. Procs GSPX. 2004; p. 27–30.

Sodium Image Denoising Based on a Convolutional Denoising Autoencoder

Simon Koppers[1], Edouard Coussoux[1], Sandro Romanzetti[2,3], Kathrin Reetz[2,3], Dorit Merhof[1]

[1]Institute of Imaging & Computer Vision, RWTH Aachen University
[2]Department of Neurology, RWTH Aachen University
[3]JARA-BRAIN Institute Molecular Neuroscience and Neuroimaging, Forschungszentrum Jülich GmbH and RWTH Aachen University
koppers@lfb.rwth-aachen.de

Abstract. Sodium Magnetic Resonance Imaging (sodium MRI) is an imaging modality that has gained momentum over the past decade, because of its potential ability to become a biomarker for several diseases, ranging from cancer to neurodegenerative pathologies, along with monitoring of tissues metabolism. One of the most important limitation to the exploitation of this imaging modality is its characteristic low resolution and signal-to-noise-ratio as compared to the classical proton MRI, which is due to the notably lower concentration of sodium than water in the human body. Therefore, denoising is a central aspect with respect to the clinical use of sodium MRI. In this work, we introduce a Convolutional Denoising Autoencoder that is trained on a training database of thirteen training subjects with three sodium MRI images each. The results illustrate that the denoised images show a strong improvement after application in comparison to the state-of-the-art Non Local Means denoising algorithm. This effect is demonstrated based on different noise metrics and a qualitative evaluation.

1 Introduction

Sodium Magnetic Resonance Imaging (sodium MRI) is an imaging modality that has the potential to become a valuable biomarker in many applications in the field of medical diagnostics [1, 2]. Because of the strict balance of sodium concentration between inner and outer cell space, sodium imaging enables a monitoring of the tissues metabolism. An increase in concentration of sodium ions in brain tissues has been shown to be potentially related to neurodegenerative diseases or inflammations of the neural system. Therefore, this imaging modality represents a tool of choice for the early diagnostic of such diseases, ideally taking place before the damages they involve have occurred.

However, sodium MRI is limited by the notably lower concentration in sodium nuclei within the human body as compared to the concentration of elements containing hydrogen, which is the nucleus involved in the classical proton MRI. For this reason, as well as because of the lower gyromagnetic ratio of sodium as compared to hydrogen, the signal-to-noise ratio (SNR) in the images is low and, consequently for this the resolution of sodium MR images is low, too. The effects of noise on such low resolution images can critically jeopardize their content, which demonstrates the crucial importance of denoising in the field of sodium MRI.

For about a decade, the domain of Deep Learning has known tremendous developments,resulting in highly efficient methods for many high level tasks in the field of computer vision [3]. The development of strategies enabling the training of more complex networks has allowed researchers to achieve impressive results in segmentation, classification, super resolution and also denoising tasks.

In this paper, a Denoising Autoencoder is applied to sodium MRI and evaluated concerning its denoising performance in comparison to the state-of-the-art non local mean algorithm [4].

2   Methods

The goal of sodium image denoising is to increase the SNR, while keeping the underlying brain structure unaffected. Our approach is to use a Denoising Autoencoder [5, 6] (DA) to predict the denoised signal based on each voxels signal and its neighboring signals. Most of the time, DAs are trained by adding noise to the original data, while being given the original uncorrupted data as target output (label). Furthermore, the learnable effect of denoising can be improved if a low-noise dataset and a high-noise dataset is available.

2.1   Denoising autoencoder

The utilized Deep Learning structure is a DA, which composes two basic blocks: First, the encoder encodes the noisy input signal into a feature vector, while the decoder part of the network tries to rebuild the input without noise based on the given feature vector. The effect of denoising can be improved, if a signal with less noise than the input is utilized as output image, while the regular noisy image is utilized as input image.

In this work, the input signal (a $5 \times 5 \times 5$ voxel neighborhood) is convoluted by 64 different $3 \times 3 \times 3$ convolutional kernels, followed by a second convolution ($3 \times 3 \times 3$ kernel size) projecting the resulting 64 feature maps onto 256 features, while only one voxel remains. Afterwards, only basic dense layers (Dense) are utilized to project the given 256 features onto 32 features and back up onto 256 features. In the end, the remaining 256 features predict the denoised signal intensity. All but the last layer utilize Rectified Linear units as activation function. The last layer uses no activation function.

An overview over the full network is given in Tab. 1.

2.2   Training

The network is trained based on a single sodium acquisition with added Gaussian noise as input, while the corresponding center voxel (label) is constructed by av-

Table 1. Topology of the DA for predicting a denoised sodium image.

#	Type	Parameters
1	3D convolution	$64 \times 3 \times 3 \times 3$
2	ReLU	—
3	3D convolution	$256 \times 3 \times 3 \times 3$
4	ReLU	—
5	Flattening	—
6	Dense	32
7	ReLU	—
6	Dense	256
7	ReLU	—
6	Dense	1

eraging all three repeated sodium acquisitions of the same subject. For training, only brain voxels, extracted with FSL's BET [7], are used. Optimization is based on the ADAM optimizer (learning rate 0.0001, batch size 128 3D patches), while the mean squared error is utilized as loss function.

Training is completed after validation performance does not improve for more than eight epochs.

3   Evaluation

In the following, we present the results of our method and a state-of-the-art denoising method, the Non Local Means (NLM) algorithm [4]. The latter calculates the average value of all pixels in the image and weights these with the similarity of the target pixel to the respective pixels. This results in a much better denoised image and a significantly lower loss of detail in the image compared to regular local denosing algorithms, e.g. Gaussian blurring and unsharpening masks [4].

For evaluation, a five-fold cross validation is performed (three groups with three subjects and two groups with two subjects). Four groups are used for training, while the remaining group is subdivided into a test and validation group, to ensure that there is no inter-subject overlap within training, validation and testing.

3.1   Materials

The dataset consists of thirteen subjects, with three sodium acquisitions each ($\approx$ 20 minutes acquisition time in total). Every sodium acquisition has an isotropic resolution of $4 \times 4 \times 4 \, mm$. Furthermore, every subject was scanned with additional calibration phantoms placed on both sides of the subject's head of known sodium concentration (Fig. 1, green circles). Based on this concentration, each scan can be re-normalized for quantitative sodium concentration measurements.

	Mean	Median	σ
NLM	1.95	1.96	0.33
DA	2.37	2.42	0.50

Table 2. Resulting relative improvement (in percent) of pSNR of the NLM and DA approach.

3.2 Results

All results are compared using the the peak SNR [8] (pSNR) defined as

$$\mathrm{pSNR(Ref, Img)} = 10\log_{10}\left(\frac{(\max(\mathrm{Ref}) - \min(\mathrm{Ref}))^2}{\mathrm{MSE(Ref, Img)}}\right) \text{ with} \qquad (1)$$

$$\mathrm{MSE(Ref, Img)} = \frac{1}{N}\sum_{\hat{x}}(\mathrm{Ref}(\hat{x}) - \mathrm{Img}(\hat{x}))^2 \qquad (2)$$

and the the Structural Similarity index [9] (SSIM) specified by

$$\mathrm{SSIM}(\hat{x}) = \frac{1}{N}\sum_{\hat{x}} l(\hat{x}) \cdot c(\hat{x}) \cdot s(\hat{x}) \qquad (3)$$

where $l(\hat{x})$ defines the similarity of the local patch luminance (brightness values), $c(\hat{x})$ defines the similarity of the local patch contrasts, while $s(\hat{x})$ defines the similarity of the local patch structures (for more information see [9]). Furthermore, Ref represents the reference image, while Img denotes the predicted denoised image. $\hat{x}$ indicates the spatial position within an image and N is the number of voxels within the utilized brain mask.

Tab. 2 and Tab. 3 presents the resulting mean, median and σ of pSNR and SSIM evaluated on the brain voxels only. It can be seen that the DA achieves a higher mean and median pSNR and SSIM. On the other side, it should be noted that σ increases, too.

	Mean	Median	σ
NLM	18.85	18.88	3.39
DA	28.75	28.93	3.85

Table 3. Resulting relative pSNR improvement (in percent) of the SSIM of the NLM and DA approach.

Furthermore, Fig. 2 shows a qualitative and exemplary slice after application of the NLM and the DA algorithm. Here, both algorithms show an improved and denoised image after application, while the NLM image results in very sharp edges with a high contrast, in comparison to DA.

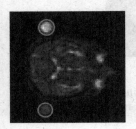

Fig. 1. Exemplary axial slice of a sodium acquisition with marked concentration bars in green.

4   Discussion

Sodium acquisitions are increasingly being included in the diagnosis and study of neurodegenerative diseases, as they can characterize degenerative processes before they are visible in standard T1 or T2 acquisitions. However, the intrinsic low SNR of this imaging modality leads to long acquisition times. To mitigate for this, low spatial resolution images are typically used within within clinical trials. In this paper, we present a denoising technique based on a DA and demonstrate its ability to outperform state-of-the-art non-deep learning techniques.

As shown in Tab. 2 and Tab. 3 the DA achieves higher mean and median values for the pSNR and the SSIM, while σ(SSIM) and σ(pSNR) increases only a little. A similar denoising performance can be seen in Fig. 2, where both algorithms show a good result. Nonetheless, the NLM seems to sharpen edges, resulting in edge artifacts, while at the same time, homogeneous areas seem to be very smooth. These effects are not visible for the DA image.

Despite these promising results, the application of deep learning comes at a cost, since it is limited by its utilized training database. Due to this, novel signals, that are not part of the training database, might result in wrongly denoised images. Although the DA was chosen as a standard deep learning architecture with only few parameters (which is due to the limited training database), it might be beneficial to train a more complex structure, if more subjects are available for training.

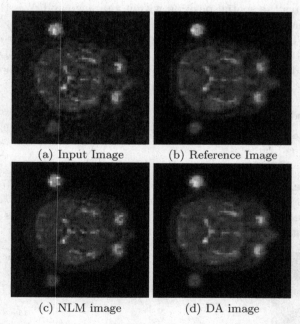

(a) Input Image   (b) Reference Image

(c) NLM image   (d) DA image

Fig. 2. Exemplary input and reference slice utilized during training and its corresponding NLM and DA denoised version (best viewed in digital version).

Overall, this work shows a feasible and practical solution for denoising sodium MRI. It is validated using quantitative and qualitative criteria.

Acknowledgement. KR is partly funded by the German Federal Ministry of Education and Research (BMBF 01GQ1402). This work was supported by the International Research Training Group 2150 of the German Research Foundation (DFG).

References

1. Madelin G, Lee JS, Regatte RR, et al. Sodium MRI: methods and applications. Prog Nucl Magn Reson Spectrosc. 2014;79:14 – 47.
2. Romanzetti S, Mirkes CC, Fiege DP, et al. Mapping tissue sodium concentration in the human brain: a comparison of MR-sequences at 9.4 tesla. Neuroimage. 2014;96:44 – 53.
3. LeCun Y, Bengio Y, Hinton G. Deep learning. Nat. 2015;521(7553):436.
4. Buades A, Coll B, Morel JM. Non-local means denoising. Image Process Line. 2011;1:208–212.
5. Vincent P, Larochelle H, Bengio Y, et al.; ACM. Extracting and composing robust features with denoising autoencoders. Procs 25th Int Conf Mach Learn. 2008; p. 1096–1103.
6. Vincent P, Larochelle H, Lajoie I, et al. Stacked denoising autoencoders: learning useful representations in a deep network with a local denoising criterion. J Mach Learn Res. 2010;11(Dec):3371–3408.
7. Smith SM. Fast robust automated brain extraction. Hum Brain Mapp. 2002;17(3):143–155.
8. Wang Z, Bovik AC. Mean squared error: love it or leave it? a new look at signal fidelity measures. IEEE Signal Process Mag. 2009;26(1):98–117.
9. Wang Z, Bovik AC, Sheikh HR, et al. Image quality assessment: from error visibility to structural similarity. IEEE Trans Image Process. 2004;13(4):600–612.

Improved X-Ray Bone Segmentation by Normalization and Augmentation Strategies

Florian Kordon[1,3], Ruxandra Lasowski[1], Benedict Swartman[2], Jochen Franke[2], Peter Fischer[3], Holger Kunze[3]

[1]Faculty of Digital Media, Furtwangen University (HFU), Germany
[2]Department for Trauma and Orthopaedic Surgery, BG Trauma Center Ludwigshafen, Germany
[3]Advanced Therapies, Siemens Healthineers Forchheim, Germany
florian.kordon@hs-furtwangen.de

Abstract. X-ray images can show great variation in contrast and noise levels. In addition, important subject structures might be superimposed with surgical tools and implants. As medical image datasets tend to be of small size, these image characteristics are often under-represented. For the task of automated, learning-based segmentation of bone structures, this may lead to poor generalization towards unseen images and consequently limits practical application. In this work, we employ various data augmentation techniques that address X-ray-specific image characteristics and evaluate them on lateral projections of the femur bone. We combine those with data and feature normalization strategies that could prove beneficial to this domain. We show that instance normalization is a viable alternative to batch normalization and demonstrate that contrast scaling and the overlay of surgical tools and implants in the image domain can boost the representational capacity of available image data. By employing our best strategy, we can improve the average symmetric surface distance measure by 36.22 %.

1 Introduction

Automatic segmentation of X-ray images is a challenging task because typically many types of X-ray systems in different scenarios need to be supported. First, the proportion of the imaged organ may vary in size and rotation, and shifts and image flips may occur. Reasons are that patients are of different size and proportion. But also the geometry of systems may be quite different, as the detector size and detector-tube distance may range from 15 cm to 40 cm and from 40 cm to 200 cm respectively. It is not always possible for a patient to move such that the body part is aligned with the system in all axes. Thus, image rotations and views on the imaged structure can slightly vary between images. Then, different contrasts between the organ and the background may occur because different tube voltage settings are used [1]. And last, an X-ray image is always a superimposition of organs, bones and objects along the ray, which means that the organ or bone of interest may be interfered by other organs or surgical instruments and implants (Fig. 1).

More recently, deep learning based solutions advance as powerful ways to tackle various problems in the medical imaging domain. For the particular task of image segmentation, fully convolutional neural networks (FCN) yield state of the art performance fueled by great representational learning power and high computational efficiency [2]. To learn the appearance and variability of different image structures, these models typically rely on a large number of training data. However, since medical image data is often limited, the sample sizes are usually not sufficient to fully account for the aforementioned image characteristics. Several strategies have been proposed to tackle this problem. If available, simulation of radiographs from appropriate 3D CT scans yields realistic results that can enlarge the available training data [3]. As shown in [4], extensive augmentation to the existing training data can enable these models to learn invariance to a broader set of image characteristics. Also, careful normalization of the input data and features in the network can alleviate covariate shift between different distributions, thus allowing for accelerated and more robust learning [5].

In this work, we draw upon a subset of these ideas and evaluate their benefit towards the problem of X-ray-based bone segmentation. To this end, we consider contrast scaling, additive noise, and the overlay of surgical tools and implants in the image domain as task-specific data augmentations that could promote practical application on clinical data. We also think of X-ray segmentation as being sensitive to different normalization techniques of the input data and network features. For this reason, we examine the input standardization methods min-max normalization and z-scoring and combine them with various potentially beneficial replacements for the widely used batch normalization (BN) [5]. Instance normalization (IN) aims to introduce invariance to image contrast by normalizing only over spatial dimensions [6]. Layer normalization (LN) and group normalization (GN) both decouple different batch examples by normalizing over spatial and channel dimensions, with the latter additionally introducing feature clusters to respect network features as structured data [7, 8]. Switchable normalization (SN) supplies a fully-learnable approach by weighting the statistics created by IN, LN, and BN, which potentially allows for an optimal normalization scenario [9]. The main contribution of the paper is to show that an ensemble of normalization and augmentation strategies can substantially improve the segmentation in the case of lateral projections of femur bones on X-ray images.

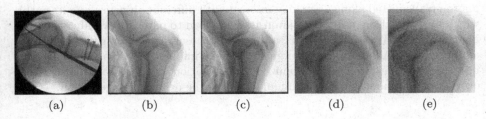

(a)   (b)   (c)   (d)   (e)

Fig. 1. Image examples representing different image characteristics. (a) depicts overlay of surgical tools and implants, (b) and (c) show different contrast settings, (d) and (e) show different noise levels.

2   Materials and methods

2.1   Formulation of input and feature normalization

Let x be some input data we want to normalize. We can formalize min-max normalization and z-scoring as $\tilde{x}_{\text{min-max}} = (x - \min(x))/(\max(x) - \min(x))$ and $\tilde{x}_{\text{z-score}} = (x - \mu)/(\sqrt{\sigma^2 + \epsilon})$ respectively. μ and σ^2 denote mean and variance of the data, whereas ϵ is a small constant for numerical stability.

To introduce a general formulation for the feature normalizations, let z_{bcij} be some pre-activation hidden feature at an arbitrary layer, represented as a vector (B, C, H, W) and indexed with $b \in [1, B]$, $c \in [1, C]$, $i \in [1, H]$, and $j \in [1, W]$. B denotes the batch dimension, C denotes the channel dimension, and (H, W) refer to the spatial height and width dimensions. Instead of directly computing the layer's activated output $a_{bcij} = g(z_{bcij})$ with an activation function g, the covered normalization strategies introduce an intermediate step of calculating a normalized representation $\tilde{z}_{bcij} = (z_{bcij} - \mu_k)/(\sqrt{\sigma_k^2 + \epsilon})$. The calculation of μ_k and σ_k^2 depends on a subset of features M_k with $k \in \{\text{IN}, \text{BN}, \text{LN}, \text{GN}\}$ (Tab. 1)

$$\mu_k = \frac{1}{|M_k|} \sum_{(b,c,i,j) \in M_k} z_{bcij} \qquad \sigma^2 = \frac{1}{|M_k|} \sum_{(b,c,i,j) \in M_k} (z_{bcij} - \mu_k)^2 \qquad (1)$$

SN builds upon the statistics computed in IN, BN, and LN to define an importance-weighted, normalized representation of the features [9]. Additionally, all covered feature normalizations introduce the trainable parameters γ and β to facilitate scaling and shifting of the layer input. That way, distribution characteristics other than $\mu = 0$ and $\sigma^2 = 1$ can be learned. Thus, the layer's activated output is calculated with $a_{bcij} = g(\gamma \tilde{z}_{bcij} + \beta)$.

2.2   Data augmentation strategies

To model different contrast settings in the image domain, we consider contrast scaling as a linear scaling of each image pixel px by $0.5 + \alpha(px - 0.5)$, $\alpha \in [0.33, 3]$. Caused by electronic readout noise and quantum mottle, radiographic images may also contain different noise levels. We approximate this by adding generated Gaussian noise which is drawn from $\sim \mathcal{N}(0, [0.01, 0.15])$. Furthermore, each photon transmitted along a ray may interact with different objects along its path, which by integration of different intensities can lead to partially or fully obscured image regions. To account for this, a randomly chosen projection generated from a proprietary CAD database of surgical tools and implants (50 images) is blended into the image region with randomized shift, rotation and surface intensity. The overlaid area amounts to a maximum of 9 % of the original image region.

2.3   Dataset

The dataset consists of 56 X-ray knee scans in lateral projection. 35 examples originate from systems with image intensifiers which leads to circularly masked

Table 1. Feature subsets used in different normalization strategies [5, 6, 7, 8, 9].

Feature normalization	Feature subset
Instance normalization (IN)	$M_{\text{IN}} = \{(i,j) \,|\, i \in [1,H], j \in [1,W]\}$
Batch normalization (BN)	$M_{\text{BN}} = \{(b,i,j) \,|\, b \in [1,B], i \in [1,H], j \in [1,W]\}$
Layer normalization (LN)	$M_{\text{LN}} = \{(c,i,j) \,|\, c \in [1,C], i \in [1,H], j \in [1,W]\}$
Group normalization (GN)	$M_{\text{GN}} = \{(c,i,j) \,|\, c \in [x_{n-1}, x_n], i \in [1,H], j \in [1,W]\}$
	Subdivision of [1,C] into G groups/subintervals
	$[x_{n-1}, x_n]$ with width $\Delta \frac{C-1}{G}$. Here, we consider G=32.

images. The remaining 21 samples are from digital radiography systems and are sometimes rotated for PACS viewing or include overlaid meta information. For each image, a ground truth segmentation mask of the femur bone was created. The data was split into three subsets for training, validation and testing with distribution ratios of 0.6/0.2/0.2. To factor in various spatial resolutions and aspect ratios present in the dataset, we applied an online data preprocessing routine which consists of rescaling with fixed aspect ratio and center-cropping to the target size of 256 × 256. For the training set, we allowed a randomized deviation of the cropping center and applied a basic set of randomized online data augmentation techniques (rotation, scaling, horizontal flipping).

2.4 Ablation study and performance metrics

The experiments were structured into three sections. First, a base model was constructed which derives from the standard U-Net architecture, but was supplemented with a dropout layer at the end of the contracting path [4]. As the standard feature normalization technique, we introduced pre-activation batch normalization layers to each network block. As for the input data, we set min-max normalization as the default. The hyper-parameters of this base model were optimized by performing 150 steps of random search limited to 120 epochs training time each, followed by manual refinement. In a second step, we evaluated the product set of both data and feature normalizations against the optimized base model, returning a total of ten combined strategies. Lastly, the two most promising strategies were used to examine the proposed augmentations. All eight strategies resulting from all possible ordered subsets of the contemplated augmentations were introduced as additional steps after the basic augmentations and were applied with a probability of $p = 0.5$ each. To allow for potentially longer training times when employing the different strategies, we raised the number of epochs to 200 for both normalization and augmentation experiments.

In all experiment stages, the model performance was measured against mean intersection over union (mIOU), average symmetric surface distance (ASD) and symmetric Hausdorff distance (HD). The mIOU score evaluated on the validation set was used as the key metric and as the main selection criteria between different steps in the ablation study [2]. To factor in potential initialization variances or outliers, the median was calculated from 20 training trials for each strategy.

3   Results

Without further modifications, the base model with BN and min-max normaliza-tion achieves a mIOU score of 0.956, 95 % CI [0.955, 0.958] (Fig. 2). It performs equally well when z-scoring is used and yields the best mIOU performance for all employed feature normalizations. The second best configuration – IN and min-max normalization – achieves a mIOU score of 0.953, [0.952, 0.956], which results in a relative deterioration of 0.31 %. The remaining normalization techniques re-turn mIOU scores of 0.938, [0.933, 0.941] (GN, min-max), 0.937, [0.933, 0.939] (SN, min-max) and 0.894, [0.886, 0.901] (LN, min-max). As regards the sur-face distance scores, the base model returns an ASD of 2.238, [1.990, 2.418] and an HD of 18.523, [16.217, 23.770]. Replacing min-max normalization with z-scoring slightly improves upon this base model's performance, returning an ASD of 2.136, [1.973, 2.579] and a HD of 17.313, [15.947, 19.404]. The combina-tion of IN and min-max normalization achieves comparable performance with an ASD of 2.157, [2.093, 2.301] and a HD of 16.729, [14.660, 18.500].

If the proposed augmentations are incorporated, most improvement can be attained by supplementing IN and min-max normalization with contrast scaling and the overlay of surgical tools and implants (Fig. 2). This configuration yields a mIOU of 0.964, [0.963, 0.965], an ASD of 1.572, [1.477, 1.650] and a HD of 11.815, [10.168, 12.991]. For the previous best configuration with BN and z-scoring, solely introducing the overlay of surgical tools and implants achieves the greatest improvement with a mIOU of 0.961, [0.960, 0.962], an ASD of 1.861, [1.706, 2.027] and a HD of 17.185, [13.790, 20.801].

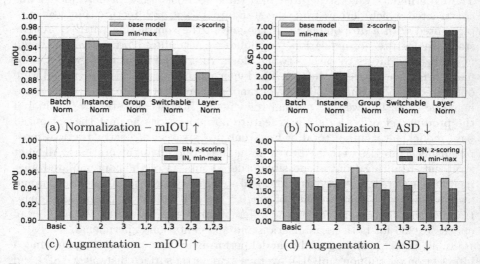

Fig. 2. Results for normalization and augmentation techniques on the validation set (1: contrast scaling, 2: overlay of surgical tools and implants, and 3: additive noise). For each metric, ↑ and ↓ indicate lower and higher is better, respectively.

4   Discussion

For the task of X-ray bone segmentation, IN shows to be a competitive feature normalization technique. The surface distance metrics' improvement of the best model that uses IN suggests a lower number of segmentation outliers, which could prove beneficial in highly contour-sensitive domains. As IN computes its statistics independently of the applied batch size, one can further think of retaining larger spatial dimensions of the input images in exchange for a smaller batch size. This potentially enables the network to learn more robust image features, though at the cost of weakening the benefits of mini-batch training. However, further evaluation on the test set shows that IN is also more susceptible to images where only a small portion of the femur bone is visible and where it is heavily obscured by medical tools. In such cases, BN is more successful due to its learned statistics over multiple images. This means that careful analysis of the target data and the employed setting is mandatory to choose the most suitable normalization strategy. Intriguingly, SN does not improve upon the base model's performance by incorporating multiple ways to learn the statistics. Ideally, in this setting, the weights for LN would drop to a small value. As we restricted the evaluation to drop-in replacement without further hyper-parameter optimization, a dedicated optimization for SN should therefore be considered in future work. In contrast to the best model with BN, where the overlay with medical tools returns the greatest relative improvement, scaling of the image contrast shows to be the most effective augmentation to be combined with IN. These augmentations do not hamper overall convergence speed and can be incorporated into the training pipeline without adding much computational overhead.

Disclaimer. The methods and information presented here are based on research and are not commercially available.

References

1. Huda W, Abrahams RB. Radiographic techniques, contrast, and noise in x-ray imaging. Am J Roentgenol. 2015;204(2):W126–W131.
2. Garcia-Garcia A, Orts-Escolano S, Oprea S, et al. A review on deep learning techniques applied to semantic segmentation. arXiv:170406857. 2017;.
3. Unberath M, Zaech JN, Lee SC, et al. DeepDRR: a catalyst for machine learning in fluoroscopy-guided procedures. arXiv:180308606. 2018;.
4. Ronneberger O, Fischer P, Brox T. U-Net: convolutional networks for biomedical image segmentation. Proc MICCAI. 2015;9351:234–241.
5. Ioffe S, Szegedy C. Batch normalization: accelerating deep network training by reducing internal covariate shift. Proc Int Conf Mach Learn. 2015;37:448–456.
6. Ulyanov D, Vedaldi A, Lempitsky VS. Instance normalization: the missing ingredient for fast stylization. arXiv:160708022. 2016;.
7. Ba JL, Kiros JR, Hinton GE. Layer normalization. arXiv:160706450. 2016;.
8. Wu Y, He K. Group normalization. arXiv:180308494. 2018;.
9. Luo P, Ren J, Peng Z. Differentiable learning-to-normalize via switchable normalization. arXiv:180610779. 2018;.

Multi-Modal Super-Resolution with Deep Guided Filtering

Bernhard Stimpel[1,2], Christopher Syben[1,2], Franziska Schirrmacher[1],
Philip Hoelter[2], Arnd Dörfler[2], Andreas Maier[1]

[1]Pattern Recognition Lab, Friedrich-Alexander-Universität Erlangen-Nürnberg
[2]Department of Neuroradiology, University Clinics Erlangen
bernhard.stimpel@fau.de

Abstract. Despite the visually appealing results, most Deep Learning-based super-resolution approaches lack the comprehensibility that is required for medical applications. We propose a modified version of the locally linear guided filter for the application of super-resolution in medical imaging. The guidance map itself is learned end-to-end from multi-modal inputs, while the actual data is only processed with known operators. This ensures comprehensibility of the results and simplifies the implementation of guarantees. We demonstrate the possibilities of our approach based on multi-modal MR and cross-modal CT and MR data. For both datasets, our approach performs clearly better than bicubic upsampling. For projection images, we achieve SSIMs of up to 0.99, while slice image data results in SSIMs of up to 0.98 for four-fold upsampling given an image of the respective other modality at full resolution. In addition, end-to-end learning of the guidance map considerably improves the quality of the results.

1 Introduction

Spatial resolution is subject to trade-offs in many medical imaging applications. For example in magnetic resonance imaging (MRI), spatial resolution must be weighed against the signal-to-noise ratio and acquisition time. A retrospective increase in resolution by post-processing measures could alleviate this problem. To this end, a vast amount of super-resolution (SR) methods have been proposed and proven in the past [1]. In general, a differentiation can be made between single and multiple image SR methods. The latter is of particular interest for medical imaging, as non-existent information in one image can be derived from another image of the same patient. Especially in diagnostics, the presence of several scans of the same patient is common. In processing these data, Deep Learning (DL) has recently developed the state of the art in SR towards a previously unknown image quality [2]. Thereby, most learning-based methods apply high-dimensional non-linear transformations that are very difficult or impossible to comprehend. If only additional information is generated, e.g. in segmentation, the lack of comprehensibility can be tolerated, as blatant errors can be quickly identified. However, if the image is modified, as is the case with super-resolution, a failure of the method cannot be detected trivially. This is a limiting factor in medical applications where no less than the lives of patients are at stake. Despite these downsides, DL-based methods are highly promising if used in an appropriate way. In combination with well understood known operators, the advantages of DL can be combined with the necessary comprehensibility [3, 4]. To transfer this to the task of super-resolution, we present the combination of the guided filter, which applies a local linear transformation to the input image, with a guidance map that is learnd end-to-end from multi-modal input.

2   Methods

2.1   The guided filter

First proposed by He et al. [5], the guided filter has been applied to a variety of tasks. Simply put, a given input image I is processed by incorporating structural information from a guidance image G. The filtering operation in this case assumes a locally linear model between the guidance and the input image. In general, the guidance map can be any given image, even the input image itself. To fully leverage the power of the guided filter, a more appropriate guide is needed. Given multiple input images from the same object, a combination of these is beneficial. However, this raises the question of how the combined guidance map is composed.

2.2   End-to-end trainable guided filter

Based on the wide range of possible applications of the guided filter as well as the ongoing success of Deep Learning, Wu et al. [6] incorporated the guided filter into a DL framework as a differentiable layer. This allows to backpropagate gradients through the filter to previous layers. We employ a convolutional neural network with the task to generate a guidance map for the guided filter based on the multi-modal input. Being able to train this generator in an end-to-end fashion enables for an optimal selection of features from all input modalities directly by the network.

The proposed pipeline consists of a guidance map generator network, for which we use a U-net-like architecture [7] with two separate encoding and a single decoding path, and the guided filtering layer.

Starting from two images, the low-resolution image I_{lr}, which is to be raised to higher resolution, and a higher-resolution image L_{hr} that serves as a guide. First, the input image I_{lr} is upsampled by bicubic interpolation to the desired output resolution as an initialization, further denoted as I_{up}. Second, I_{lr} and L_{hr} are fed into the generator network in order to extract the best possible combined representation G. Finally, the learned guidance map G and the upsampled input I_{up} are processed by the guided filter, resulting in the high-resolution output I_{hr}. By this, only (locally) linear processing steps are applied to the computed output image. A graphical representation of the pipeline is shown in Fig. 1.

Optimization is performed using a feature matching (FM) loss [8] based on the VGG-19 network [9].

3   Experiments

For evaluation, on the one hand multi-modal MRI data is used in the form of 8 tomographic T1 and T2 flair datasets with a spatial resolution of 256 x 256. On the other hand, 13 cone-beam MR and X-ray projections at a resolution of 512 x 512 are processed. All experiments are performed on clinical patient datasets provided by the Department of Neuroradiology, University Clinics Erlangen (MR: 1.5 T MAGNETOM Aera / CT: SOMATON Definition, Siemens Healthineers, Erlangen / Forchheim, Germany). Of each combination of modalities two corresponding patient dataset pairs are reserved for final testing. Image registration is done using 3D slicer [10]. The forward projections are taken from the work on hybrid MR/CT imaging by [11, 4, 12] and are generated using the CONRAD framework [13]. The low resolution images are artificially created by nearest neighbor downsampling by a factor of 4, resulting in a resolution of 64 x 64 for the tomographic and 128 x 128 for the projection data. For quantitative evaluation, we compute the mean squared error (MSE) and multi-scale structural similarity (MS-SSIM) measures. To avoid optimistic bias by the large homogeneous air regions, all background pixel are ignored for the evaluation metrics.

4   Results

The proposed approach was evaluated in comparison with bicubic upsampling and guided filtering using only the high-resolution image L_{hr} as guidance. The results are presented in Tab. 1. Exemplary qualitative results with their respective inputs are shown in Fig. 4. Furthermore, in Fig. 3 a region of interest can be seen to better observe the differences in the fine details.

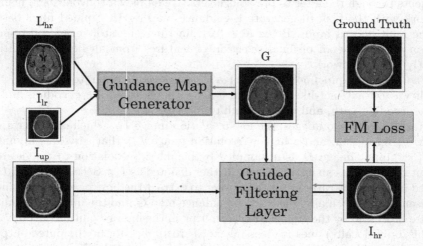

Fig. 1. The proposed guided filtering pipeline. Black arrows indicate the order of processing steps and orange arrows the gradient flow.

Table 1. Evaluation metrics of the proposed multi-modal guided filter.

CT & MRI Projection Images ($128 \times 128 \rightarrow 512 \times 512$)			
	Bicubic	GF w/o learned guidance	GF w learned guidance
MSE	0.0019 ± 0.001	0.0873 ± 0.0398	0.0005 ± 0.0001
MS-SSIM	0.97 ± 0.00	0.74 ± 0.04	0.99 ± 0.003
Tomographic T1 & T2 MRI images ($64 \times 64 \rightarrow 256 \times 256$)			
	Bicubic	GF w/o learned guidance	GF w learned guidance
MSE	0.0997 ± 0.0526	0.1506 ± 0.0493	0.0138 ± 0.0077
MS-SSIM	0.89 ± 0.04	0.63 ± 0.13	0.98 ± 0.01

5 Discussion

The quantitative and qualitative results show clear improvement of the proposed guided filtering pipeline compared to the reference method. Especially when observing the differences between the bicubic and the proposed upsampling method for the tomographic images in Fig. 4(a) and 4(b), respectively, the improved performance of the guided filter upsampling becomes apparent. The proposed framework captures fine details that are present in the guidance map which can not be estimated from the low-resolution input alone. Furthermore, the end-to-end learned guidance map clearly benefits the processing, as indicated in Tab. 1. This comes with the additional advantage that the optimal guidance map can be learned individually for each task and each combination of inputs. The learned guidance maps are already close to the desired high-resolution output images (Fig. 4(e)). However, due to the high-dimensional transforms applied in the computation of these, the required comprehensibility is not given. In con-

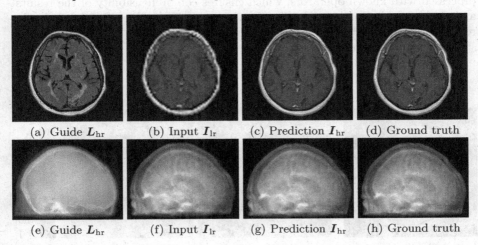

(a) Guide L_{hr} (b) Input I_{lr} (c) Prediction I_{hr} (d) Ground truth

(e) Guide L_{hr} (f) Input I_{lr} (g) Prediction I_{hr} (h) Ground truth

Fig. 2. Results of the guided filtering process. T1 & T2 MRI image pairs (a)-(d) and CT & MRI projection images (e)-(h).

Fig. 3. Comparison of the proposed GF results with bicubic upsampled images.

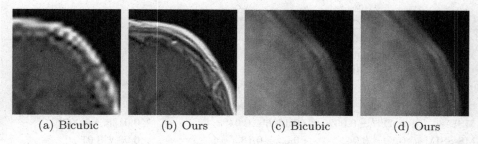

(a) Bicubic   (b) Ours   (c) Bicubic   (d) Ours

trast, when only used as guidance, the modifications to the input images can be reduced to locally linear operations.

For future work, the proposed pipeline needs to be evaluated more thoroughly against a variety of comparable methods. In addition, we want to compare our method with state-of-the-art deep learning super-resolution methods, although these are not in line with our fundamental considerations regarding comprehensibility of the results. Furthermore, we would like to apply the proposed approach to other tasks that can be addressed by the guided filter, e.g., denoising.

6   Conclusion

We presented a guided filtering pipeline for multi-modal medical image super-resolution. The proposed approach has two key points. First, it solves the problem of the unknown best combination of multi-modal inputs by learning a task-optimal guidance map directly from the data. Second, the actual data is only processed with known operators, which ensures comprehensibility of the results and simplifies the implementation of guarantees. The achieved results closely resemble the ground truth data which is substantiated by the low error and high structural similarity measures.

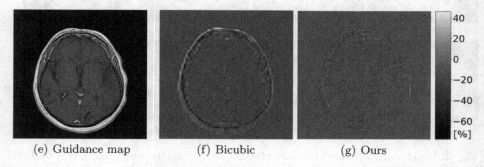

(e) Guidance map   (f) Bicubic   (g) Ours

Fig. 4. An exemplary guidance map (a). Difference maps of the bicubic (b) and guided filtering (c) upsampled images w.r.t the ground truth.

Acknowledgement. This work has been supported by the project P3-Stroke, an EIT Health innovation project. EIT Health is supported by EIT, a body of the European Union. Furthermore, we thank the NVIDIA Corporation for their hardware donation.

References

1. Köhler T. Multi-frame super-resolution reconstruction with applications to medical imaging. Friedrich-Alexander-Universität Erlangen-Nürnberg; 2018.
2. Wang Y, Perazzi F, McWilliams B, et al. A fully progressive approach to single-image super-resolution. IEEE Conf Comput Vis Pattern Recognit Work. 2018; p. 864–873.
3. Maier A, Schebesch F, Syben C, et al. Precision learning: towards use of known operators in neural networks. Proc ICPR. 2017;Available from: http://arxiv.org/abs/1712.00374.
4. Syben C, Stimpel B, Lommen J, et al. Deriving neural network architectures using precision learning: parallel-to-fan beam conversion. Proc Ger Conf Pattern Recognit. 2018;.
5. He K, Sun J, Tang X. Guided image filtering. IEEE Trans Pattern Anal Mach Intell. 2013;35(6):1397–1409.
6. Wu H, Zheng S, Zhang J, et al. Fast end-to-end trainable guided filter. IEEE Conf Comput Vis Pattern Recognit. 2018;.
7. Ronneberger O, Fischer P, Brox T. U-net: convolutional networks for biomedical image segmentation. Proc MICCAI. 2015; p. 234–241.
8. Johnson J, Alahi A, Fei-Fei L. Perceptual losses for real-time style transfer and super-resolution. arXiv:160308155. 2016;.
9. Simonyan K, Zisserman A. Very deep convolutional networks for large-scale image recognition. arXiv:14091556. 2015;.
10. Pieper S, Halle M, Kikinis R. 3D slicer. Proc ISBI. 2004;2:632–635.
11. Stimpel B, Syben C, Würfl T, et al. MR to X-ray projection image synthesis. Proc Fifth Int Conf Image Form X-Ray Comput Tomogr. 2017;.
12. Lommen JM, Syben C, Stimpel B, et al. MR-projection imaging with perspective distortion as in X-ray fluoroscopy for interventional X/MR-hybrid applications. Proc 12th Interv MRI Symp. 2018; p. 54.
13. Maier A, Hofmann HG, Berger M, et al. CONRAD: a software framework for cone-beam imaging in radiology. Med Phys. 2013;40(11).

Semi-Automatic Cell Correspondence Analysis Using Iterative Point Cloud Registration

Shuqing Chen[1]*, Simone Gehrer[2]*, Sara Kaliman[2], Nishant Ravikumar[1],
Abdurrahman Becit[1], Maryam Aliee[2], Diana Dudziak[3], Rudolf Merkel[4],
Ana-Sunčana Smith[2,5], Andreas Maier[1]

[1]Pattern Recognition Lab, FAU Erlangen-Nürnberg, Germany
[2]PULS Group, Theo. Physics I, FAU Erlangen-Nürnberg, Germany
[3]Department of Dermatology, University Hospital Erlangen, Germany
[4]ICS 7: Biomechanics, Forschungszentrum Jülich GmbH, Germany
[5]Division of Physical Chemestry, Institute Ruđer Bošković, Croatia
*Both contributed equally.
shuqing.chen@fau.de

Abstract. In the field of biophysics, deformation of *in-vitro* model tissues is an experimental technique to explore the response of tissue to a mechanical stimulus. However, automated registration before and after deformation is an ongoing obstacle for measuring the tissue response on the cellular level. Here, we propose to use an iterative point cloud registration (IPCR) method, for this problem. We apply the registration method on point clouds representing the cellular centers of mass, which are evaluated with a Watershed based segmentation of phase-contrast images of living tissue, acquired before and after deformation. Preliminary evaluation of this method on three data sets shows high accuracy, with 82 % - 92 % correctly registered cells, which outperforms coherent point drift (CPD). Hence, we propose the application of the IPCR method on the problem of cell correspondence analysis.

1 Introduction

Epithelial and other types of tissues are constantly exposed to stress, which is affecting the cell shape. The mechanism of this response is not understood, and progress lies on deconvolving the response of individual cells comprising the tissue. This requires sophisticated and automated image analysis techniques. Here, we induce an affine deformation of a 2D tissue model to relate the macroscopic deformation of the tissue to changes on the cellular level for a large number of cells in an automated fashion.

In our experiments, MDCK II cells (Madin Darby Kidney Cells) were grown as confluent epithelial cell layers on fibronectin(FN)-coated Polydimethylsiloxane (PDMS), and subjected to uniaxial stress through the underlying substrate. With existing methods it is only possible to investigate the average cell shape changes in the distributions over all cells for large tissue deformations. However, establishing the correspondence of every single cell is not yet possible for statistical relevant sample sizes.

The cell correspondence problem can also be formulated as a cell tracking problem, which often relays on cell detection based on computer vision algorithms [1, 2] and a series of time frames as input. However, image registration has been seldom employed for this purpose. Nonetheless, recent studies showed that image registration is potent for aligning cell nuclei [3] and feasible for tracking of single cells imaged with phase-contrast [4].

In this work, we propose a novel approach based on Watershed segmentation and iterative point cloud registration (IPCR), to find the cellular correspondences in the micrographs before and after deformation, such that shape changes may be investigated for each cell independently. By this we present, to the best of our knowledge, the first cell correspondence analysis algorithm using point cloud registration.

2 Materials and methods

2.1 Cell stretching and image acquisition

Clusters of MDCK II monolayers (about 8,000 cells) were stretched using FN-coated PDMS substrates and a cell-stretching device [5] (Fig. 1a). Samples were imaged before and subsequently after deformation in phase-contrast tile scans (Axiovert 200M, $10\times/0.25$ Achroplan, both Zeiss, pixel size: 0.8μ m $\times$ 0.8μ m)[6]. Resulting images were background corrected [7] and stitched using ImageJ [8].

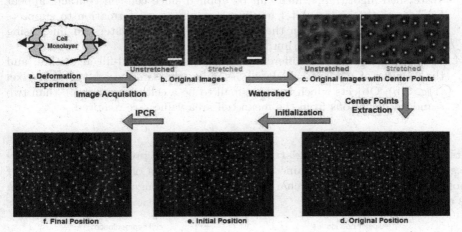

Fig. 1. The workflow of the proposed approach. a) Scheme of the deformation experiment. b) The original images, left: unstretched; right: stretched for 30 %. Scale bar 50 μm. c) Zoomed-in images with center points. d) Original position of the two point clouds. e) Initial position after manual placement. f) Best matching after the registration. The unstretched and the stretched images are denoted with red and green, respectively.

2.2   Semi-automatic cell correspondence analysis

The workflow of the proposed approach to the cell correspondence analysis problem is illustrated in Fig. 1. The approach consists of two steps, elaborated below: (i) Cell centroid coordinates before and after stretching are obtained by segmentation. These centroids represent the images as point clouds, for subsequent steps. (ii) The spatial relationship of the point clouds is initialized by manual placement using a visual representation. Finally, we obtain the spatial relationship and therefore, cellular correspondence using IPCR.

Cell segementation Cell segmentation is implemented using MATLAB [9]. As an input, the program can take either an image of a cell monolayer or a stitched image showing a whole cell cluster.

1. If the input is a whole cell cluster, the edge of the cluster is found using Otsu's method [10], so that single cells and dirt outside the cluster are excluded. Within the current imaging approach slightly lower threshold levels (90 % of the calculated level) provided the best outline of the cell cluster (Fig. 2a).
2. Small objects as well as the holes in the cell layer are removed by the area-opening-procedure. The border of the cell cluster is recognized using a flood-fill algorithm and used as a mask for further image analysis.
3. For the segmentation of single cell shapes within the mask, we used the Watershed algorithm, which can be applied since cell-cell contacts appear brighter in the image. After appling H-minima transformation to suppress all insignificant minima in the image, we obtain the watershed lines using the Fernand Meyer algorithm [11].
4. Cells are recognized as different objects with the flood-fill algorithm, and their center of mass is calculated assuming the same weight of each pixel (Fig. 2 b). Objects which are too small to be a cell (deviate more than two standard deviations from the mean cell area value) are removed.

Iterative point cloud registration As described previously, the cell correspondences should be obtained based on the clouds of the extracted center points. Fig. 3 shows the flowchart of our registration algorithm. The algorithm is described in the following:

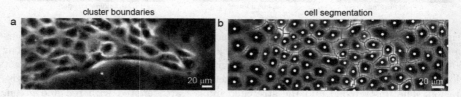

Fig. 2. Segmentation results. a) Segmented border (red) of a typical cell cluster. b) Cell segmentation (red) and corresponding centers of cell mass (white dots).

1. With a visualization of the extracted 2D point clouds assuming $\mathbf{A} = \{\mathbf{a_1}, ..., \mathbf{a_M}\}$ as the source and $\mathbf{B} = \{\mathbf{b_1}, ..., \mathbf{b_N}\}$ as the target or the reference, an initial position $\mathbf{T^0}$ is obtained manually by moving the source cloud close to the target cloud.
2. The initial point matching $\mathbf{A_c^0}$ and $\mathbf{B_c^0}$ is generated according to the initial transformation $\mathbf{T^0}$ based on k-d tree nearest neighbor (NN) search [12]. Due to the outlier rejection in the NN search, the matched point clouds are equal to or smaller than the original point clouds, i.e. $\mathbf{A_c} \subseteq \mathbf{A}$ and $\mathbf{B_c} \subseteq \mathbf{B}$
3. The transformation matrix $\mathbf{T}$ is updated to achieve optimal alignment of the two reciprocal point clouds $\mathbf{A_c}$ and $\mathbf{B_c}$
4. The point matching is recalculated using the new transformation matrix.
5. Step 3 and Step 4 are repeated until the termination criterion is fulfilled.

We used the Fast Library for Approximate Nearest Neighbors (FLANN) [12] for the k-d tree NN search. Covariance Matrix Adaptation Strategy (CMA-ES) [13] is utilized as the optimizer to update the transformation between the point clouds. Because the image was stretched, we assumed that the transformation is affine and the variation can be constrained with translation and scaling. The cost function of our optimization problem is defined with Euclidean distances of the reciprocal points (Eq. 1). We also used the average Euclidean distance in the termination criterion of the iterative algorithm to determine whether the best point matching is achieved

$$f = \frac{M \cdot N}{K^3} \sum_{k=1}^{K} \|\mathbf{T} \cdot \mathbf{a_{c,k}} - \mathbf{b_{c,k}}\| \tag{1}$$

where K is the amount of the reciprocal pairs, M and N are the number of points of the source and the target, $K \leq M$ and $K \leq N$.

3   Results

The proposed approach for cell correspondence analysis was evaluated with three data sets. Each data set contains two images before and after the deformation (Fig. 1b). Tab. 1 summarizes the information of the evaluated results of these three data sets. Cells (U/S) records the total number of cells of the unstretched (U) and stretched (S) images. The proposed approach is compared with another major type of point cloud registration algorithm – the coherent point drift (CPD) algorithm [14]. *Found* shows the calculated correspondences using FLANN [12]

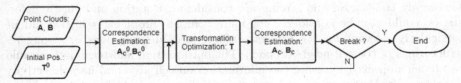

Fig. 3. Flowchart of the proposed IPCR method.

Table 1. Information and results of the evaluated data sets.

Data	Cells (U/S)	deform.	CPD [14] found [%]	eval.	cor.	Acc. [%]	Proposed found [%]	eval.	cor.	Acc. [%]
Set 1	160/156	30.0 %	91.0	142	137	87.8	91.0	142	140	89.7
Set 2	170/158	20.3 %	86.1	136	52	32.9	92.4	146	145	91.8
Set 3	1264/900	20.3 %	88.2	301	69	20.2	88.4	289	267	81.7

after the registration in percentage of the maximum of possible correspondences. Eval. and correct records the number of evaluated pairs, and out of those the correctly identified ones. The proposed approach obtained $88.4\% - 92.4\%$ reciprocal cell pairs. The calculated accuracy, according to Eq. 2, is $81.7\% - 91.8\%$

$$\text{Acc.} = \text{found} \times \frac{\text{Correct correspondences}}{\text{Evaluated cells}} \tag{2}$$

4 Discussion

We propose a novel approach based on the Watershed algorithm and IPCR to identify correspondences in the practical analysis of cells in tissue. We report 81.7 % to 91.8 % of correctly aligned cells in the preliminary evaluation and outperform CPD (with default parameter settings), which suggests that our approach is feasible for cell correspondence analysis. For the data set 1 with 30 % deformation, both methods performed similarly. Comparing the registration of different sized data sets (2 and 3), the proposed method obtained more correct reciprocal cell pairs in both cases. An important observation is that CPD provides high accuracy at the center of the input, declining with the distance to the center. The reason could be that CPD supposes the point sets are distributions built by a Gaussian Mixture Model (GMM). This may be due the manual initialization used in this study and the uniform distribution term incorporated within the GMM by CPD, designed to accommodate outliers and missing correspondences. However, minimal missing correspondences and outliers were present in the data used in this study. Consequently, CPD is inferred to over-constrain the registration process, and the here proposed approach thus resulted in higher accuracy.

It is important to note that only a baseline is provided in this work. Currently, the deformation is assumed to be affine, as appropriate for the given experiment, where only translation and scaling are considered. Rotation and elastic deformation could also be considered for more complex problems, which could be particularly relevant for tissues' that exhibit large deformations or strong restructurings of the cell neighborhoods. The optimization and termination could be further improved by using the information on cell area and its connectivity to other cells. Furthermore, the manual initialization could be replaced by an automatic method, which would be useful for large data sets. For the analysis of tissues over long time scales, the algorithm should be augmented to account for cell death and division (i.e. missing correspondences). In the context of these challenges, image registration seems a particularly suitable approach.

Acknowledgement. This work has partly been supported by the European Research Council to ASS (ERC StG 2013-337283, MEMBRANESACT), by the German Research Foundation to ASS and DD (RTG 1962), and by the Emerging Field Initiative of the FAU Erlangen-Nürnberg: Big-Thera to AM, ASS and DD.

References

1. Mualla F, Schöll S, Sommerfeldt B, et al. Automatic cell detection in bright-field microscope images using SIFT, random forests, and hierarchical clustering. IEEE Trans Med Imaging. 2013;32(12):2274–2286.
2. Mualla F, Schöll S, Sommerfeldt B, et al. Unsupervised unstained cell detection by SIFT keypoint clustering and self-labeling algorithm. Med Image Comput Comput Assist Interv. 2014; p. 377–384.
3. De Vylder J, De Vos WH, Manders EM, et al. 2D mapping of strongly deformable cell nuclei-based on contour matching. Cytometry A. 2011;79A(7):580–588.
4. Hand A, Sun T, Barber D, et al. Automated tracking of migrating cells in phase-contrast video microscopy sequences using image registration. J Microsc. 2009;234(1):62–79.
5. Faust U, Hampe N, Rubner W, et al. Cyclic stress at mHz frequencies aligns fibroblasts in direction of zero strain. PLoS One. 2011;6(12):e28963.
6. Gehrer S. Stress-strain relation in reconstituted tissue. Friedrich-Alexander-Universität Erlangen-Nürnberg; 2016.
7. Sternberg SR. Biomedical image processing. Comput. 1983;16:22 – 34.
8. Preibisch S, Saalfeld S, Tomancak P. Globally optimal stitching of tiled 3D microscopic image acquisitions. Bioinform. 2009;25(11):1463.
9. Kaliman S, Jayachandran C, Rehfeldt F, et al. Limits of applicability of the voronoi tessellation determined by centers of cell nuclei to epithelium morphology. Front Physiol. 2016;7.
10. Otsu N. A threshold selection method from gray-level histograms. IEEE Trans Syst Man Cybern. 1979;9(1):62–66.
11. Meyer F. Topographic distance and watershed lines. Sign Process. 1994;38(1):113 – 125.
12. Muja M, Lowe DG. Fast approximate nearest neighbors with automatic algorithm configuration. VISAPP. 2009; p. 331–340.
13. Hansen N. The CMA evolution strategy: a comparing review. Towards New Evol Comput. 2006; p. 75–102.
14. Myronenko A, Song X. Point set registration: coherent point drift. IEEE Trans Pattern Anal Mach Intell. 2010;32(12):2262–2275.

Pediatric Patient Surface Model Atlas Generation and X-Ray Skin Dose Estimation

Xia Zhong[1], Philipp Roser[1,3], Siming Bayer[1], Nishant Ravikumar[1]
Norbert Strobel[2], Annette Birkhold[2], Tim Horz[2], Markus Kowarschik[2],
Rebecca Fahrig[2], Andreas Maier[1,3]

[1]Pattern Recognition Lab, FAU Erlangen-Nürnberg
[2]Siemens Healthcare GmbH, Forchheim Germany
[3]Erlangen Graduate School in Advanced Optical Technologies (SAOT)
xia.zhong@fau.de

Abstract. Fluoroscopy is used in a wide variety of examinations and procedures to diagnose or treat patients in modern pediatric medicine. Although these image guided interventions have many advantages in treating pediatric patients, understanding the deterministic and long term stochastic effects of ionizing radiation are of particular importance for this patient demographic. Therefore, quantitative estimation and visualization of radiation exposure distribution, and dose accumulation over the course of a procedure, is crucial for intra-procedure dose tracking and long term monitoring for risk assessment. Personalized pediatric models are necessary for precise determination of patient-X-ray interactions. One way to obtain such a model is to collect data from a population of pediatric patients, establish a population based generative pediatric model and use the latter for skin dose estimation. In this paper, we generate a population model for pediatric patient using data acquired by two RGB-D cameras from different views. A generative atlas was established using template registration. We evaluated the registered templates and generative atlas by computing the mean vertex error to the associated point cloud. The evaluation results show that the mean vertex error reduced from 25.2 ± 12.9 mm using an average surface model to 18.5 ± 9.4 mm using specifically estimated pediatric surface model using the generated atlas. Similarly, the dose estimation error was halved from $10.6 \pm 8.5\%$ using the average surface model to $5.9 \pm 9.3\%$ using the personalized surface estimates.

1 Introduction

In modern pediatric radiology, fluoroscopy is used to provide the physicians dynamic and functional information of the patients' internal organs, both in diagnostic and minimally invasive surgery. However, as an ionizing radiation based imaging modality, the use of fluoroscopy is associated with radiation related risks such as radiation-induced cancer. A retrospective study by Pearce [1] showed a noticeably increased risk of leukemia and brain cancer when accumulated dose reached a certain level in children. Therefore it is desirable to reduce

X-ray exposure adhering to the as low as reasonably achievable (ALARA) principle, particularly in pediatric patients, who are more sensitive to X-rays than adults. One way to help facilitate dose reduction in the interventional suite is to use digital patient twins to better model and monitor X-ray dose exposure. An interesting practical application for such models is to keep track of the dose deposition in the skin. Skin entrance dose estimation often comprises two steps: (1) identification of the irradiated skin area, and (2) dose calculation based on a forward projection of an online-measured dose-related quantity such as dose-area-product from the X-ray source onto the skin surface. Previous studies have shown progressive improvements concerning the accuracy of skin dose estimation, but also highlight the importance of an accurate patient model [2]. An interesting practical question is, how accurate a patient model has to be, such that the skin dose estimate is reliable. This forms the basic motivation for the current study, with the focus on pediatric patients. The associated task is challenging as the anatomy and physiology of children exhibits a significantly higher degree of variation relative to adults. Models of pediatric patients are typically generated using MRI (or in rare cases CT) scans, referred to as computation or reference phantoms. While such phantoms are highly detailed and accurate, they are difficult to obtain on a large scale as they usually require very high resolution data and significant manual post-processing, e.g. for segmentation. With the introduction of RGB-D cameras, using depth data to construct surface models has become increasingly popular. While most efforts have been aimed at modeling adults [3, 4, 5], Hesse et al. [6] investigated methods to generate infant body models, using RGB-D image sequences.

In this work, we propose a method to build a generative atlas using two RGB-D cameras. Using this atlas, a patient specific pediatric model can be estimated using patient height and weight as input data. We evaluated the model both in terms of model estimation accuracy, and its impact on skin dose estimation.

2 Materials and methods

2.1 RGBD imaging setup and data acquisition

Two Microsoft Kinect V2 cameras were used to acquire RGBD data from two fixed, but different viewing angles. Children ($n = 20$) were asked to stand in front

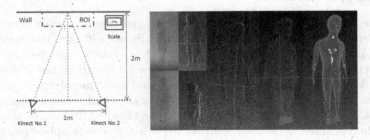

Fig. 1. Data acquisition setup (left) and processing pipeline (right).

of a wall in the target region of interest (ROI). Cameras were mounted on two tripods and oriented such that the target ROI (complete child) was located in the ISO center. The angle between the two cameras was set to be approximately 30deg. An illustration of the acquisition setup is shown in Fig. 1, left side. The RGBD cameras are calibrated jointly using a calibration phantom to determine distortion correction and obtain the intrinsic as well as the extrinsic camera parameters. Besides the RGBD data, we further collected meta data (gender, height, weight and age) of the children. In order to get most accurate height and weight information, measurements were performed shortly before the image acquisition. Gender and age of the children was inquired from the parents. The data acquisition was voluntary and followed the rules set out by the European General Data Protection Regulation. Each data set acquired and processed has an associated consent form with signatures of both parents and the child, if necessary.

2.2 Preprocessing

The data preprocessing pipeline is illustrated in Fig. 1. First, the point cloud of a patient is reconstructed using both depth images from the two cameras. Two point clouds are reconstructed separately using associated undistorted depth images and the intrinsic camera matrix. These two point clouds are then aligned using the extrinsic camera matrices. As the tripods may have moved accidentally during the acquisition, we added an extra correction step performing a rigid registration using coherent point drift (CPD) [7] to ensure that the point clouds are aligned. Subsequently, the two point clouds of each child are merged. Next, we determined the wall and floor planes using RANSAC with plane fitting and removed these from the data. As the backs of the patients and the bottom of their feet were occluded in the acquisition setup, we used the calculated wall and floor planes to fill in the missing information. As not all patients were positioned next to the wall, we had to manually align the reference wall planes to obtain the missing data. Finally, we manually removed remaining artifacts, e.g., wide clothes obstructing the body silhouette. The extracted region was adjusted for cases where patients were positioned outside the target ROI.

2.3 Template fitting

Template fitting was used to extract a structured mesh for each preprocessed point cloud, for atlas generation. The MakeHuman[1] software was used to initialize a patient *reference* template. An iterative scheme was then used to fit the reference to the cleaned-up point cloud. In each iteration, the reference was registered to each point cloud using an affine, and subsequently, non-rigid transformation (using CPD). As clothing and pose of the children varied significantly in the training data, a high outlier rate was used in the CPD registration. CPD tries to find a globally optimal solution when fitting the template to the point

---

[1] http://www.makehumancommunity.org/

cloud by performing a non-rigid deformation. Since the head-to-body-ratio of children, however, changes with age, we decided to treat head and body trunk separately.

Afterwards, the reference was again fitted to the separately registered point clouds to ensure smoothness of the model. At the end of each iteration, the reference was updated by calculating the mean shape of all fitted meshes. This fitting process converged after a few iterations, and we took the result for each point cloud as the associated ground truth mesh.

2.4 Atlas generation

The goal of atlas generation is to learn a generative model and estimate a personalized surface, based on a given height and weight of the child. For this purpose, we used the ground truth meshes to compute a statistical shape model using Principal Component Analysis (PCA), where P^c encodes the modes of variation and b_i^c encodes the associated shape parameters. We then computed the PCA space of the associated height and weight data. Unfortunately, the measured data in the acquired datasets suffered from rank deficiency, making a regression of shape parameters $b_i^c = f(h_i, w_i)$ in native PCA space insufficient to generate a model having correct height h_i and weight w_i. Therefore, we used the mode of variation P^a learned from the adult CEASAR [8] database as an extra term. Our aim was to find the associated shape parameters b^a for a given height h_i and weight w_i such that

$$x_i = \bar{x} + P^c b_i^c + P^a b_i^a \tag{1}$$

$$\arg\min_{b^a} = \sum_i (\lambda_1 \|\rho V(x_i) - w_i\| + \lambda_2 \|H(x_i) - h_i\|) + \|\nabla b^a\| \tag{2}$$

where ρ denotes the approximate body mass density of children, $V(\cdot)$ describes the calculation of the input mesh volume, and $H(\cdot)$ represents the calculation of the height of the input mesh, respectively. The gradient of the shape parameter ensures smooth adaption. Minimizing this equation resulted in generation of an estimated surface model which is in good agreement with the ground truth and coherent with the associated measured data.

2.5 Skin entrance dose estimation

For validation purposes, we computed the accumulated skin entrance dose for each surface model, focused on a central body region. The goal was not to simulate an actual interventional setup, but to focus on differences in skin dose estimation resulting from the use of different models. The surface models were placed within a virtual model of the imaging setup (source–object–detector) for the dose simulations, comprising a homogeneous projection and view geometry of the X-ray source and the model matrix of the patient, specifying its orientation and position with respect to the X-ray beam. Based on the resulting model-view-projection matrix, each mesh face was forward projected onto the detector plane if at least one associated vertex was positioned within the X-ray beam and the face normal pointed towards the X-ray source making sure that only those surfaces were considered that received radiation. The corresponding distance to the X-ray source was given by the last homogeneous coordinate of each vertex. Applying barycentric depth interpolation, the triangle in the image plane was rasterized and the depth map was constructed iteratively [9]. The skin entrance dose was then calculated by forward projecting a dose-related quantity measured at the X-ray emitter onto the area of irradiation, taking additional correction terms into account [2]. We evaluated the percentage error of the skin entrance dose introduced by both surface estimation methods: 1) using an average surface model, 2) using personalized surface models. Both types of surface models were based on the atlas data. The template fitted to the original point cloud served as ground truth.

3   Evaluation and results

In total, we gathered 20 point cloud sets with associated measurements. We first evaluated the accuracy of the atlas generation pipeline by overlaying the atlas-based estimate with the associated 3D point cloud and calculating the minimal distance for each vertex. We performed a leave-one-out cross validation in which the estimate was rigidly registered to the associated point cloud using CPD. An illustration of color coded mean vertex error of the *reference*, estimate and *ground truth*, is shown in Fig. 2. Using only the reference, an average distance of 25.2 ± 12.9 mm was achieved. The ground truth had an average distance of 15.3 ± 8.7 mm. A mean vertex error of 18.5 ± 9.4 mm was achieved using the estimate. The percentage error of the skin entrance dose using the template model (for each sample compared to its ground truth) was estimated to 10.6 ± 8.5 %. The percentage error using models generated by the atlas (for each sample compared to its ground truth) was 5.9 ± 9.3 %.

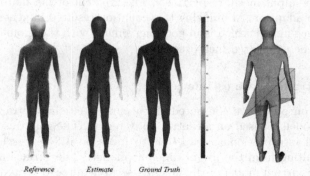

Reference   Estimate   Ground Truth

Fig. 2. An illustration of mean vertex distance in mm to its merged point cloud using the reference template late (left), estimation based on metadata (middle) and the fitted template. Right: Visualization of dose estimation setup.

4 Discussion

The proposed statistical atlas complements our adult atlas derived from the CEASAR database. Both atlases yield comparable accuracy. Although the average error of approximately 2 cm will still contribute to a (skin) dose estimation error, the proposed atlas is still an improvement when compared to a setup involving only one single representation, (average) reference model, for all pediatric cases. Our statistical atlas could also be used as a first estimate of a continuously adapting model which refines itself after each new source of information, e.g., provided by successive MRI scans. A possible improvement of the modeling pipeline would be to use a more robust point set registration method than CPD. Although CPD introduces an outlier ratio, the underlying Gaussian mixture model can not effectively model the point cloud in the present of extreme or large percentage of outliers. Despite the successful application of the adults' modes of variation to the children's atlas, more representative modes of variation of the children might improve the accuracy of the model further. In this atlas, we used height and weight measurements only. We were not able to account for gender and age of the children due to the rank deficiency in the dataset. This was caused by the limited amount of training data collected. In future work, we hope to be able to gather more data such that we can incorporate this information as well, to further reduce the estimation error.

Acknowledgement. We gratefully acknowledge the support of Siemens Healthineers, Forchheim, Germany. Note that the concepts and information presented in this paper are based on research, and they are not commercially available.

References

1. Pearce MS, et al. Radiation exposure from CT scans in childhood and subsequent risk of leukaemia and brain tumours: a retrospective cohort study. Lancet. 2012;380(9840):499–505.
2. Johnson PB, et al. Skin dose mapping for fluoroscopically guided interventions. Med Phys. 2011;38(10):5490–5499.
3. Zhong X, et al. Generation of personalized computational phantoms using only patient metadata. Proc IEEE NSS/MIC. 2017;.
4. Zhong X, et al. A machine learning pipeline for internal anatomical landmark embedding based on a patient surface model. Int J Comput Assist Radiol Surg. 2018;10:1–9.
5. Wu Y, et al.; Springer. Towards generating personalized volumetric phantom from patients surface geometry. Proc MICCAI. 2018; p. 171–179.
6. Hesse N, et al.; Springer. Learning an infant body model from RGB-D data for accurate full body motion analysis. MICCAI. 2018; p. 792–800.
7. Myronenko A, Song X. Point set registration: coherent point drift. IEEE Trans Pattern Anal Mach Intell. 2010;32(12):2262–2275.
8. Robinette KM, et al.; IEEE. The CAESAR project: a 3-D surface anthropometry survey. 3D Digit Imaging Model. 1999; p. 380–386.
9. Catmull E. A subdivision algorithm for computer display of curved surfaces. Utah Univ Salt Lake City School Comput. 1974;.

Blind Rigid Motion Estimation for Arbitrary MRI Sampling Trajectories

Anita Möller[1], Marco Maass[1], Tim J. Parbs[1], Alfred Mertins[1]

[1]Institute for Signal Processing, Universität zu Lübeck
moeller@isip.uni-luebeck.de

Abstract. In this publication, a new blind motion correction algorithm for magnetic resonance imaging for arbitrary sampling trajectories is presented. Patient motion during partial measurements is estimated. Exploiting the image design, a sparse approximation of the reconstructed image is calculated with the alternating direction method of multipliers. The approximation is used with gradient descent methods with derivatives of a rigid motion model to estimate the motion and extract it from the measured data. Adapted gridding is performed in the end to receive reconstruction images without motion artifacts.

1 Introduction

Artifacts caused by patient motion result in diagnostically unusable images measured by magnetic resonance imaging (MRI). These artifacts appear especially as ghost replications of the object or image blurring. In many cases, motion can be avoided by a motionless patient. But especially the motion of organs like lung, liver, and heart can not be stopped for a long time and also swallowing can not be suppressed effectively. To overcome these artifacts, techniques are developed to either adapt the measurement process to the motion or compensate motion afterwards.

In contrast to other method, blind motion estimation uses only information about the motion hidden in the measurement. The main idea is not to restrict oneself to periodical motion but also be capable of compensating spontaneous motion. Based on the knowledge about the sampling trajectories many methods were developed to estimate the performed motion. Then, it is extracted from the measurement data to reconstruct images without artifacts. One popular technique was proposed for rotated blade sequences by Pipe et al. [1] and is implemented in current MR scanners. There, motion is estimated from several partial measurements based on their correlation.

Former research showed that MR images can effectively be represented in sparse domains. Sparsification reduces the artifacts appearing in those representations. This was used to blindly estimate motion in [2]. The new proposed algorithm measures the MRI k-space on arbitrary trajectories and combines the ideas of sparsifying images and gradient descent algorithms. This leads to an image reconstruction algorithm with very high reduction of motion artifacts.

2 Materials and methods

In MRI, as the k-space contains sampled frequency coefficients, it can be interpreted as Fourier transform of the MR image. More exactly, one measurement of the whole k-space is composed of partial measurements at intervals in time specified by trajectories. Let $\boldsymbol{x}(\boldsymbol{r}) \in \mathbb{R}^{o \times m}$ be a two dimensional MR image with spatial coordinates $\boldsymbol{r} = [\boldsymbol{r}_1, \boldsymbol{r}_2, \dots, \boldsymbol{r}_M] \in \mathbb{R}^{2 \times M}$, $M = om$ and $\boldsymbol{r}_i = [r_{i,1}, r_{i,2}]^T, i \in \{1, 2, \dots, M\}$ with coordinate ranges $r_{i,1} \in [0, o-1], r_{i,2} \in [0, m-1]$

The Fourier transform of the image is described by $\mathcal{F}\boldsymbol{x}$. Parts of the k-space are sampled in consecutive time intervals indexed by $n = 1, 2, \dots, N \in \mathbb{N}$ The read out is so fast that no motion occurs during these intervals. Let $\mathcal{S}(\boldsymbol{k}_n)$ be a sampling operator at frequency coordinates $\boldsymbol{k}_n$ belonging to all trajectory points measured at time n. The frequency coordinates of the samples are defined by $\boldsymbol{k}_n = [\boldsymbol{k}_{n,1}, \boldsymbol{k}_{n,2}, \dots, \boldsymbol{k}_{n,P_n}] \in \mathbb{R}^{2 \times P_n}$ with two-dimensional coordinates $\boldsymbol{k}_{n,q} = [k_{n,q,1}, k_{n,q,2}]^T, q \in \{1, 2, \dots, P_n\}$ in the ranges $k_{n,q,1} \in \left[-\frac{o-1}{2}, \frac{o-1}{2}\right], k_{n,q,2} \in \left[-\frac{m-1}{2}, \frac{m-1}{2}\right]$ With it, the partial measurement $\boldsymbol{y}_n(\boldsymbol{k}_n) \in \mathbb{C}^{P_n}$ with $P_n \in \mathbb{N}$ being the number of samples measured at this time n is given by $\boldsymbol{y}_n(\boldsymbol{k}_n) = \mathcal{S}(\boldsymbol{k}_n)\mathcal{F}\boldsymbol{x}$

If patients move during a complete MR scan, the partial measurements represent a motion corrupted image each. This motion is modeled by the operator $\mathcal{T}_{\boldsymbol{\theta}_n}$, where $\boldsymbol{\theta}_n \in \mathbb{R}^{\Theta}, \Theta \in \mathbb{N}$ contains all motion parameters necessary to describe the object motion from the first measurement at $n = 1$ to time n. In total, the partial measurement model is given by $\boldsymbol{y}_n(\boldsymbol{k}_n) = S(\boldsymbol{k}_n)\mathcal{F}\mathcal{T}_{\boldsymbol{\theta}_n}\boldsymbol{x}$ and the complete measurement is $\boldsymbol{y}(\boldsymbol{k}) = [\boldsymbol{y}_1(\boldsymbol{k}_1), \boldsymbol{y}_2(\boldsymbol{k}_2), \dots, \boldsymbol{y}_N(\boldsymbol{k}_N)]$ with $\boldsymbol{k} = [\boldsymbol{k}_1, \boldsymbol{k}_2, \dots, \boldsymbol{k}_N]$ Then, the reconstruction problem for the measured image $\hat{\boldsymbol{x}} \in \mathbb{R}^{o \times m}$ from all partial measurements $\boldsymbol{y}_n(\boldsymbol{k})_n$ can be formulated as

$$\hat{\boldsymbol{x}} = \arg\min_{\boldsymbol{x}} \sum_{n=1}^{N} \|\mathcal{S}(\boldsymbol{k}_n)\mathcal{F}\mathcal{T}_{\boldsymbol{\theta}_n}\boldsymbol{x} - \boldsymbol{y}_n(\boldsymbol{k}_n)\|_2^2 + \frac{1}{\sigma^2}\Phi(\boldsymbol{x}) \tag{1}$$

with a regularization term $\Phi(\boldsymbol{x})$ and $0 < \sigma \in \mathbb{R}$.

2.1 Rigid motion model

To model patient motion, we restrict ourselves to rigid motion. Therefore, we need three motion parameters $\boldsymbol{\theta}_n = [\beta_{n,1}, \beta_{n,2}, \alpha_n]$ in two dimensions. The translation operator is given by $\mathcal{D}_{\theta_{n,1},\theta_{n,2}}$ and the rotation is described by $\mathcal{R}_{\alpha_n}$. Then, the complete motion operator is given by $\mathcal{T}_{\boldsymbol{\theta}_n}\boldsymbol{x} = \mathcal{D}_{\beta_{n,1},\beta_{n,2}}\mathcal{R}_{\alpha_n}\boldsymbol{x}$

Translationmodel From [2], for a shift $\beta_{n,i} = \delta_{n,i} + \gamma_{n,i}$ with $\delta_{n,i} \in \mathbb{N}, \gamma \in (0, 1], i \in \{1, 2\}$, it is known that the translation transform is given by

$$\mathcal{D}_{\beta_{n,1},\beta_{n,2}}\boldsymbol{x} = D_{\gamma_{n,1}}D_1^{\delta_{n,1}}\boldsymbol{x}\left(D_1^{\delta_{n,2}}\right)^T D_{\gamma_{n,2}}^T \tag{2}$$

with convolution matrices $D_{\gamma_{n,i}}$ realising subpixel shift and D_1 realising full pixel circular shifts of the image.

Rotation model The rotation of the image is described with a rotation matrix $R_{\alpha_n} \in \mathbb{R}^{2\times2}$ which rotates the coordinates r of the image x. Afterwards, the image is interpolated back onto the unrotated coordinates by barycentric interpolation $I(x(R_{\alpha_n}r), r)$ [3] combined with Delaunay triangulation [4], to cope with arbitrary spatial grids. In total, the rotation model is described by

$$\mathcal{R}_{\alpha_n}x = I(x(R_{\alpha_n}r), r) \tag{3}$$

2.2 Nonequidistant sampling scheme

To allow for any arbitrary sampling trajectory, the operator $\mathcal{S}$ is able to sample any point $k_{n,q} \in \mathbb{R}^{2\times1}$ in frequency domain. This sampling can be formulated as nonequidistant discrete Fourier transform (NDFT) [5]

$$y_n(k_{n,q}) = \mathcal{S}(k_{n,q})\mathcal{F}x(r) = \sum_{i=1}^{M} x(r_i)e^{-2\pi j k_{n,q}^T r_i}, \ q = 1, 2, \ldots, P_n \tag{4}$$

2.3 Regularization

Generally, MR images consist of clear structures and edges and should not show noise. Especially, motion artifacts like ghosting appear as noise. So, the reconstructed images are supposed to be sparse in the wavelet domain. Therefore, the regularization term is chosen as $\Phi(x) = \|\mathcal{W}x\|_1$ with $\mathcal{W}$ being the wavelet transform. In the proposed setup, especially Daubechies wavelets are efficient.

2.4 Motion estimation gradient

Motion estimation is performed in a three-step iterative algorithm. It is based on the assumption that MR images can be sparsely represented in the wavelet domain. For each partial measurement n, separate motion parameters $\hat{\theta}_n$ are estimated. The following algorithmic steps are iterated for each partial measurement separately.

Sparsifying by alternating direction method of multipliers (ADMM)
The ADMM [6] solves (1) for fixed motion parameters $\hat{\theta}_n$. It converges to the sparsest image $\hat{x}$ representing partial measurements $y_{n\in\Upsilon}$ whereby Υ contains all indexes n for measurements y_n with already estimated $\hat{\theta}_n$ and the index of the currently considered measurement.

Problem (1) is split into two separate minimization problems and is iteratively updated by

$$\hat{x}_{d+1} = \arg\min_x \sum_{n\in\Upsilon} \|\mathcal{S}(k_n)\mathcal{F}\mathcal{T}_{\theta_n}x - y_n(k_n)\|_2^2 + \frac{1}{\lambda^2}\|x - \bar{x}_{d+1}\|_2^2$$

$$\bar{x}_{d+1} = \hat{v}_d - u_d \tag{5}$$

$$\hat{v}_{d+1} = \arg\min_v \|\mathcal{W}v\|_1 + \frac{\sigma^2}{\lambda^2}\|v - \bar{v}_{d+1}\|_2^2, \quad \bar{v}_{d+1} = \hat{x}_{d+1} + u_d \tag{6}$$

$$u_{d+1} = u_d + \hat{x}_{d+1} - \hat{v}_{d+1} \tag{7}$$

with $\lambda, \sigma \in \mathbb{R}$, $\boldsymbol{u}_d, \boldsymbol{v}_d \in \mathbb{R}^{o \times m}$ and iteration index $d \in \mathbb{N}$. The measurement fitting problem (5) is solved by a conjugate gradient method [7] using the inverse NDFT (INDFT) [6]. The sparsifying step (6) is performed by soft thresholding.

Motion estimation by quasi-Newton gradient descent Gradients of the motion models (2), (3) with respect to $\beta_{n,1}, \beta_{n,2}$, and α_n are optimized in a quasi-Newton gradient descent with backtracking line search to estimate the motion. The Boyden, Fletcher, Goldfarb, and Shanno update rule [7] is used. The translation gradient is additionally parameterized by convolution with a Gaussian model.

Three gradient descents are calculated on the sparse image $\hat{\boldsymbol{x}}$ until an update for $\hat{\boldsymbol{\theta}}_{n,A_n}$ with $A_n \in \mathbb{N}$ being the iteration number per partial measurement is given. First, the rotation gradient is evaluated to get a first estimation for $\hat{\alpha}_{n,a}, a = 1, 2, \ldots, A_n \in \mathbb{N}$ With a sparse image temporarily rotated by $\hat{\alpha}_{n,a}$, the translation estimation gradient is applied in the quasi-Newton manner for both directions $\hat{\beta}_{n,1}^a, \hat{\beta}_{n,2}^a$ Finally, starting from the former estimations, all three motion parameters are estimated in one gradient for rotation and translation.

Motion update The estimated motion is added to a global motion $\hat{\boldsymbol{\theta}}_n = \hat{\boldsymbol{\theta}}_{n,A_n} = \sum_{a=1}^{A_n} \hat{\boldsymbol{\theta}}_{n,a}$ The sampling trajectory coordinates per partial measurement are updated by rotation with $\hat{\alpha}_{n,A_n}$, and image translation $[\hat{\beta}_{n,1,A_n}, \hat{\beta}_{n,2,A_n}]$ is updated in its frequency coefficients by phase shifts.

2.5 Image reconstruction

Finally, the global translation $[\hat{\beta}_{n,1}, \hat{\beta}_{n,2}]$ per partial measurement n is corrected by a phase shift in k-space. Afterwards, the global rotation per partial measurement is compensated by rotating the frequency coordinates by the estimated angle $\hat{\alpha}_n$ with $\hat{\boldsymbol{k}}_n = R_{\hat{\alpha}_n} \boldsymbol{k}_n$ In total, we get translation corrected frequency coefficients $\hat{\boldsymbol{y}}_n(\hat{\boldsymbol{k}}_n)$ which belong to rotated sampling coordinates in k-space.

The final reconstruction is done by gridding to avoid blurring caused by the INDFT. We follow the gridding scheme of Pipe et al. [8]. With it, the reconstruction is described by

$$\tilde{\boldsymbol{y}}(\boldsymbol{k}_g) = \left(\left(\left(\hat{\boldsymbol{y}}\left(\hat{\boldsymbol{k}}\right) w_\omega\left(\hat{\boldsymbol{k}}\right) \right) * c\left(\hat{\boldsymbol{k}}\right) \right) g(\boldsymbol{k}_g) \right) *^{-1} c(\boldsymbol{k}_g) \tag{8}$$

with $\boldsymbol{k}_g \in \mathbb{R}^{2 \times g}$ being new grid coordinates with the same ranges as $\boldsymbol{k}$. The weighting function $w_\omega(\boldsymbol{k})$ is calculated iteratively by $w_\omega(\boldsymbol{k}) = w_{\omega-1}(\boldsymbol{k})/(w_{\omega-1}(\boldsymbol{k})* c(\boldsymbol{k}))$, $w_0(\boldsymbol{k}) = 1, \omega \in \mathbb{N}$. With it, sampling coefficients are weighted by an area density compensation function to equalize the sample contribution to the new sampled coefficients.

The kernel $c(\boldsymbol{k})$ was analytically designed as described in [9] to optimize the reconstructed image in a circular field of view (FOV). It is given by

$$c(\boldsymbol{k}_{n,q}) = \left(\frac{J_1\left(\frac{m}{2}\pi |\boldsymbol{k}_{n,q}|\right)}{m\pi |\boldsymbol{k}_{n,q}|} \right)^2 \tag{9}$$

with J_1 denoting the Bessel function of first kind and order.

By convolution with the sampling function $g(\boldsymbol{k}_g)$ the data is sampled onto a new grid $\boldsymbol{k}_g$. In contrast to former time consuming propositions by Johnson et al. [9], we calculated all convolutions effectively using KD-trees [10].

Deapodization as inversion of the kernel convolution is realized in the image domain by dividing by the pseudoinverse of the kernel to remove aliased sidelobes of the image kernel. If the grid $\boldsymbol{k}_g$ is Cartesian, the reconstructed image $\tilde{\boldsymbol{x}}$ is gained by inverse discrete Fourier transform of $\tilde{\boldsymbol{y}}$.

2.6   Test setup

As the algorithm is built for arbitrary sampling trajectories, we exemplarily used periodically rotated overlapping parallel lines with enhanced reconstruction (PROPELLER) to evaluate the proposed algorithm. The k-space is divided into rectangular blades of the same size consisting of parallel lines. The blades are rotated around the k-space center in uniform angles. Pipe proposed the blades to contain m equidistant samples per line and $l = \frac{\pi m}{2N}$ lines for a circular FOV [11]. The motion was modeled as an autoregressive moving average process with maximal amplitude given to simulate a smooth patient motion for each motion parameter. It is sampled at N positions to extract each $\boldsymbol{\theta}_n$. Test images were the Shepp-Logan phantom in a FOV with a diameter of $m = 160$ and Brainweb simulations [12] in a FOV with a diameter of $m = 455$.

3   Results

Two reconstruction examples are given in Fig. 1. The Brainweb image was transformed by smaller motion and image details are reconstructed. The Shepp-Logan phantom was corrupted by large motion. No image, only motion artifacts are visible in the corrupted scene, but the image is reconstructed very well. Only a few gridding artifacts are visible. In Tab. 1, the mean percental improvement of the image quality measures peak signal-to-noise ratio (PSNR), structural similarity (SSIM), and mutual information (MI) calculated between the motion corrected and ground truth Shepp-Logan phantoms. The results for several numbers of partial measurements, maxima of translation and rotation are shown. High rates of improvement are reached. For Brainweb, similar results were gained.

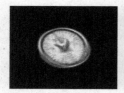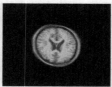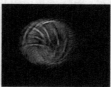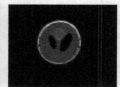

Fig. 1. Left to right: Brainweb image corrupted by motion with $\beta_{n,1}, \beta_{n,2} \leq 5, \alpha_n \leq \frac{\pi}{6}, N = 5$; motion compensated Brainweb image; Shepp-Logan phantom corrupted with $\beta_{n,1}, \beta_{n,2} \leq 30, \alpha_n \leq \frac{\pi}{6}, N = 8$; motion compensated Shepp-Logan phantom.

N	Trans	Rot	PSNR	SSIM	MI
5	5	$\pi/4$	4.35	2.87	8.50
8	10	$\pi/6$	6.73	4.97	23.99
5	30	$\pi/4$	6.73	4.82	28.08
6	30	$\pi/4$	8.08	5.32	30.06
6	30	$\pi/6$	9.74	5.36	23.28

Table 1. Percental improvement of the quality measures PSNR, SSIM, MI for N partial measurements with maximum translation (Trans) and maximum rotation angle (Rot) on the Shepp-Logan phantom.

4 Discussion

The motion compensation algorithm reaches reconstructions without motion artifacts and with a lot image details even for large motion. For small motion, image details are reconstructed even better. Only gridding artifacts remain in the images caused by low resolution. Overall, image quality measures are highly improved. A higher number of partial measurements comes with better motion compensation even if the number of samples per measurement gets smaller. With this blind motion compensation algorithm a new design for motion compensation for arbitrary sampling trajectories is given. Improvements could be reached by expansion to natural elastic motion and further reduction of gridding artifacts.

Acknowledgement. This work has been supported by the German Research Foundation under Grant No. ME 1170/11-1.

References

1. Pipe JG, Gibbs WN, Li Z, et al. Revised motion estimation algorithm for PRO-PELLER MRI. Magn Reson Med. 2014;72(2):430–437.
2. Möller A, Maaß M, Mertins A. Blind sparse motion MRI with linear subpixel interpolation. Proc BVM. 2015; p. 510–515.
3. Hormann K. Barycentric interpolation. Approximation Theory XIV: San Antonio. 2014; p. 197–218.
4. Aurenhammer F, Klein R, Lee DT. Voronoi Diagrams and Delaunay Triangulations. WORLD SCIENTIFIC; 2013.
5. Keiner J, Kunis S, Potts D. Using NFFT 3: a software library for various nonequispaced fast fourier transforms. ACM Trans Math Softw. 2009;36(4):19:1–19:30.
6. Parikh N, Boyd S. Proximal algorithms. Found Trends Optim. 2014;1(3):127–239.
7. Nocedal J, Wright SJ. Numerical Optimization. 2nd ed. New York: Springer; 2006.
8. Pipe JG, Menon P. Sampling density compensation in MRI: rationale and an iterative numerical solution. Magn Reson Med. 1999;41(1):179–186.
9. Johnson KO, Pipe JG. Convolution kernel design and efficient algorithm for sampling density correction. Magn Reson Med. 2009;61(2):439–447.
10. Bentley JL. Multidimensional binary search trees used for associative searching. Commun ACM. 1975;18(9):509–517.
11. Pipe JG. Motion correction with PROPELLER MRI: application to head motion and free-breathing cardiac imaging. Magn Reson Med. 1999;42(5):963–969.
12. Cococsco CA, Kollokian V, Kwan RKS, et al. BrainWeb: online interface to a 3D MRI simulated brain database. Neuroimage. 1997;5:425.

Maximum Likelihood Estimation of Head Motion Using Epipolar Consistency

Alexander Preuhs[1], Nishant Ravikumar[1], Michael Manhart[2],
Bernhard Stimpel[1], Elisabeth Hoppe[1], Christopher Syben[1],
Markus Kowarschik[2], Andreas Maier[1]

[1]Pattern Recognition Lab, Friedrich-Alexander-Universität Erlangen-Nürnberg
[2]Siemens Healthcare GmbH, Forchheim, Germany
alexander.preuhs@fau.de

Abstract. Open gantry C-arm systems that are placed within the interventional room enable 3-D imaging and guidance for stroke therapy without patient transfer. This can profit in drastically reduced time-to-therapy, however, due to the interventional setting, the data acquisition is comparatively slow. Thus, involuntary patient motion needs to be estimated and compensated to achieve high image quality. Patient motion results in a misalignment of the geometry and the acquired image data. Consistency measures can be used to restore the correct mapping to compensate the motion. They describe constraints on an idealized imaging process which makes them also sensitive to beam hardening, scatter, truncation or overexposure. We propose a probabilistic approach based on the Student's t-distribution to model image artifacts that affect the consistency measure without sourcing from motion.

1 Introduction

Modern C-arm systems enable 3-D imaging of the head in an interventional environment. This is of high relevance in neuroradiology, where a 3-D reconstruction allows to distinguish an ischemic from hemorrhagic stroke. The patients benefit from reduced time-to-therapy [1] but the open gantry system and the interventional setting constrain the acquisition speed compared to conventional Computed Tomography (CT). With prolonged scan time, involuntary movements of patients constitute a major challenge for high quality image reconstruction.

This gives rise to a strong need for motion compensation algorithms [2]. In recent years, consistency conditions have been shown to be promising in this context [3, 4]. Besides the compensation of motion, consistency measures are heavily used in cone-beam CT, as they provide a mathematical model constraining the imaging process. The most commonly applied consistency measure uses Grangeat's theorem to judge the pairwise consistency of two projections.

The measure was successfully applied for the correction of a variety of acquisition artifacts. Beam hardening can be corrected by projection linearization using a polynomial model. The parameters for the model are found by optimizing for Grangeat's consistency [5, 6]. Hoffmann et al. used Grangeat's consistency to estimate parameters of an additive scatter model [7]. The consistency measure can also be used to estimate missing data due to truncation for field of view reconstruction [8] and possibly to the closely related problem of overexposure correction [9]. The most widely use of Grangeat's consistency is the estimation of geometry information that is distorted either due to rigid patient motion or geometry jitter [3, 4, 10]. The reason for its wide applicability is the sensitivity of the consistency measure to a variety of image artifacts. Thus, when we use the consistency measure to compensate for motion, we also measure the inconsistency induced by other sources. In this work, we propose to use a statistical model to handle inconsistencies that are not originating from motion artifacts.

2   CIV look-up-table

In cone-beam imaging, a line profile l on the detector plane is created by attenuated X-ray beams within a plane p connecting the X-ray source and l. Grangeat's theorem describes a transformation, to find a common value — we denote it as Consistency Intermediate Value (CIV) — that can be computed either from l, or the 3-D Radon value indexed by p [11]. Formally, the derivative of the 3-D Radon value in the normal direction of p equals a transformed value of l. As a consequence, any pair of epipolar lines can be used as a consistency measure by computing their respective CIVs, which must be equal. All CIVs can be precomputed as a look-up-table (LUT) by a concatenation of cosine-weighting, Radon transform and derivative. As a result, from each projection we obtain a CIV look-up-table as depicted in (Fig. 1).

Using the geometry information, we can sample CIVs [11] as visualized in (Fig. 1). Here, the dark blue dotted line corresponds to a correct sampling, where

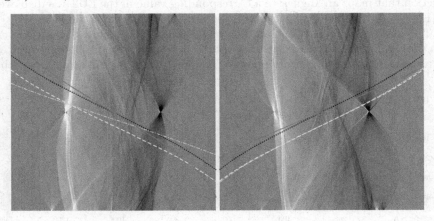

Fig. 1. LUT of two projections containing CIVs and corresponding lines visualizing the sampling of redundancies based on the given geometry information. The CIVs along corresponding lines in the left and right LUT, e.g. along the dotted lines, should be equal (Fig. 2 for a visualization of line profile). True geometry (dotted), z translation (dashed), x rotation (chained) and y translation (solid).

the geometry information is consistent with the acquired projection data. The profile of the sampled line is shown in (Fig. 2). If the geometry information is corrupted then the sampling pattern changes, as visualized by the solid line in (Fig. 1). The corresponding sampling profile is shown in (Fig. 2). Due to the misalignment, the profiles sampled from both LUTs, corresponding to two projections, do not match anymore. This is used to restore the correct geometry by minimizing the difference between two profiles and in turn maximizing the consistency. However, the profiles of two projections with perfect geometry will not match exactly (Fig.2), because other acquisition artifacts reduce the consistency. We propose to model these artifacts using a probabilistic approach.

3   Student's t-distribution-based maximum likelihood estimation for consistency optimization

Instead of assuming two CIVs to be equal, we propose a Bayesian description of the matching problem. We assume that the sampled CIV of projection a is a random variable x, distributed according to a Student's t-distribution with mean μ, variance σ and a shape factor ν

$$p(x|\mu,\sigma,\nu) = \frac{\Gamma(\frac{\nu+1}{2})}{\sqrt{\nu\pi}\,\Gamma(\frac{\nu}{2})\,\sigma}\left(1 + \frac{(x-\mu)^2}{\nu\,\sigma^2}\right)^{-\frac{\nu+1}{2}} \tag{1}$$

where Γ is the gamma function. We use a t-distribution, because it can model our inherently outlier-affected sampling process (Fig. 3). We assume that the mean of the random variable is the CIV of our second projection image b described by $S_b(h(\kappa))$. Here S_b is the LUT generated from projection b, and $h(\cdot)$ defines a function that maps an angle κ to a corresponding value in the LUTs as displayed in (Fig. 1). A detailed explanation on the function $h(\cdot)$ can be found in [11].

The motion compensation can then be formulated by finding the parameters of a probability density function that results in the greatest likelihood, or alternatively minimizing the negative log-likelihood. By setting the random variable

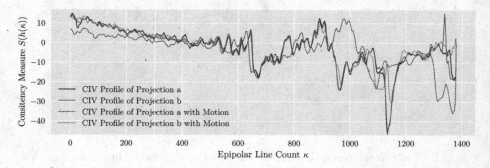

Fig. 2. Profiles along the LUTs for correct and motion-affected geometry. The profiles are sampled along the true geometry and the geometry affected by a translation in y direction as depicted in (Fig. 1).

x as $S_a(h(\kappa))$ the maximum likelihood is defined by

$$\min \sum_\kappa - \ln\left(p(x|\mu, \sigma, \nu)\right) = \min \sum_\kappa \frac{\nu + 1}{2} \ln\left(1 + \frac{(S_a(h(\kappa)) - S_b(h(\kappa)))^2}{\nu \sigma^2}\right)$$
(2)

For similar objects (e.g. head) and a given system, the distribution will always be similar. Thus, the unknown parameters ν and σ can be estimated from a motion free prior scan (not identical to the scanned object) by accumulating the distances within the CIVs given by $\sum_\kappa S_a(h(\kappa)) - S_b(h(\kappa))$. In a second step we fit a Student's t-distribution to the data. This is depicted in (Fig. 3), where we can see that the t-distribution properly fits to the data: outliers are modeled by its approximately constant tails. For comparison, fitting a Gaussian distribution leads to a very high standard deviation ($\sigma = 29$) due to the outliers.

4   Experiments and results

4.1   Experimental Setup

To evaluate our method, we compare our norm, derived as the log-likelihood of a Student's t-distribution ($\sigma = 0.398$, $\nu = 0.8228$) with the L^2 norm, which is the log-likelihood assuming a Gaussian distribution and the more robust L^1 norm. We apply them for the compensation of axial motion (z) modeled with splines. Thus, each projection is shifted in the z direction by the amount of the spline at that projection index. The spline shape is controlled by 12 nodes, whose values are determined randomly in the range of ± 0.5 mm. We use z-motion, because z-translations produce inconsistencies. In contrast, motions within the acquisition plane do not necessarily violate the consistency measure [3, 4]. We show our results on three phantoms (Fig. 4.1), acquired with a robotic C-arm system (Artis zeego, Siemens Healthcare GmbH, Germany).

4.2   Motion Compensation

We use a simplex method to find the motion-compensated geometry. We iteratively optimize each node of a spline separately, assuming all other spline nodes

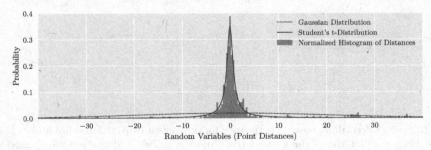

Fig. 3. Histogram of distances between corresponding CIVs from two projections (Fig. 2) and fitted probability density functions.

constant. For each dataset, we model a different motion trajectory. The induced motion trajectory is displayed in (Fig. 5) for all the three datasets, with the estimated motion curves using the respective norms.

4.3   Results

The motion-estimated reconstruction using the proposed method is displayed in (Fig. 4.1) together with the motion-affected reconstruction. The mean distance between the estimated and ground truth motion parameters are displayed in (Tab. 1). Using the proposed norm, we achieve the best results in restoring the motion parameters. The second best estimation is achieved using the robust L^1 norm. Using the L^2 norm the consistency and the motion parameters can only be poorly approximated. A visual inspection of the parameters is provided in (Fig. 5). The L^2 norm especially fails to approximate the areas at the beginning and end of the trajectory. The motion structure in the middle is approximated in its structure, although, with a great offset.

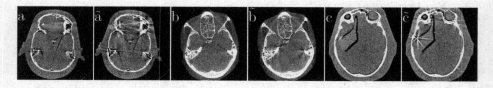

Fig. 4. Central slices of three reconstructed anthropomorphic head phantoms (HU [-200,400]). Motion-compensated reconstruction using the proposed method (a,b,c) and reconstruction with motion artifacts ranging from ± 0.5 mm ($\tilde{a},\tilde{b},\tilde{c}$).

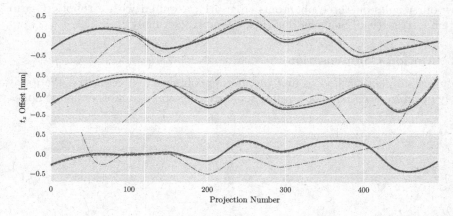

Fig. 5. Splines describing motion trajectory for datasets a (top), b (middle) and c (bottom). Each subplot shows the ground truth motion (solid) and the estimated motion using the proposed norm (dotted), the L^1 norm (dashed) and the L^2 norm (chained).

Dataset	a [mm]	b [mm]	c [mm]
Proposed	**0.0057**	**0.0044**	**0.0048**
L^1	0.0152	0.0158	0.0077
L^2	0.5044	0.6167	0.4268

Table 1. Mean distance between estimated and ground truth motion curves.

5   Conclusion

We propose a statistical description for evaluating the consistency of a trajectory. We model the consistency value as a Student's t-distribution and find the optimal geometry by minimizing the negative log-likelihood. Consequently, we derive a robust norm for the comparison of consistency values, insensitive to outliers which naturally arise due to physical effects. The proposed solution outperforms the L^1 and L^2 norm. The L^2 norm is very sensitive to outliers which pose it improper. In the current approach, we fixed the parameters of the t-distribution. Each projection pair reveals a different outlier-characteristic due to the scanned object. Thus, the precision might be enhanced by estimating projection pair dependent parameters for the Student's t-distribution.

Disclaimer. The concepts and information presented in this paper are based on research and are not commercially available.

References

1. Psychogios M, Behme D, Schregel K, et al. One-stop management of acute stroke patients: minimizing door-to-reperfusion times. Stroke. 2017;.
2. Müller K, Maier A, Lauritsch G, et al. Image artefact propagation in motion estimation and reconstruction in cardiac C-arm CT. Proc PMB. 2014;.
3. Preuhs A, Maier A, Manhart M, et al. Double your views: exploiting symmetry in transmission imaging. Proc MICCAI. 2018;.
4. Frysch R, Rose G. Rigid motion compensation in C-arm CT using consistency measure on projection data. Proc MICCAI. 2015;.
5. Abdurahman S, Frysch R, Bismark R, et al. Beam hardening correction using cone beam consistency conditions. IEEE Trans med Imaging. 2018;.
6. Würfl T, Maaß N, Dennerlein F, et al. Epipolar consistency guided beam hardening reduction-ECC 2. Fully 3D. 2017;.
7. Hoffmann M, Würfl T, Maaß N, et al. Empirical scatter correction using the epipolar consistency condition. CT-Meet. 2018;.
8. Punzet D, Frysch R, Rose G. Extrapolation of truncated C-arm CT data using grangeat-based consistency measures. CT-Meet. 2018;.
9. Preuhs A, Berger M, Xia Y, et al. Over-exposure correction in CT using optimization-based multiple cylinder fitting. Proc BVM. 2015;.
10. Debbeler C, N, Elter M, et al. A new CT rawdata redundancy measure applied to automated misalignment correction. Fully 3D. 2013;.
11. Aichert A, Berger M, Wang J, et al. Epipolar consistency in transmission imaging. IEEE Trans Med Imaging. 2015;.

Retrospective Blind MR Image Recovery with Parametrized Motion Models

Tim J. Parbs, Anita Möller, Alfred Mertins

Institut für Signalverarbeitung, Universität zu Lübeck
parbs@isip.uni-luebeck.de

Abstract. In this paper, we present an alternating retrospective MRI reconstruction framework based on a parametrized motion model. An image recovery algorithm promoting sparsity is used in tandem with a numeric parameter search to iteratively reconstruct a sharp image. Additionally, we introduce a multiresolution strategy to restrict the numeric complexity. This algorithm is then tested in conjunction with a simple motion model on simulated data and provides robust and fast reconstruction of sharp images from severely corrupted k-spaces.

1 Introduction

In the context of medical imaging, magnetic resonance imaging (MRI) is particularly sensitive to patient movement during data acquisition. Even though the scanning process was sped up considerably during recent years through improvements of scanner hardware and image recovery algorithms, the duration of a full scan often is prohibitively long even for cooperative patients. In addition, some involuntary movements -- such as pulsatile expansions and contractions due to blood flow or intestinal peristalsis – are impractical to stop for a scan.

Autofocussing recovery algorithms, used to reduce these motion artefacts, require only the data measured in a conventional scan and approximate motion and recover the sharp image by minimizing some error metric after the scan is finished. Algorithms utilizing autofocussing do not require specialized scanner hardware nor do they influence the measurement or increase acquisition time. Generally, these approaches utilize the gradient of an error function for image updates while regularizing the motion parameters over time (e.g., in [1]). However, up to this point, blindly retroactively removing nonaffine motion remains an open challenge. As these models might not be readily differentiable, prior approaches employing gradients are not readily applicable.

We propose a general framework for such an algorithm that allows us to fit arbitrary parametrized motion models in a blind MRI reconstruction. We employ a novel regularization scheme using path searching algorithms to find suitable time-dependent parameter sets. By iteratively approximating the image using a sparse recovery approach and numerically updating the motion model, the unknown motion is compensated effectively.

2 Methods

Let $\mathbf{x} \in \mathbb{R}^{M^2}$ be a vectorized square image and $D_{\boldsymbol{\theta}}$ a known motion model. Generally, $D_{\boldsymbol{\theta}}$ can be understood as a linear transform matrix of size $M^2 \times M^2$ with an underlying structure compactly described by a set of parameters $\boldsymbol{\theta} \in \mathbb{R}^T$.

In MRI, read-out trajectories through k-space are acquired nearly instantly. If we measure N trajectories described by k-space coordinate vectors $\mathbf{f}_n$ with $n \in \{0, 1, \ldots N-1\}$, we are interested in the deformation of the image $D_{\boldsymbol{\theta}}\mathbf{x}$ at N points in time and therefore affected by N distinct motion parameter sets $\boldsymbol{\theta}_n$.

The whole measurement can be described with a k-space data vector $\mathbf{y} = [\mathbf{y}_0, \ldots, \mathbf{y}_{N-1}]^T$. Each $\mathbf{y}_n \in \mathbb{C}^{U_n}$ represents a partial measurement of the k-space acquired by the trajectory through frequency coordinates $\mathbf{f}_n$ with a number of captured coefficients $U_n \ll M^2$ defined by $\mathbf{y}_n = \mathfrak{F}_{\mathbf{f}_n} D_{\boldsymbol{\theta}_n} \mathbf{x}$. In this, $\mathfrak{F}_{\mathbf{f}_n}$ is a partial Fourier transform which can be expressed as a $\mathbb{C}^{U_n \times M^2}$ matrix.

Disregarding $D_{\boldsymbol{\theta}}$ in the reconstruction of $\mathbf{x}$ will lead to ghosting artifacts which degrade image quality and, in the worst case, will make the resulting image unfit for medical evaluation. The exact recovery of $\mathbf{x}$ requires the approximation of the underlying motion. In blind MRI image reconstruction, where no additional data is acquired, we are left with the partial measurements $\mathbf{y}_n$ and the corresponding $\mathbf{f}_n$ and tasked with the simultaneous approximation of both image and the motion through $\boldsymbol{\Theta} = \{\boldsymbol{\theta}_0, \ldots \boldsymbol{\theta}_{N-1}\}$.

2.1 Optimization scheme

The objective function of our reconstruction problem can generally be – and, in comparable approaches, is – expressed as

$$f_{\tilde{\boldsymbol{\Theta}}, \tilde{\mathbf{x}}} = \sum_{n=0}^{N-1} \|\mathfrak{F}_{\mathbf{f}_n} D_{\tilde{\boldsymbol{\theta}}_n} \tilde{\mathbf{x}} - \mathbf{y}_n\|_2^2 \tag{1}$$

for a fixed measurement $\mathbf{y}$. To jointly approximate image and motion parameters we split the optimization problem into an alternating algorithm in which we iteratively reduce the artifacts corrupting $\mathbf{y}$ and fit the motion model to better describe the updated image. Beginning with some arbitrary starting points $\mathbf{x}^0$ and $\boldsymbol{\Theta}^0$ we seek an updated image through

$$\mathbf{x}^{k+1} = \operatorname*{argmin}_{\tilde{\mathbf{x}}} f_{\boldsymbol{\Theta}^k, \tilde{\mathbf{x}}} + \alpha \, \mathcal{R}_x(\tilde{\mathbf{x}}) \tag{2}$$

where $k \in \{0, 1, \ldots K-1\}$ is the current iteration with a maximum number of iterations K. Since the problem is ill-posed, $\mathcal{R}_x$ is a regularization term for the image with Lagrange multiplier α. We then seek an updated motion parameter set through

$$\boldsymbol{\Theta}^{k+1} = \operatorname*{argmin}_{\tilde{\boldsymbol{\Theta}}} f_{\tilde{\boldsymbol{\Theta}}, \mathbf{x}^{k+1}} \text{ s.t. } \tilde{\boldsymbol{\Theta}} \in \Psi \tag{3}$$

which fits the parameter set to the updated image. Since acquisition time in MRI is generally short, we expect that the motion state does not change too much between consecutive time steps. To quantify this change, we define a distance function $\phi(\cdot, \cdot)$ which is used as a difference measure of parametrized motion states. Using this, we define a set of admissible motion parameter sets

$$\Psi = \{\boldsymbol{\Theta} \mid \phi(\boldsymbol{\theta}_n, \boldsymbol{\theta}_{n-1}) < \tau \ \forall n \in \{1, \ldots, N-1\}\} \tag{4}$$

with a maximally allowed distance between time steps τ.

We will now describe the two update steps and their motivation in greater detail while providing some implementation details.

2.2   Image reconstruction

The optimization probem in Eq. (2) is regularly found in literature and research concerning sparse data recovery. In the latter, the regularization term is chosen so that structure of the underlying data is exploited and a solution is chosen which is sparse in a transform basis.

Using this approach, we chose $\mathcal{R}_x(\mathbf{x}) = \|\mathbf{W}\mathbf{x}\|_1$, where $\mathbf{W} \in \mathbb{R}^{M^2 \times M^2}$ is an invertible wavelet transform matrix. It is well known from literature that natural images can be represented sparsely in the wavelet domain. Since the ghosting artifacts afflicting the image reduce its sparsity, we can expect to improve image quality by this approach.

Thus, Eq. (2) is an unconstrained convex optimization problem which can be solved in numerous ways. Because of the size of the involved system matrices, algorithms requiring system matrix inversion are not feasible for larger images. We instead use the (scaled) alternating direction method of multipliers (ADMM)[2] to find a solution iteratively.

Using the ADMM framework, the problem can be decomposed into an alternating algorithm consisting of the three sub-steps

$$\mathbf{u}^{j+1} = \underset{\tilde{\mathbf{u}}}{\operatorname{argmin}} \sum_{n=0}^{N-1} \|\mathfrak{F}_{\mathfrak{f}_n} D_{\tilde{\boldsymbol{\theta}}_n} \tilde{\mathbf{u}} - \mathbf{y}_n\|_2^2 + \frac{\lambda}{2} \|\tilde{\mathbf{u}} - (\mathbf{v}^j + \mathbf{w}^j)\|_2^2 \tag{5}$$

$$\mathbf{v}^{j+1} = \mathcal{T}_{\alpha/\lambda}\left(\mathbf{W}\left(\mathbf{u}^{j+1} + \mathbf{w}^j\right)\right), \quad \mathbf{w}^{j+1} = \mathbf{w}^j + \mathbf{u}^{j+1} - \mathbf{W}^{-1}\mathbf{v}^{j+1} \tag{6}$$

starting from some arbitrary $\mathbf{u}^0$, $\mathbf{w}^0$ and $\mathbf{v}^0$ with j denoting the iteration and λ being the penalty parameter of the augmented Lagrangian. With a soft-thresholding function $\mathcal{T}_z(\cdot)$ with threshold z, the updates for $\mathbf{v}^{j+1}$ and $\mathbf{w}^{j+1}$ are trivial. The update of $\mathbf{u}^{j+1}$ can be solved using convex optimization – we used a conjugate gradient descent to find an update.

2.3   Motion update

The optimization of $\boldsymbol{\Theta}$ is unfortunately not straight-forward for arbitrary motion models $D_{\boldsymbol{\theta}}$. Since we seek a general solution independent of the underlying motion model, we cannot optimize using convex optimization.

The objective function Eq. (1) however can be split into a number of N smaller problems by splitting the sum. For a fixed measurement and image approximation we end up with

$$\hat{f}_{\boldsymbol{\theta}}^{n} = ||\mathfrak{F}_{\mathbf{f}_{\mathbf{n}}}^{H} \mathbf{y}_{n} - D_{\boldsymbol{\theta}} \mathbf{x}^{k+1}||_{2}^{2} \tag{7}$$

By defining a search space for the parameter set, we can then numerically evaluate every *partial* objective function $\hat{f}_{\boldsymbol{\theta}}^{n}$ on possible values for $\boldsymbol{\theta}_n$ and look for the set that minimizes Eq. (1) while being in Ψ.

To sample the partial objective function with respect to $\boldsymbol{\theta}$, we create a parameter lattice $\Omega \subset \mathbb{R}^{T}$. We approximate a maximum absolute value G_t and a step size γ_t for each value in the parameter representation $\boldsymbol{\theta}_t$, so that we end up with

$$\Omega = \left\{ \sum_{t=0}^{T-1} a_t \boldsymbol{\theta}_t \mid a_t \in \{-G_t, -G_t + \gamma_t, \ldots, G_t\} \right\} \tag{8}$$

The parameters G_t and γ_t are crucial for the algorithm, as they define the maximum value for every parameter as well as its resolution.

Using a linear index $v \in \{0, 1, \ldots, V-1\}$ with $V = \prod_{t=0}^{T} \left\lceil \frac{2G_t}{\gamma_t} \right\rceil$ we then calculate the error term for every motion state $\boldsymbol{\omega}_v$ on the lattice and collect them into a matrix $\mathbf{Q} \in \mathbb{R}^{N \times V}$ with entries $q_{n,v} = \hat{f}_{\boldsymbol{\omega}_v}^{n}$.

The update of $\boldsymbol{\Theta}^k$ reduces to a path search problem through $\mathbf{Q}$. We use a modified variant of the Viterbi algorithm [3], but other path search algorithms might be applicable as well.

For the path search algorithm, we initialize a path storage $p_{0,v} = v$, state transition sets $\beta_v = \{\boldsymbol{\omega}_h \mid \phi(\boldsymbol{\omega}_v, \boldsymbol{\omega}_h) \leq \tau\}$, and a path error matrix $\mathbf{E} \in \mathbb{R}^{N \times V}$ with entries $e_{0,v} = q_{0,v}$. We then update paths and error matrix by

$$\tilde{p}_v = \operatorname*{argmin}_{c \in \beta_v} [e_{n-1,c}], \quad e_{n,v} = e_{n-1,\tilde{p}_v} + q_{n,v}, \quad p_{n,v} = [p_{n-1,v}, \tilde{p}_v] \tag{9}$$

while iterating through $n = \{1, \ldots, N-1\}$. The optimal path $p_{j,N-1}$ corresponding to the smallest $e_{N-1,v}$ then defines the updated motion parameter set by $\boldsymbol{\Theta}^{k+1} = \{\boldsymbol{\omega}_{p_{j,0}}, \ldots, \boldsymbol{\omega}_{p_{j,N-1}}\}$. This formulation allows us to find the optimal path in $\mathcal{O}(VN)$, once $\mathbf{Q}$ is calculated.

Due to the nature of $\mathbf{Q}$, accurately approximating a large number of parameters in a big region would be infeasible using this approach. However, if the partial objective functions are smooth enough for a step size γ_t we can utilize a different approach. Refining the grid between iterations by progressively lowering G_t and γ_t and centring the search space on $\boldsymbol{\Theta}^{k-1}$ – that is, evaluating $q_{n,v} = \hat{f}_{(\boldsymbol{\omega}_v - - \boldsymbol{\theta}_n^{k-1})}^{n}$ – yields a multiresolution approach. This approach will fail if the partial objective function changes too rapidly for a step size γ_t, which depends on the motion model and the underlying image.

Regardless whether the grid is refined or not, the update formulation comes with a slight caveat: The resulting motion set is ambiguous in that every $\boldsymbol{\Theta}$ which fulfills $\mathbf{y}_n = \mathfrak{F}_{\mathbf{f}_n} D_{\boldsymbol{\theta}_n} D_{\boldsymbol{\xi}} \mathbf{x}$ is a possible solution. In essence, we cannot directly influence the stating state of $\mathbf{x}$, which might still be warped with a constant bias motion $D_{\boldsymbol{\xi}}$. Although this might be unproblematic in practical situations, we circumvent this problem after the final iteration of the algorithm. Modifiying $\boldsymbol{\Theta}^{K-1}$ with a bias term $\boldsymbol{\kappa} \in \mathbb{R}^T$ yields a final set $\hat{\boldsymbol{\Theta}} = \{\boldsymbol{\theta}_0^{K-1} - \boldsymbol{\kappa}, \ldots, \boldsymbol{\theta}_{N-1}^{K-1} - \boldsymbol{\kappa}\}$ so that $D_{\hat{\boldsymbol{\theta}}_0}\mathbf{I} = \mathbf{I}$ and the image at $n = 0$ is recovered.

2.4 Test setup

Up to this point, we have outlined a reconstruction framework for arbitrary motion. The model used during recovery are part of ongoing research. However, we evaluate the performance using a simple model to provide preliminary results.

We used PROPELLER [4] (Periodically Rotated Overlapping ParallEL Lines with Enhanced Reconstruction) as a k-space acquisition scheme with 50 blades. Translational movements of the underlying image between blade acquisitions were used to corrupt the measured k-space. This motion model results in a very small set of parameters ($T = 2$) and an intuitive parameter distance function $\phi(\boldsymbol{\theta}_a, \boldsymbol{\theta}_b) = \|\boldsymbol{\theta}_a - \boldsymbol{\theta}_b\|_2$. As a base image, we used a simulated tomography of the human brain [5] with a size of 150×150 pixels.

Approximately smooth random motion curves were used with a varying maximum amplitude of $\boldsymbol{\theta}_{\max}$.

Preliminary numerical evaluations show the partial objective functions to be almost convex in a region around the true minimum. Therefore, we utilize multiresolution and refine the lattice between iterations. Starting with a maximum allowed motion of $G_t = 30$ pixels and step size $\gamma_t = 3$ for both parameters, both were halved every three iterations. The maximum number of iterations was fixed to $K = 18$. The starting step size was found to be inconsequential and fixed to $\gamma_t = 3$. The maximum parameter distance τ was set to $2/10 \cdot G_t$.

Parameters concerning image recovery were chosen empirically – we used a separable wavelet transform with a Daubechies mother wavelet, a shrinking parameter $\alpha = 1/2$ and an ADMM penalty parameter of $\lambda = 1$.

For error measurements we used an l_2-norm between base image and reconstruction to quantify the recovery error as well as the structural image similarity measure (SSIM) and total variation (TV) for artefact quantisation.

3   Results

Fig. 1 shows the simulated data prior to the algorithm and after its final iteration. Sharp images are recovered even from harshly corrupted k-spaces, while the iterative approach allows for the improvement of images with $\boldsymbol{\theta}_{\max} > G_t$. We expect the image to further improve with more iterations of the algorithm.

Fig. 2 shows the error measurements at the last iteration of the algorithm (after about 5 minutes) for different $\boldsymbol{\theta}_{\max}$. As expected, the l_2-error is robustly decreased for all $\boldsymbol{\theta}_{\max}$, yielding near perfect results for small movements while SSIM is increased. Note that PROPELLER oversamples central regions of k-space while undersampling edge regions, which in itself yields an l_2-error even for unmoving subjects. Although preliminary, these results indicate robust performance of both the base algorithm and its multiresolution expansion.

Fig. 1. Corrupted image and reconstruction for two maximal motion amplitudes.

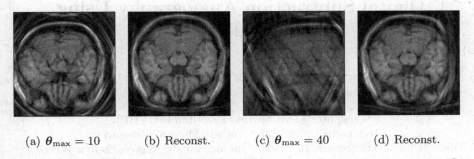

(a) $\theta_{max} = 10$ (b) Reconst.   (c) $\theta_{max} = 40$ (d) Reconst.

Fig. 2. Error values for images before (cross) and after (square) reconstruction.

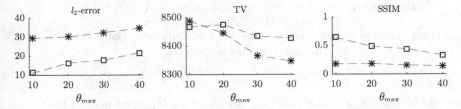

4 Discussion

In our algorithm, the parameter set of an a-priori defined motion model is approximated using partially sampled k-spaces. It can be used to find a robust approximation of both sharp image and corrupting motion simultaneously. Although it can be computationally intensive, we propose a scheme to find a good solution with a reduced number of numeric evaluations using multiresolution. The development of suitable low-parametric motion models is subject of ongoing research.

Acknowledgement. This work has been supported by the German Research Foundation under Grant No. ME 1170/11-1.

References

1. Loktyushin A, Nickisch H, Pohmann R, et al. Blind retrospective motion correction of MR images. Magn Reson Med. 2013;70(6):1608–1618.
2. Parikh N, Boyd S. Proximal algorithms. Found Trends Optim. 2014;1(3):127–239.
3. Forney GD. The viterbi algorithm. Proc IEEE. 1973;61:268 – 278.
4. Pipe JG. Motion correction with PROPELLER MRI: application to head motion and free-breathing cardiac imaging. Magn Reson Med. 1999;42(5):963–969.
5. Cocosco CA, Kollokian V, Kwan RKS, et al. BrainWeb: online interface to a 3D MRI simulated brain database. NeuroImage. 1997;5:425.

Model-Based Motion Artifact Correction in Digital Subtraction Angiography Using Optical-Flow

Sai Gokul Hariharan[1,2], Christian Kaethner[2], Norbert Strobel[2,3],
Markus Kowarschik[1,2], Julie DiNitto[4], Rebecca Fahrig[2,5], Nassir Navab[1,6]

[1]Computer Aided Medical Procedures (CAMP),
Technische Universität München, Munich, Germany
[3]Fakultät für Elektrotechnik, Hochschule für angewandte Wissenschaften Würzburg-
Schweinfurt, Schweinfurt, Germany
[4]Siemens Medical Solutions, Hoffman Estates, USA
[5]Pattern Recognition Lab, Friedrich-Alexander-Universität Erlangen-
Nürnberg (FAU), Erlangen, Germany
[6]Whiting School of Engineering, Johns Hopkins University, Baltimore, USA
saigokul.hariharan@tum.de

Abstract. Digital subtraction angiography is an important method for
obtaining an accurate visualization of contrast-enhanced blood vessels.
The technique involves the digital subtraction of two X-ray images, one
with contrast filled vessels (fill image) and one without (mask image).
Unfortunately, artifacts that are introduced due to the subtraction of
misaligned mask and fill images may potentially degrade the diagnostic value of an image. The techniques used for correcting such artifacts
involve the use of affine image registration techniques for aligning the
mask and fill images and image processing techniques for suppressing the
artifacts. Although affine registration techniques often yield acceptable
results, they may fail when the imaged object undergoes 3D transformations. The techniques used for suppressing artifacts may cause blurring,
when a projection image can no longer be corrected using a globally uniform motion model. In this paper, we have introduced an optical-flow
based local motion compensation approach, where pixel-wise deformation fields are computed based on an X-ray imaging model. A visual
inspection of the results shows a significant improvement in the image
quality due to a reduction in the artifacts caused by misregistrations.

1 Introduction

Digital subtraction angiography (DSA) is an important technique to enable a
detailed structure assessment of blood vessels without the potentially compro-
mising effect of anatomical background information. The technique is based on a
digital subtraction of a non-contrast-enhanced native image (mask image) from
a corresponding image with contrast-enhanced vascular structures (fill image).
To account for the exponential attenuation of the imaged object, the digital

subtraction is usually carried out after applying a logarithmic transformation on the mask and fill images. Unfortunately, if the mask and the fill images are not spatially aligned, e.g., due to patient motion, DSA images may be affected by misalignment artifacts. When these artifacts are present in regions with contrast enhanced vascular structures, the diagnostic value of the images may be compromised.

Commonly used approaches to correct such artifacts involve the application of geometrical transformations accounting for shifts caused by patient movement [1, 2, 3]. Deuerling-Zheng et al. [4] have proposed and analyzed methods to detect local motions in DSA sequences and the application of pixel-shifting and block matching to correct motion artifacts. Ionasec et al. [5] have presented a method for a rigid motion compensation that optimizes the physical position and orientation of a C-arm X-ray device using an image based registration approach. Since X-ray images are projections of 3D objects, it may not be possible to accurately represent a 3D motion using 2D affine transformations. Moreover, due to a variation in the amount of noise present in images acquired at different dose levels, current techniques may have a significantly decreased performance, particularly at low-dose levels. Extensive calibrations and parameter tuning may be required to adapt the techniques to different dose levels. In this paper, we propose the use of a novel optical-flow based approach to perform a deformable registration of the mask and the fill images. The approach relies on a realistic X-ray imaging model to reduce the influence of noise on the registration process and therefore allows a robust application even at varying dose levels.

2 Materials and methods

X-ray images are corrupted by noise from various sources, e.g., Poisson noise, electronic noise and quantization noise. Depending on the imaging situation, different gains are applied [6]. In this section, we have presented an algorithm designed to minimize the impact of the signal-dependent noise on the outcome of an image registration. After stabilizing the noise variance to a known constant based on an image formation model, we have computed the deformation vectors.

2.1 Image formation and noise model

We have made use of the imaging model proposed in [7]. According to the model, X-ray images are corrupted by signal-dependent quantum noise and signal independent electronic noise. The model can be represented by

$$y[i,j] = \alpha \cdot x[i,j] + h + \eta[i,j] \tag{1}$$

where $y[i,j]$, $x[i,j]$ and $\eta[i,j]$ represent the observed gray value, quanta and electronic noise at the particular location $[i,j]$, respectively, and α and h represent the system gain and the system offset, respectively. The quantum noise associated with x can be approximated using a Poisson distribution and the electronic noise η can be approximated using a Gaussian distribution with a specific standard deviation σ. The overall signal-dependent noise may negatively influence optimization problems, such as denoising and registration, when applied in the image domain. This may, in turn, result in undesirable artifacts. In order to remove the signal dependency of the overall noise present in the images, we use the generalized Anscombe transform (GAT) [8] on the images to transform the noise in the images to unit variance σ_n^2 More formally, we apply the GAT on y_m (mask image) and y_f (fill image) to obtain Y_m and Y_f, respectively.

2.2   Deformable registration of mask and fill images

An affine 2D transformation in the projection space may not be sufficient to represent either a change in the 3D orientation of an object or in the angulation of an imaging device. A better representation of the geometrical situation and therefore a better registration, can be achieved by estimating pixel-wise deformation vectors. For this, we have used the optical flow estimation approach proposed in [9], which is based on minimizing the objective function

$$E(u_i, v_j) = \int \left(\sqrt{(Y_m(p + w_p) - Y_f(p))^4 + \epsilon} + \lambda \sqrt{(|\nabla u|^2 + |\nabla v|^2)^2 + \epsilon} \right) dp \tag{2}$$

in the continuous spatial domain, where $p = (i, j)$ is the image lattice, $w_p(p) = (u_i(p), v_j(p))$ represents the underlying flow field and $u_i(p)$ and $v_j(p)$ represent the horizontal and vertical components of the flow field associated with the pixel location $[i, j]$, respectively, λ is a parameter that controls the importance of the regularization term and $\epsilon = 10^{-6}$ Since the objective is highly non-convex, a coarse-to-fine refining scheme on a dense Gaussian pyramid with image warping can be used to avoid local minima [9]. In order to obtain the flow fields, an iterative reweighted least squares approach can be applied on a discretized formulation of Eq. 2. The deformed pixel elements in the mask image can then be computed from the flow fields by

$$Y_m'[i, j] = g(Y_m[i + u, j + v]) \tag{3}$$

where Y_m' and $g(.)$ represent the transformed mask and a cubic interpolation function, respectively. Even though the solution is expected to converge to a minimum, it may be difficult to achieve, when there are significant differences between the images used in the registration. In such cases, the algorithm might compute incorrect deformation fields for the mask images, which may result in anatomical artifacts, such as missing or blurred vessels in DSA images. To reduce this effect, we propose a correction mechanism that depends on the similarity of the local means of the input mask and the transformed mask and the local standard deviations of the transformed mask and the fill images in regions without contrast agent. This similarity measure can be represented by

$$e^{-w_{\sigma_{i,j}} \times w_{\mu_{i,j}}} < \tau \tag{4}$$

with $w_{\sigma_{i,j}} = |\sigma(\mathbf{y}_{m_{i,j}}' - \mathbf{y}_{f_{i,j}}) - \sqrt{2} \times \sigma_n|$ and $\mathbf{w}_{\mu_{i,j}} = |\mu(\mathbf{y}_{m_{i,j}}' - \mathbf{y}_{m_{i,j}})|$

where $\mathbf{y'_{m_{i,j}}}$, $\mathbf{y_{m_{i,j}}}$ and $\mathbf{y_{f_{i,j}}}$ represent $k \times k$ regions around $Y'_{m_{i,j}}$, $Y_{m_{i,j}}$ and $Y_{f_{i,j}}$, respectively, σ_n and τ represent the standard deviation of noise in Y_m and a threshold for distinguishing between acceptable and unacceptable registrations, respectively, and $\sigma(.)$ and $\mu(.)$ represent functions for calculating the standard deviation and the mean of a region, respectively. In order to choose τ independent of the used X-ray dose, we have scaled the noise variance stabilized images to the same range and modified σ_n accordingly. When $w_{\mu_{i,j}}$ and $w_{\sigma_{i,j}}$ in Eq. 4 are close to zero, the transformation may not introduce artifacts since $\mathbf{y'_{m_{i,j}}}$ is expected to be similar to $\mathbf{y_{m_{i,j}}}$ and well registered with $\mathbf{y_{f_{i,j}}}$. Otherwise, the registration may not be accurate. In order to prevent such misregistrations in Y'_m from influencing the computed DSA images, especially on regions involving contrast agent, we use the corresponding regions in Y_m instead of Y'_m to compute the final motion compensated mask Y^*_m as shown below

$$Y^*_m[i,j] = \begin{cases} Y'_m[i,j] & \text{if } e^{-w_{\sigma_{i,j}} \times w_{\mu_{i,j}}} < \tau \\ Y_m[i,j] & \text{otherwise} \end{cases} \tag{5}$$

Finally, an inverse generalized Anscombe transform [10] is applied to $Y^*_m[i,j]$ to transform it back to the image domain. The DSA is then computed for y_f using the computed motion compensated mask y^*_m

2.3 Material

In order to validate the proposed method, we have used X-ray images of an anthropomorphic brain phantom, where a contrast agent can be manually injected (Fig. 1). The mask and fill images have been acquired at 100% and 12% of the standard dose level. During the acquisition, we have introduced realistic deformations commonly observable in real clinical scenarios.

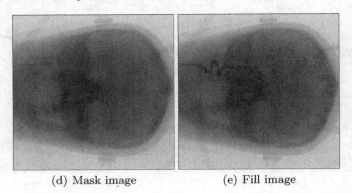

(d) Mask image   (e) Fill image

Fig. 1. Visualization of a mask and a fill image acquired at standard dose level.

3   Results

In Fig. 2, we have presented the DSA images computed with and without applying the proposed motion compensation on the mask image for 100% and 12% of the standard dose level. For this, we have empirically estimated the values of $\tau = .00001$ and $k = 21$ by analyzing the obtained deformation fields for the two image sequences acquired at different dose levels. It can be seen that the motion artifacts visible in Fig. 2(a) and Fig. 2(c), especially around the borders of the skull and the tubes used for simulating blood vessels, can be successfully reduced by the proposed approach (Fig. 2(b) and Fig. 2(d)). On the other hand, in all the DSA images presented in Fig. 2, a significant amount of noise can be observed in some regions that are associated with low gray values in the mask image (Fig. 1(d)). Please note that a very narrow gray level window width has been chosen to highlight misalignment artifacts.

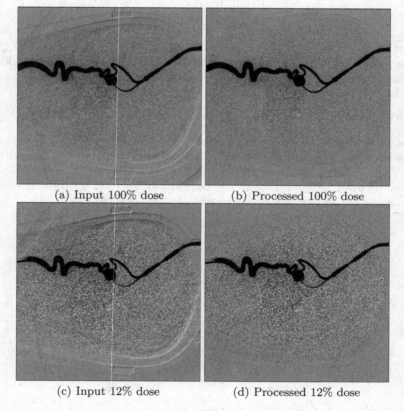

(a) Input 100% dose   (b) Processed 100% dose

(c) Input 12% dose   (d) Processed 12% dose

Fig. 2. Visualization of DSA images acquired at 100% and 12% of the standard X-ray dose level. In the case of (a) and (c), no motion compensation has been applied, and for (b) and (d), the proposed motion compensation approach has been applied.

4 Discussion and conclusion

In this paper, we have proposed an X-ray dose independent motion compensation approach to align corresponding contrast-enhanced (fill) and non-contrast-enhanced X-ray (mask) images, where the deformation fields are computed in the generalized Anscombe transform domain using an optical-flow based approach and subsequently refined based on a realistic X-ray imaging model. This allows for a significant reduction in the applied X-ray dose that is otherwise required to prevent the negative influence of noise on registration algorithms. Although, the impact of signal dependent non-stationary noise is still prominently visible in some parts of the computed DSA images, it can be reduced using denoising algorithms. Therefore, if the proposed motion compensation approach is combined with suitable denoising algorithms, a further reduction in the artifacts and the X-ray dose may be possible. In our future work, we will evaluate the performance of the proposed algorithm on clinical X-ray sequences and also focus on improving the performance of the proposed approach by constraining the optimization of the optical-flow algorithm using physiologically motivated regularizing terms.

Acknowledgement. This work was supported by Siemens Healthineers AG. The concepts and results presented in this paper are based on research and not commercially available.

References

1. Buzug TM, Weese J. Image registration for DSA quality enhancement. Comput Med Imaging Graph. 1998;22(2):103–113.
2. Meijering EH, Zuiderveld KJ, Viergever MA. Image registration for digital subtraction angiography. Int J Comput Vis. 1999;31(2-3):227–246.
3. Bentoutou Y, Taleb N, El Mezouar MC, et al. An invariant approach for image registration in digital subtraction angiography. Pattern Recognit. 2002;35(12):2853–2865.
4. Deuerling-Zheng Y, Lell M, Galant A, et al. Motion compensation in digital subtraction angiography using graphics hardware. Comput Med Imaging Graph. 2006;30(5):279–289.
5. Ionasec RI, Heigl B, Hornegger J. Acquisition-related motion compensation for digital subtraction angiography. Comput Med Imaging Graph. 2009;33(4):256–266.
6. Hariharan SG, Strobel N, Kaethner C, et al. A photon recycling approach to the denoising of ultra-low dose X-ray sequences. Int J Comput Assist Radiol Surg. 2018;13(6):847–854.
7. Hariharan SG, Strobel N, Kowarschik M, et al. Simulation of realistic low dose fluoroscopic images from their high dose counterparts. Procs BVM. 2018; p. 80–85.
8. Starck JL, Murtagh FD, Bijaoui A. Image Processing and Data Analysis: the Multiscale Approach. Cambridge University Press; 1998.
9. Liu C. Beyond pixels: exploring new representations and applications for motion analysis. Doctoral Thesis. 2009;.
10. Makitalo M, Foi A. Optimal inversion of the generalized anscombe transformation for poisson-Gaussian noise. IEEE Trans Image Process. 2013;22(1):91–103.

MedicVR

Acceleration and Enhancement Techniques for Direct Volume Rendering in Virtual Reality

Ingrid Scholl[1], Alex Bartella[2], Cem Moluluo[1], Berat Ertural[1], Frederic Laing[1], Sebastian Suder[1]

[1]MASCOR Institute, FH Aachen
[2]Clinic for Oral and Maxillofacial Surgery, Uniklinik RWTH Aachen
scholl@fh-aachen.de

Abstract. Further developments of the medical virtual reality application MedicVR were achieved by new approaches to direct volume rendering with the HTC Vive head mounted display. Even though the necessary real-time performance for a smooth interactive experience is accomplished by the shader technologies, the rendered image quality and performance is influenced by several parameters. We propose in this paper multiple technological upgrades to our application including: Lens Matched Shading, interactive volume clipping, semi-adaptive sampling, global illumination in direct volume rendering with shadow rays as well as an optimisation method for shadow rays and multiple light source integration. The quality of the rendered images is increased while keeping impact on performance at minimal levels. The application is currently used in study and planning in the field of dentofacial surgery.

1 Introduction

Direct volume rendering (DVR) techniques can be used to visualise surfaces from volume data sets. The DVR ray casting algorithm can be massively parallelized using the graphics processor units (GPU). Hadwiger et al. [1] presented a single-pass fragment shader based approach. Hänel et al. [2] evaluated acceleration techniques for volume data visualisation within immersive virtual environments (IVE). Mastmeyer et al. [3, 4] developed a CUDA based DVR to simulate a visuo-haptic VR training and planning system. It was shown that a sufficient performance in IVEs remains a challenge. MedicVR [5] (www.medicvr.de) is a virtual reality application and is based on the new shader technology for interactive real-time volume rendering in virtual reality. What are the requirements for the DVR ray casting in virtual reality? A high-quality image pair must be calculated at optimally 90 frames-per-second (FPS) to allow a comfortable and smooth experience, while avoiding motion-sickness. Exemplary, in case of the HTC Vive each rendering image requires a resolution of 1080×1020 pixel. This results in about 233.280.000 integrated rays per second. The following sections will describe how acceleration techniques are used and enhancement methods are integrated in the shading pipeline for MedicVR. The results summarise performance measurements in frames-per-second with and without the respective feature and the resulting quality of the visualisation.

2   Materials and methods

MedicVR imports standardised DICOM data files from computer tomography or magnetic resonance tomography. The DVR algorithm complexity correlates with the number of rays, the number of samples per ray, the design of the transfer function and the amount of rays intersecting the volume. The visualisation for IVEs requires highly optimised algorithms to maintain a stable frame rate, while assuring a high quality rendering output for medical application. The following subsections describe applied improvement methods to MedicVR.

2.1   Lens matched shading for direct volume rendering

Lens Matched Shading (LMS) [6] is a technique used to improve performance and image quality by taking advantage of physical properties of HMDs. Due to lens distortion of the rendered image, the shading rate distribution does not match the lens profile. Fig. 1a shows how the central region in the focus of the lens is under-sampled, while the periphery is significantly super-sampled. With LMS the viewport is divided into four sub regions, each being distorted according to certain lens parameters. For each viewport LMS modifies the homogeneous w component of each vertex in clip-space before perspective division with $w' = w + Ax + By$ with A, B being the lens parameters. Fig. 1b shows the projective viewport correction. Fig. 1c, 1d show the effect before and after LMS. No difference can be seen through the lens, but LMS reduces the total number of rays in DVR and increases performance while focusing the image quality to the centre point.

2.2   Volume clipping with the virtual reality plane-tool

An interactive clipping plane is introduced in MedicVR for clipping of the rendered volume in three dimensional space. The clipping plane enables the user

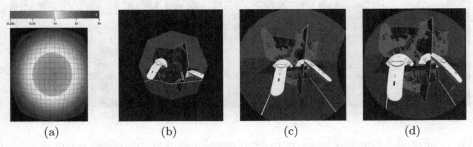

(a)   (b)   (c)   (d)

Fig. 1. Lens matched shading (LMS): shading rate without LMS (a); projective viewport correction (b), before LMS (c), and after LMS (d).

to view the inner structures of the volume by placing a plane tool in the IVE onto the volume. The resulting cut into the volume reveals internal features and coherences, otherwise obscured by higher opacities. The challenge of projecting a two dimensional cut of the volume onto a plane is solved by determination of the position of a sampling point on the plane so that the influence on the rendering integral is nullified for all points in front of the plane. The geometric properties of the dot product can be used to calculate the facing direction of a plane spanned by its normal vector towards a certain point. Multiplying the result of this calculation with the source value of the sampling point reduces the value to zero if the sampling point is in front of the plane. As such further computation on the sampling point can be skipped.

Fig. 2 shows the clipping plane combined with different visualisations. Sampling points in front of the plane are not included in ray integration.

2.3   Shadow ray diffuse culling (SRDC)

To assist the depth perception of volumetric data we integrated a gradient-based Blinn-Phong shading model and accelerated it by a gradient map [7] computed in a preprocessing-step (Fig. 3a).

When using a global illumination model in virtual reality, additional challenges occur in comparison to a desktop based solution. Due to the high degree of interaction and constant movements any preprocessing-steps relying on a fixed position of the light sources, the volume or the camera become impractical.

For global illumination of volumetric data MedicVR introduces the new technique shadow ray diffuse culling (SRDC) which is based on shadow rays by Ropinski et al. [8] combined with the Blinn-Phong shading model (Fig. 3b).

SRDC checks if the diffuse component of the Blinn-Phong shading model equals to zero. If given the sample position lies in the shadow and only the ambient component contributes to the shading. By exploiting this information the amount of emitted shadow rays can be reduced noticeably (Fig. 3c).

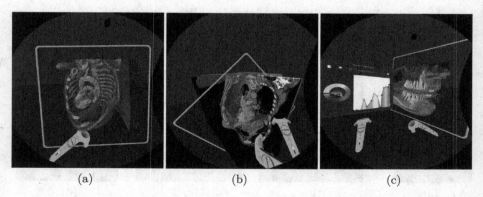

(a)   (b)   (c)

Fig. 2. Clipping Plane (turquoise rectangle) on different visualisations.

Fig. 3. SRDC: Exploitation of the diffuse light intensity from the Blinn-Phong shading model to accelerate shadow rays. (a) Blinn-Phong shading model, (b) Blinn-Phong shading model combined with shadow rays and (c) shadow rays but no shadowing (light blue), shadow rays with shadowing (dark blue), SRDC reduced shadow rays (green).

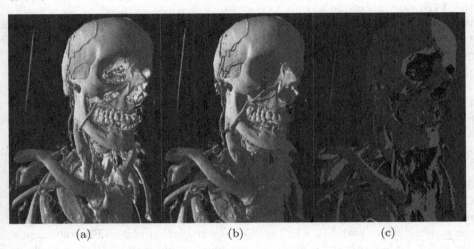

| (a) | (b) | (c) |

2.4 Semi-adaptive sampling

When using the first hit method [1] for direct volume rendering with medical image data a conspicuous noise is visible. This phenomenon is caused by the ray-casting rays entering and sampling the different tissues on slightly different depths. Hence the density on the sample point differs from the neighbouring pixels. This problem is especially recognisable on low sample rates (Fig. 4b), but also occurs on very high sample rates (Fig. 4a). Sampling between the first hit sample and the previous sample with additional correction samples results in a much higher sampling rate only in the important section of the ray-casting

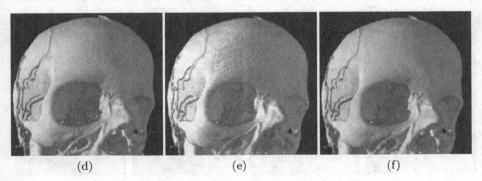

| (d) | (e) | (f) |

Fig. 4. Semi-adaptive sampling in first hit with correction steps. Panle (a), (b), and (c) show 1024 samples without correction, 128 samples without correction, and 128 samples with 20 correction steps, respectively.

Table 1. Average FPS for shadow rays 0, 150 and 500 samples with 1 or 3 light sources, LMS on or off and sample rate 512 or 1024. LMS improves the FPS rate about 30 % in case of no shadow rays. The performance decreases with the number of light sources.

light sources	LMS on off	sample rate	Shadow rays 0	rays 150	FPS 500
1	on	512	93	54	45
1	off	512	60	45	34
1	on	1024	62	36	27
1	off	1024	40	27	19
3	on	512	92	23	16
3	off	512	60	17	12

ray. Therefore the surface can be represented more accurate and the noise is significantly reduced, even at a much lower overall sample rate (Fig. 4c).

3 Results

The methods were implemented using OpenGL shading language GLSL and C++ on a NVIDIA GTX 1080 graphics card with 8 GB GDDR5X RAM and rendered at the native resolution of the HTC Vive. For the evaluation we used the manix dataset with $512 \times 512 \times 460$ voxel resolution and 16 Bit color depth per voxel. Unless otherwise noted an optimal sample rate of 1024 is used. A stable 1D transfer function is used for all measurements where more than 90 % iso values have an opacity value > 0. During the performance measurement we use a stable visualisation considering the whole volume data. Tab. 1 shows the average FPS rate over 1024 measurements.

With semi-adaptive sampling in first hit we achieved heavy noise reduction with lower sample rates (128 samples, 20 correction) and higher performance (58 FPS to 92 FPS in average) reaching almost the exact same image when using a much higher rates (1024 samples).

Using SDRC a performance gain was observed when using the same parameters by enableing and disableing SDRC in accumulate and first hit. Performance increased by 10 FPS in average in accumulate and 3 FPS in first hit.

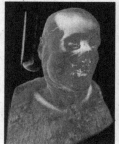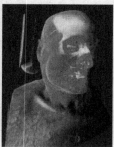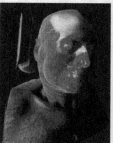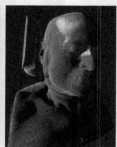

Fig. 5. Increasing the shadow ray sample rate increases the depth perception and realism of the scene while still being useable in VR at lower rate. Shadow ray sample rate from left: 0/50/150/500.

The quality of the rendered images is increased while keeping impact on performance at minimal levels. The application is currently used in study and planning in the field of dentofacial surgery. The three dimensional visualisation of the data in MedicVR acts as an auxiliary tool for the surgeon in order to understand the structural relationships and internal properties of the study case, serving as a new medium in medical education as well as in academical training. The interactive clipping plane is intensively used for preoperative planing and gives the surgeon an interactive real-time visualisation of the patient inner structures.

4 Discussion

Key concepts to MedicVR are high quality medical visualisation methods combined with the requirements of a smooth and interactive virtual reality application. Further developments into visualisation, usability and performance have been integrated into MedicVR for a better user experience and increased productivity. LMS takes advantage of the lens distortion of HMDs to significantly reduce the amount of rendered pixels and focus the computation power where it is needed. The image quality is increased while rendered pixels are reduced by about 40 %. The clipping plane tool serves as an arbitrary anatomical plane in the virtual reality. The presented method allows the user to explore the volume interactively, while showing no impact on the performance. In further developments, we will integrate more new VR hardware acceleration techniques. In the end, we want to improve the usability for the clinical use cases.

References

1. Engel K, Hadwiger M, Kniss J, et al. Real-time volume graphics. CRC Press; 2006.
2. Hänel C, Weyers B, Hentschel B, et al.; IEEE. Interactive volume rendering for immersive virtual environments. IEEE VIS Int Workshop 3DVis. 2014; p. 73–74.
3. Mastmeyer A, Fortmeier D, Handels H. Direct haptic volume rendering in lumbar puncture simulation. Med Meet Virtual Real 19: NextMed. 2012;173:280–286.
4. Fortmeier D, Mastmeyer A, Schröder J, et al. A virtual reality system for PTCD simulation using direct visuo-haptic rendering of partially segmented image data. IEEE J Biomed Health Inform. 2016;20(1):355–366.
5. Scholl I, Suder S, Schiffer S. Direct volume rendering in virtual reality. Procs BVM. 2018; p. 297–302.
6. Edward L. Lens matched shading and unreal engine 4 integration Ppart 1; 2018. [Accessed 26-10-2018]. [Online]. Available from: https://developer.nvidia.com/lens-matched-shading-and-unreal-engine-4-integration-part-1.
7. Levoy M. Display of surfaces from volume data. IEEE Comput Graph Appl. 1988;(3):29–30.
8. Ropinski T, Kasten J, Hinrichs. Efficient shadows for GPU-based volume raycasting. WSCG Full Pap. 2008; p. 17–24.

Efficient Web-Based Review for Automatic Segmentation of Volumetric DICOM Images

Tobias Stein[1], Jasmin Metzger[1], Jonas Scherer[1], Fabian Isensee[1],
Tobias Norajitra[1], Jens Kleesiek[2], Klaus Maier-Hein[1], Marco Nolden[1]

[1]Division of Medical Image Computing, German Cancer Research Center (DKFZ)
[2]Division of Radiology, German Cancer Research Center (DKFZ)
t.stein@dkfz-heidelberg.de

Abstract. Within a clinical image analysis workflow with large data sets of patient images, the assessment, and review of automatically generated segmentation results by medical experts are time constrained. We present a software system able to inspect such quantitative results in a fast and intuitive way, potentially improving the daily repetitive review work of a research radiologist. Combining established standards with modern technologies creates a flexible environment to efficiently evaluate multiple segmentation algorithm outputs based on different metrics and visualizations and report these analysis results back to a clinical system environment. First experiments show that the time to review automatic segmentation results can be decreased by roughly 50% while the determination of the radiologist is enhanced.

1 Introduction

Nowadays, medical images are a backbone of medical diagnosis and therefore omnipresent in the clinical environment. Reasons are decreasing imaging cost and concomitant. Therefore, it is a challenge in radiology to keep up with analyzing and reviewing a large amount of image data. Experienced radiologists develop an impressive intuition in how to classify medical images without further do. This approach is however restricted to a qualitative analysis. However, quantitative analysis, which is an essential part of clinical decision making, requires a voxelwise segmentation of the image. Well-proven automatic segmentation methods exist, namely statistical shape models and deep neural networks, that could significantly simplify and speed-up this task.

The time of radiologists is usually constrained and entailed to high costs. This cost can be reduced by a system that allows to review and rework image segmentations time-efficiently. Such a system can improve the clinical workflow of a radiologist regarding the certainty of his decisions. The system shall be designed to support radiologists as well as researchers with the task of creating a reliable and valid ground truth with less supervisor interaction when multiple segmentations for one image exist.

A system, which supports quantitative image analysis profits from quantitative imaging (QI). QI aims to extract quantifiable features from medical images within systematic and routine measurements to assess and track the severity of a patients condition. Automatic workflows can then summarize the feature results into useful reports for radiologists.

Common standards like DICOM (Digital Imaging and Communication in Medicine) are established to transfer image data interoperable in a clinical environment. To preserve clinical information like text or measurements in a structured way, DICOM offers the Structured Report (SR) while segmentations are properly stored in DICOM Segmentation (SEG) objects. In this context, the work of Herz et al. has published open source tools to enable the use of suitable DICOM data objects for quantitative image analysis [1]. They present a solution to interoperate with commonly used data formats in imaging research.

Not only interoperability is important for modern DICOM-based systems, but also the environment and its technology where image data is reviewed today. The web technology must be leveraged to meet the shift to the mobile era, meaning DICOM support for browsers on modern devices [2]. As DICOMweb is now a stable standard, next-generation technologies like image analytics and machine learning are enabled. Imaging is more ubiquitous with improved access to imaging and reduced cost of interoperability by DICOMweb [2]. Although DICOMweb exists since 2003, more recent publications are not using it, but instead, focus on HTML5 based viewers [3, 4]. These works convert DICOM images into PNG or JPEG and sent them to the client by Ajax or web sockets.

In summary, this work aims to combine the advantages of previous work. Referring to a standardized REST-API, with DICOMweb shall avoid the overhead of custom services which are handling metadata. In addition to that, modern HTML5 technology is used to leverage the power of today's browsers. The system shall follow established standards, scalable calculations by virtualization and easy integration in a web environment.

2   Materials and methods

The proposed system is now named as Segmentation Review System (SRS). In a brief overview, the top level workflow with its components is explained. The image server sends images to the website's included DICOM viewers. The website provides tools to support the decision whether a segmentation rework is necessary. This reworking process takes place within an established desktop application with a variety of imaging and viewing tools. Finally, the image server saves the reworked segmentation and a separate evaluation result database logs the reworking event.

2.1   Architecture and tools

The SRS consists of two components which both represent a web server (Fig. 1). The technology used for the web server is implemented in Python. Reasons for this decision are its fast and straight-forward way to configure a simple web server. The decision for the REST-Service framework falls to Django[1], as it offers a well-proven REST package. The frontend web server is implemented as light-weight Flask[2] application. Flask supports the idea of a zero-footprint viewer more than Django because it has less unnecessary features. The tools for displaying and interacting with image data on the frontend are implemented in JavaScript. The libraries dcm.js and dicomweb-client.js[3] are valuable for the implementation of querying and handling DICOM data. The library cornerstone.js[4] fulfills the actual interaction and image display task. To support a virtualized environment for the components triggered by the REST-API, Docker is chosen. It represents a state-of-the-art and a well-established choice in virtualization. The tool EvaluateSegmentation of the VISCERAL project[5] supports the calculation of metrics. The following component and context diagram displays the design of the architecture and the tool decisions (Fig. 1).

Fig. 1. The system boundary encloses components within the SRS, represented by a dashed line. The systems in context are the rework desktop application and a PACS server as discussed previously. The libraries for the frontend and the containerized tools, executed by the REST-Service, are highlighted.

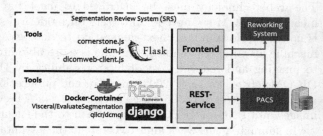

2.2   Segmentation evaluation

As discussed earlier, Docker executes the evaluation in a virtualized environment. The pixel data is converted from DICOM Segmentation (SEG) to Nrrd as common researcher format, to align with existing tools like the EvaluateSegmentation. The selection of metrics for the evaluation follows an established guideline [5], while EvaluateSegmentation tool performs the calculation. The evaluation of two segmentation volumes consists of calculating a set of different kind of metrics on each slice where segmented areas exist in both volumes. Overlap-based metrics like Dice, are used in combination with distance-based metrics like the Hausdorff distance. All metrics are normalized and weighted by a known correlation resulting in a slice similarity score. Every slice score contributes to a volume score. In addition to a single value, a local dissimilarity map (LDMap)

---

[1] https://www.djangoproject.com/
[2] http://flask.pocoo.org/
[3] Pieper et al., https://github.com/dcmjs-org
[4] https://github.com/cornerstonejs/
[5] http://www.visceral.eu/resources/evaluatesegmentation-software/

[6] is calculated for each slice. This map uses a modified Hausdorff distance with an adjusted window-size to catch local distances between segmentation contours and its spatial layout. It is stored as DICOM Parametric Map (PM) object.

The segmentation evaluation workflow starts with two DICOM SEG objects. The evaluation results (metrics, DICOM PM), calculated in a new Docker container, are documented in a DICOM Structured Report (SR) which contains all referenced DICOM objects in the composite context. The dcmqi tool [1] performs the data conversion, for example, DICOM to Nrrd, and the DICOM SR creation. A new Docker container simplifies the necessary metadata generation used by the dcmqi tool.

The browser receives the objects by encoded unique identifiers (UID) in a URL like stated in the IHE Invoke Image Display profile[6]. This profile gives a standard mechanism to request images for displaying them on a viewer. The profile connects image-aware systems like the analysis page and non-image-aware systems like a management page. The proposed web application can process a URL like "?requestType=SEG_EVAL&studyUID=...&srStudyUID=..." containing the type of request, the study UID, and the UID of the structured report. The analysis page parses the mentioned input parameters and fetches the SR series at first. In parallel, the composite context of the SR is extracted and the metrics are parsed. The composite context reveals the series UID of the base image, two SEG and one PM object. After the image base series is fetched, the other DICOM series are fetched asynchronously and displayed since loaded.

2.3 Experiment

For the experiment, two segmentation results of organ segmentation on abdominal CT volume scans are compared. Each scan contains about 100 up to 150 slices. A U-Net based approach called nnU-Net from Isensee et al. [7] is compared against a shape model method from Norajitra et al. [8]. The system evaluation design is built on two different setups of the analysis view displayed in Fig. 2. One cycle (Setup 1) is done without supporting tools like the LDMap in the middle, the slider background on the left and a function which makes the viewport display the region of interest. This cycle represents the usual workflow. Another cycle (Setup 2) is done with supporting tools. We measure the time when the page is loaded until a decision is made. Possible choices are the result of one algorithm or the need for rework. The data for the experiment consists of 45 image series including 30 kidneys and 15 livers.

3 Results

The results consists of the implementation of the web page and its infrastructure (Subsec. 2.1). A screenshot of the viewing page is displayed in Fig. 2.

In addition to that, the system was evaluated by one radiologist and one medical student to show its use for experts (Subsec. 2.3). The results of both

---

[6] http://www.ihe.net/uploadedFiles/Documents/Radiology/IHE_RAD_Suppl_IID.pdf

experts are averaged. The number of datasets at which the experts made the same decision with and without tools is 32 of 45 which is about 71% of all cases. The time improvement result of this evaluation is shown in Fig. 3. It reveals that in 35 of 45 cases, the experts were faster with our tools than without. In some cases, for example, 7, 18, and 24 a time improvement with about 150% is remarkable, meaning a factor of 2.5. The average time improvement factor over all datasets is 1.53.

4   Discussion

The radiologist states, he is able to make decisions more target-oriented with our tools, especially with the region of interest function for kidneys. A better comprehension of the segmentation differences can be assumed. The time improvement for the decision is quite variable. This variation is caused by dataset-related characteristics, like vessels or fat tissue which are sometimes segmented by only one of the methods. It also depends on the size and variability of the organ. Fig. 3 shows a higher time improvement on the rather smaller kidney within the first 30 datasets than on the larger liver. A considerable trend to a time improvement with tools is noticeable with an average proportion of 78% of the cases, where the decision was made faster with tools. This trend of faster decision making is also confirmed by the average time improvement factor per case of 1.53 which splits the time needed for a review session in half.

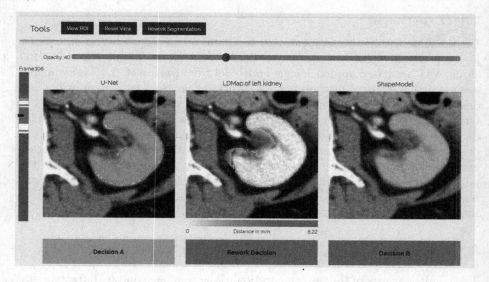

Fig. 2. Analysis web page. The middle viewer displays the dissimilarities between the left and right segmentation in a LDMap. At the left border, a frame slider with a highlighted background is displayed, indicating areas with a high deviation based on the combined metrics. The tools are displayed on top and the decision buttons are displayed below.

Fig. 3. Time improvement to decide between the three choices without tools against with tools on average over both experts. The background marks the left group as kidneys and the right as livers.

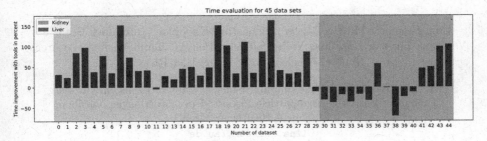

This work has successfully shown that DICOMweb and HTML5 technology together can bring DICOM data in a large number to the browser. The proposed application is easily accessible for a radiologist, which can save time using the mentioned tools while reviewing segmentations. The usage of DICOM enables segmentation analysis as a routine operation in nearly any clinical environment. Future use cases will include an integration with the training part of the underlying segmentation methods to investigate the potential of a tight feedback loop for active learning based on medical expert input.

References

1. Herz C, et al. dcmqi: an open source library for standardized communication of quantitative image analysis results using DICOM. Cancer Res. 2017;77.
2. Genereaux BW, et al. DICOMweb: background and application of the web standard for medical imaging. J Digit Imaging. 2018;31.
3. Monteiro EJM, et al. A DICOM viewer based on web technology. IEEE 15th Int Conf e-Health Netw, Appl Serv (Healthcom). 2013; p. 167–171.
4. Ellerweg R, et al. Architecture of a web-based DICOM viewer showing segmentations and simulations. IEEE 18th Int Conf e-Health Netw, Appl Serv (Healthcom). 2016; p. 1–5.
5. Taha AA, et al. Metrics for evaluating 3D medical image segmentation: analysis, selection, and tool. BMC Med Imaging. 2015;15.
6. Baudrier E, et al. Binary-image comparison with local-dissimilarity quantification. Pattern Recognit. 2008;41.
7. Isensee F, et al. nnU-Net: self-adapting framework for u-net-based medical image segmentation. arXivorg. 2018;.
8. Norajitra T, Maier-Hein KH. 3D statistical shape models incorporating landmark-wise random regression forests for omni-directional landmark detection. IEEE Trans Med Imaging. 2017; p. 155–168.

Abstract: Phase-Sensitive Region-of-Interest Computed Tomography

Lina Felsner[1], Martin Berger[3], Sebastian Kaeppler[1], Johannes Bopp[1], Veronika Ludwig[2], Thomas Weber[2], Georg Pelzer[2], Thilo Michel[2], Andreas Maier[1], Gisela Anton[2], Christian Riess[1]

[1]Pattern Recognition Lab, Computer Science, Univ. of Erlangen-Nürnberg
[2]Erlangen Centre for Astroparticle Physics, Univ. of Erlangen-Nürnberg
[3]Siemens Healthcare GmbH
lina.felsner@fau.de

X-ray Phase-Contrast Imaging (PCI) is a novel imaging technique that can be implemented with an grating interferometer. PCI is compatible with clinical X-ray equipment, and yields in addition to an absorption image also a differential phase image and a dark-field image. Computed Tomography (CT) of the differential phase can in principle provide high-resolution soft-tissue contrast. Recently, grating-based PCI took several hurdles towards clinical implementation by addressing, for example, acquisition speed, high X-ray energies, and system vibrations. However, a critical impediment in all grating-based systems lies in limits that constrain the grating diameter to few centimeters. Such a small field of view is a major challenge, since the object is typically larger, which leads to truncation in the projection images and therefore artifacts in the reconstruction.

In our work, we propose a system and a reconstruction algorithm to correct for phase truncation artifacts, and to obtain quantitative phase values in a clinically compatible way [1]. We propose to perform a phase-sensitive region-of-interest CT within a full-field absorption CT. An attenuating collimator can be used to mount the gratings, leading to less dose in the peripheral region outside of the gratings. Furthermore we propose an algorithm to correct for the phase value truncation by using the absorption information. Our method first performs a segmentation of the materials, which allows to obtain an estimate of their respective phase values. Then, a non-truncated sinogram is extrapolated from the truncated sinogram and the estimated phase values.

Our method is robust, and shows high-quality results on simulated data and on a biological mouse sample. The work is a proof of concept showing the potential to use PCI in CT on large specimen, such as humans, in clinical applications.

References

1. Felsner L, Berger M, Kaeppler S, et al. Phase-sensitive region-of-interest computed tomography. Proc MICCAI. 2018;1:37–144.

Joint Multiresolution and Background Detection Reconstruction for Magnetic Particle Imaging

Christine Droigk, Marco Maass, Corbinian Englisch, Alfred Mertins

Institute for Signal Processing, University of Lübeck
droigk@isip.uni-luebeck.de

Abstract. Magnetic particle imaging is a tracer-based medical imaging technology that is quite promising for the task of imaging vessel structures or blood flows. From this possible application it can be deduced that significant areas of the image domain are related to background, because the tracer material is only inside the vessels and not in the surrounding tissue. From this fact alone it seems promising to detect the background of the image in early stages of the reconstruction process. This paper proposes a multiresolution and segmentation based reconstruction, where the background is detected on a coarse level of the reconstruction with only few degrees of freedom by a Gaussian-mixture model and transferred to finer reconstruction levels.

1 Introduction

Magnetic particle imaging (MPI) is a tracer-based medical imaging method which was published in 2005 [1]. It is based on the nonlinear magnetization behavior of super-paramagnetic iron-oxide particles (SPIOs). The goal is to ascertain the SPIOs' distribution inside a volume, e.g. the distribution inside the vessel structure of a patient. Therefore, MPI scanners measure the induced voltage from the SPIOs' distribution by their change of magnetization. Fortunately, only SPIOs around the vicinity of the field free point (FFP) can significantly contribute to the voltage signal due to the nonlinear magnetization of those [2]. The FFP is the position where the different magnetic fields cancel each other out and this point is in MPI periodically moved, e.g. by a Lissajous trajectory, over the field of view. However, for two- and three-dimensional MPI there is no closed-form solution known so far for the system function, which relates the measured signal to the SPIOs distribution and vice versa [3]. This is the reason that the system function is normally approximated by a linear model. The resulting matrix models the spatio-temporal relationship and is called system matrix.

MPI offers a relatively high spatial and temporal resolution. To exploit the full spatial resolution, the system matrix has to be large in size. Unfortunately, solving the linear inverse problem becomes quite slow for dense system matrices. To speed up the reconstruction process, different matrix compression strategies were developed [4, 5]. The main idea is based on the usage of transforms, like the discrete cosine transform (DCT), to compress the system matrix. Recently, a simultaneous compression and multiresolution formulation for the system matrix was proposed. The authors also presented a multiresolution reconstruction procedure based on this formulation [6].

With the new formulation of the system matrix, a level-wise background segmentation and image reconstruction is proposed. The idea to exclude regions without SPIOs inside the reconstruction is based on the work in [7]. A quite similar idea was presented in [8], but there the background information was coming from an additional magnetic resonance image scan and is used for structural prior information. For the background segmentation a Gaussian mixture model (GMM) is used, which has also been successfully applied in positron emission tomography [9]. It will be shown that the background segmentation will help to significantly improve the particle distribution reconstruction at finer resolution levels.

2   Materials and methods

2.1   Multiresolution reconstruction

Due to page limitation the description is shortened to the necessary parts of the multiresolution system matrix approach from [6]. Let $S^\ell \in \mathbb{C}^{M \times K_\ell}$ be the low-resolution system matrix (low-pass approximation on the $(\ell - 1)$-th level of the discrete wavelet transform (DWT)) with $K_\ell = \left\lceil \frac{N_x}{2^\ell} \right\rceil \cdot \left\lceil \frac{N_y}{2^\ell} \right\rceil$ where $\lceil \cdot \rceil$ denotes the ceiling operator and N_x, N_y are the numbers of pixels in x and y direction. Then the transform matrix $T_\ell \in \mathbb{R}^{K_\ell \times K_\ell}$ denotes one stage of the DWT+DCT. The DWT+DCT decomposition is mathematically described by $S_T^\ell = S^\ell T_\ell$. The level-wise particle distribution reconstruction is defined as follows

$$c^\ell = \underset{c \in \mathbb{R}_+^{K_\ell}}{\operatorname{argmin}} \| S_T^\ell T_\ell^{-1} c - f \|_2^2 + \lambda^2 \| c \|_2^2 \tag{1}$$

where $\lambda > 0$ is the regularization factor $f \in \mathbb{C}^M$ defines the measured frequency components, which are derived from the voltage signal T_ℓ^{-1} is the inverse DWT+DCT and $c^\ell \in \mathbb{R}_+^{K_\ell}$ denotes the unknown particle distribution on the resolution stage ℓ. Preknowledge about the background pixels can be obtained by a segmentation on the coarser level reconstruction and then transferred to the finer resolution levels. Let $\mathbb{B}$ denote the set of background pixel indices and $\mathbb{P} = \{c \in \mathbb{R}_+^{K_\ell} | \forall i \in \mathbb{B} : c_i = 0\}$ then the problem in (1) can be reformulated to the easier problem

$$c^\ell = \underset{c \in \mathbb{P}}{\operatorname{argmin}} \, | S_T^\ell T_\ell^{-1} c - f |_2^2 + \lambda^2 \| c \|_2^2 \tag{2}$$

This problem is solved by an iterative shrinkage thresholding algorithm [10].

2.2   Background detection

To separate foreground and background pixels a thresholding with a variable threshold at each level is used. The threshold is obtained by estimating the probability density function of the foreground and background pixels with a GMM. The obtained mask is postprocessed by some morphological operations.

It is assumed that both the reconstructed particle distribution of the background and the foreground pixels follow a Gaussian distribution. Mean, standard deviation and mixture weights are estimated by a GMM. For the approximated density follows $p(x|\theta) = \sum_{i=1}^{K} \lambda_i f(x|\mu_i, \sigma_i)$, with $\theta = (\mu, \sigma)$ the parameter vector, $f(x|\mu, \sigma)$ the probability density function of the normal distribution with mean μ and standard deviation σ, and K the number of components. In this paper $K = 2$ is used under the assumption that contained structures share a similar concentration of the tracer. The weights λ_i can be seen as the estimation of the a-priori probability P_i. Then the threshold can be obtained by a maximum a-posteriori estimation, which is a solution of $P_1 f(x|\mu_1, \sigma_1) = P_2 f(x|\mu_2, \sigma_2)$. In the case of two solutions, the one between μ_1 and μ_2 is the desired one. Now the thresholding is performed and a binary mask is obtained. Small areas of foreground are deleted by morphological operations and then the structures are extended to preserve foreground. The obtained mask is used to set background pixels to zero during the reconstruction process. This procedure is repeated at each level and in this way the mask is refined step by step. After a successfull masking the amount of background pixels that are not set to zero decreases. For this reason only concentrations $c_k > 0$ are used for the GMM estimation. Besides, if the masking is nearly perfect, there only exists a single cluster of concentration values. This results for the GMM in two means which are close together. For detection of this case, it was tested whether $2 \cdot \min(\mu_1, \mu_2) < \max(\mu_1, \mu_2)$ is satisfied. If this is not fulfilled, no further thresholding is performed at this level.

2.3   Test setup

For the simulation of the MPI scanner the Langevin model of paramagnetism was used. The simulated MPI scanner has the frequency ratio of $f_x/f_y = 32/33$ with $f_x = 25.25$ KHz for the acceleration fields. This ratio results in a Lissajous FFP-trajectory with a repetition time of 1.27 ms. For the gradient fields in both spatial directions gradients up to a strength of 1.25 Tm^{-1} were used. The simulated system matrix was sampled for both receive channels up to a frequency of 1.3 MHz, which corresponds to 2×817 frequency components for a real-valued voltage signal. For the Langevin model a particle size of 30 nm and body temperature was assumed. The field of view had a size of 5×5 cm^2.

The multiscale segmentation reconstruction algorithm was tested on different concentration phantoms with different SNRs. In view of an application in the field of visualization of the blood flow, vessel structures were used as phantoms. Each phantom had a size of 250×250 pixels. The background had the value 0 while the concentration in the structures was 1.

For comparison purposes, also a reconstruction without foreground segmentation was performed [6], which is referred to as the baseline. A variation, where the thresholding method was used at the last level after completed reconstruction, is also included. The root mean square error (RMSE) and the structural similarity index (SSIM) [11] are used as measurements for comparison.

An RMSE near to zero shows a low difference in the concentration levels, while an SSIM near to one shows highly similar structures. A 9/7 wavelet decomposition in four levels was used.

3   Results

In Fig. 1 the ground truth concentrations and the reconstructed concentrations for an SNR of 20 dB for all compared approaches are shown. It can be observed that the proposed approach deletes background noise and delivers less blurring around the edges of the vessels than the other reconstruction results.

Fig. 2 shows the results of RMSE and SSIM for the different phantoms and methods in dependence of the SNR. The regularization parameter λ was chosen to produce the best RMSE or SSIM, respectively. It can be observed that the SSIM value of the proposed method is significantly higher for all phantoms and all SNRs than the value of the baseline. For most SNRs, advantages can be seen in comparison to the thresholded baseline method as well. The RMSE of the postprocessed baseline is better than the original baseline results for all phantoms and all SNRs. The results for the proposed method with regard to the

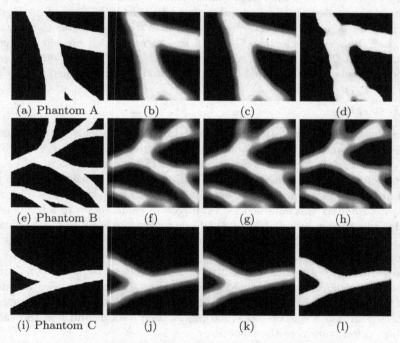

(a) Phantom A   (b)   (c)   (d)

(e) Phantom B   (f)   (g)   (h)

(i) Phantom C   (j)   (k)   (l)

Fig. 1. Best reconstructions of the three phantoms for the tested methods and an SNR of 20 dB. The left column shows the ground truth. In the middle, the reconstructions of the baseline and the thresholded baseline are depicted. On the right the final results of the proposed method are shown.

RMSE for phantom B and C is equal or better than the other approaches. For high SNRs and for phantom A a worsening can be seen.

4   Discussion

It could be observed that the proposed method provides a reconstruction with improved SSIM compared to standard reconstruction and even to postprocessed reconstructions. It works well for different structures and improves especially the SSIM while delivering a similar RMSE in most cases. With increasing SNR the RMSE value becomes unexpectedly worse. Fig. 3 shows the estimation of the multilevel thresholded approach and the result for the baseline method. At some areas at the borders of the vessels the foreground is underestimated and as a consequence high estimations of the concentration appear at the border and lead to a high RMSE value, though in the authors' perception the quality of this estimation is better. To avoid this phenomenon, the strong enhancement at the mask boundaries could be used to detect mismasked areas and expand the mask around these edges. The enhancement of the SSIM is due to the suppression of the background noise in areas without tracer concentration and the generation of sharp edges. This disembogues in a more homogenous concentration inside the object. Our further research is directed towards a speeding up of the reconstruction process using the obtained masks. Instead of setting the background to zero in each step, the calculations at these positions are not neccessary and could be skipped. This could result in a faster reconstruction.

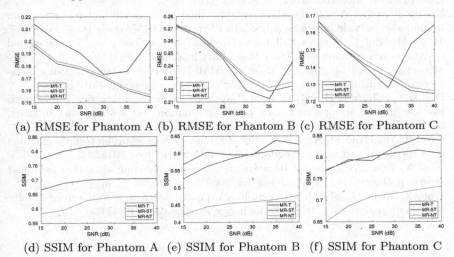

(a) RMSE for Phantom A (b) RMSE for Phantom B (c) RMSE for Phantom C

(d) SSIM for Phantom A   (e) SSIM for Phantom B   (f) SSIM for Phantom C

Fig. 2. RMSE and SSIM for the tested phantoms and different methods. The proposed method with foreground segmentation is referred to as MR-T, the baseline is MR-NT, and the postprocessed baseline is MR-ST. For each method and for each SNR the regularization parameter with the best result among the tested values was used.

Fig. 3. Particle distribution estimation of phantom B with an SNR of 40 dB with the proposed method (a) and the baseline system (b).

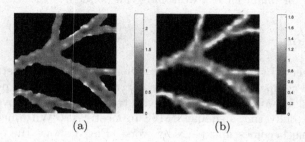

(a)   (b)

Acknowledgement. This work was supported by the German Research Foundation under grant number ME 1170/7-1.

References

1. Gleich B, Weizenecker J. Tomographic imaging using the nonlinear response of magnetic particles. Nature. 2005;435(7046):1214–1217.
2. Knopp T, Buzug TM. Magnetic Particle Imaging: An Introduction to Imaging Principles and Scanner Instrumentation. Berlin/Heidelberg: Springer; 2012.
3. Rahmer J, Weizenecker J, Gleich B, et al. Signal encoding in magnetic particle imaging: properties of the system function. BMC Med Imaging. 2009;9(4):4.
4. Lampe J, Bassoy C, Rahmer J, et al. Fast reconstruction in magnetic particle imaging. Phys Med Biol. 2012;57(4):1113–1134.
5. Knopp T, Weber A. Local system matrix compression for efficient reconstruction in magnetic particle imaging. Adv Math Phys. 2015;2015(Article ID 472818):1–7.
6. Maass M, Mink C, Mertins A. Joint multiresolution magnetic particle imaging and system matrix compression. Int J Magn Part Imaging. 2018;4(2).
7. Siebert H, Maass M, Ahlborg M, et al. MMSE MPI reconstruction using background identification. Proc Int Workshop Magn Part Imaging. 2016; p. 58.
8. Bathke C, Kluth T, Brandt C, et al. Improved image reconstruction in magnetic particle imaging using structural a priori information. Int J Magn Part Imaging. 2017;3(1).
9. Layer T, Blaickner M, Knäusl B, et al. PET image segmentation using a gaussian mixture model and markov random fields. EJNMMI Phys. 2015;2(1).
10. Beck A, Teboulle M. A fast iterative shrinkage-thresholding algorithm for linear inverse problems. SIAM J Imaging Sci. 2009;2(1):183–202.
11. Wang Z, Bovik AC, Sheikh HR, et al. Image quality assessment: from error visibility to structural similarity. IEEE Trans Image Process. 2004;13(4):600–612.

Abstract: Double Your Views: Exploiting Symmetry in Transmission Imaging

Alexander Preuhs[1], Andreas Maier[1], Michael Manhart[2], Javad Fotouhi[3],
Nassir Navab[3], Mathias Unberath[3]

[1]Pattern Recognition Lab, Friedrich-Alexander-Universität Erlangen-Nürnberg
[2]Siemens Healthcare GmbH, Forchheim, Germany
[3]Computer Aided Medical Procedures, Johns Hopkins University
alexander.preuhs@fau.de

For a plane symmetric object we can find two views – mirrored at the plane of symmetry – that will yield the exact same image of that object. In consequence, having one image of a plane symmetric object and a calibrated camera, we can automatically have a second, virtual image of that object if the 3D location of the symmetry plane is known. In this work, we show for the first time that the above concept naturally extends to transmission imaging and present an algorithm to estimate the 3D symmetry plane from a set of projection domain images based on Grangeat's theorem. We then exploit symmetry to generate a virtual trajectory by mirroring views at the plane of symmetry. If the plane is not perpendicular to the acquired trajectory plane, the virtual and real trajectory will be oblique. The resulting X-shaped trajectory will be data-complete, allowing for the compensation of in-plane motion using epipolar consistency [1].

Utilizing Grangeat's theorem, we can measures the pairwise consistency of two projections by comparing corresponding epipolar lines. The theorem explains a transformation of the projection images, such that two values must match if they correspond to two epipolar lines. This value equals a transformation of the object mass within the epipolar plane – i.e. the derivative of the Radon transform. It directly follows, that inconsistency induced by a rigid object motion within the epipolar plane cannot be detected, as the object mass within the epipolar plane is not affected. In a circular trajectory, most of the measurable epipolar planes are parallel to the acquisition plane, limiting the detectable inconsistencies to motion that steps out of the acquisition plane. As a result, out-plane motion is well compensable while in-plane motion remains an open challenge.

This limitation can be mitigated by the X-shaped trajectory. This enables epipolar planes in more directions and it is shown that with an adequate tilde between the acquisition plane and the plane of symmetry, in-plane motion becomes well detectable.

References

1. Preuhs A, Maier A, Manhart M, et al. Double your views: exploiting symmetry in transmission imaging. Proc MICCAI. 2018; p. 356–364.

3D-Reconstruction of Stiff Wires from a Single Monoplane X-Ray Image

Katharina Breininger[1], Moritz Hanika[2], Mareike Weule[2], Markus Kowarschik[2], Marcus Pfister[2], Andreas Maier[1]

[1]Pattern Recognition Lab, Friedrich-Alexander-Universität Erlangen-Nürnberg, Erlangen, Germany
[2]Siemens Healthcare GmbH, Forchheim, Germany
katharina.breininger@fau.de

Abstract. of preoperative data with intraoperative fluoroscopic images has been shown to reduce contrast agent, radiation dose and procedure time during endovascular repair of aortic aneurysms. However, the quality of the fusion may deteriorate due to often severe deformations of the vasculature caused by instruments such as stiff wires. To adapt the preoperative information intraoperatively to these deformations, the 3D positions of the inserted instruments are required. In this work, we propose a reconstruction method for stiff wires that requires only a single monoplane acquisition, keeping the impact on the clinical workflow to a minimum. To this end, the wire is segmented in the available X-ray image. To allow for a reconstruction in 3D, we then estimate a virtual second view of the wire orthogonal to the real projection based on vessel centerlines from a preoperative computed tomography. Using the real and estimated wire positions, we reconstruct the catheter using epipolar geometry. We achieve a mean modified Hausdorff distance of 4.1 mm between the 3D reconstruction and the true wire course.

1 Introduction

of preoperative data with intraoperative images has proven its benefits in a number of minimally invasive procedures. One example is endovascular aortic repair (EVAR) for aortic aneurysms, during which stent grafts are inserted under fluoroscopic guidance to reduce the risk of aneurysm rupture. Visualization of the aorta and branching vessels extracted from preoperative computed tomography angiography (CTA) on the intraoperative images can aid navigation and can help to reduce the amount of contrast agent needed during the intervention [1]. The guide wires and stents inserted during the procedure, however, can deform the vasculature and the utility of the preoperative information deteriorates. On the other hand, these instruments can be assumed to lie within the aorta and the iliac arteries, and are visible in the fluoroscopic images without contrast injection. Accordingly, information about their position can be used to correct for deformations and restore the usefulness of the fusion. To allow for a correction based on the instruments, the 3D course of the instrument has to be known.

3D reconstruction of instruments from fluoroscopic images has been addressed repeatedly using biplane systems or two projections [2, 3]. Acquiring a second projection, however, may heavily impact the interventional workflow during EVAR as repositioning of the C-arm is required. Reconstruction from a single image requires additional information, for example in form of a preoperative model of the anatomy. In previous work on reconstruction from one view [4, 5, 6], the anatomy under investigation is assumed not to be heavily impacted by the inserted wires. In contrast to this, the vessels and especially the iliac arteries are deformed during EVAR due to the stiffness of the inserted wires [1], requiring a different approach. Finite element modeling has been investigated to estimate guide wire position for EVAR preoperatively [7], however, computation times are prohibitively long for intraoperative estimation.

In this work, we propose a method to reconstruct the 3D position of guide wires based on the segmentation of a single monoplane acquisition of the respective instrument. To this end, we utilize prior information in form of a vessel segmentation from preoperative CT. Based on the segmentation, more specifically the vessel centerlines, we estimate a virtual second projection of the wire to approximate the depth. Using the real and virtual projection of the guide wire, we reconstruct the 3D positions as described in [2]. The reconstruction error in 3D is evaluated by comparing our estimation to biplane reconstructions of the stiff wire and ground truth acquired from cone-beam CT (CBCT).

2   Materials and methods

Given a registered preoperative segmentation and the 2D image, the reconstruction of the 3D wire course can be divided into three steps as follows: 1) segmentation of the wire in the available monoplane image, 2) estimation of a virtual

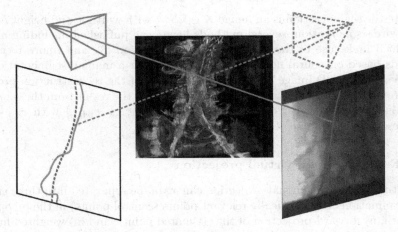

Fig. 1. Visualization of set-up. The wire is segmented (solid red line) in one X-ray image from an angulation of approximately 45° LAO/RAO. A virtual second projection of the wire (dotted red line) is estimated based on the preoperative CT (solid green line).

second view of the device and 3) reconstruction of the wire using the real and virtual wire course as biplane information. The main contribution of this work is step 2). The set-up is depicted in Fig. 1. In the following, we will describe the data we use in this work, as well as the three steps in more detail.

2.1   Data

Prerequisite for the proposed method is a preoperative CT and corresponding 3D centerlines of the vessels in which the stiff wire is inserted, namely the aorta, the common and external iliac artery, and the femoral artery. We evaluate our method using data from 16 patients who underwent EVAR at Sahlgrenska Hospital, Gothenburg, Sweden. For each patient, a preoperative CTA was segmented using in-house prototype software. During the procedure, an X-ray image is acquired that shows the area around the iliac bifurcation before the stent is deployed with the stiff wire in place. This is done at an angulation of approximately 45° RAO for the left and 45° LAO for the right iliac artery. At this angulation, the iliac bifurcation is generally well defined in contrast-enhanced acquisitions which allows for accurate stent placement. We obtained this data from an intraoperative CBCT that was originally acquired for 3D image guidance. Each patient had a stiff wire and optionally a delivery device inserted in at least one iliac artery at the time of the CBCT. Projection images from 45° LAO/RAO were extracted from the corresponding projection run. The wires inserted in the left and right iliac artery were annotated manually in these projection images and in the 3D reconstruction. The preoperative CT and the intraoperative CBCT were registered semi-automatically with focus on the lower vertebrae of the spine.

2.2   2D segmentation

Input to the segmentation is an image $\mathbf{X} \in \mathbb{R}^{w \times h}$ with width w and height h. For guide wire segmentation, several methods have been published, including methods which make use of the preoperative segmentation [8], and, more recently, methods based on neural networks [9]. We opted for a manual segmentation of the device in the 2D image to avoid mixing errors of the reconstruction process and errors in the segmentation. With either method, the result from the segmentation is a sequence of 2D coordinates $W_{2D} = \{\boldsymbol{v}_{w1}, \ldots, \boldsymbol{v}_{wn_A}\}$ with $\boldsymbol{v}_{wi} \in \mathbb{R}^2$ that describes the course of the device in $\mathbf{X}$.

2.3   Estimation of a virtual projection

The estimation of the virtual projection can again be separated into three steps: i) determination of anatomically relevant points (control points) in the preoperative data, ii) forward-projection of the estimated points, and iii) weighted fitting of a polynomial function through these points. The selected points in step i) and the weights in step iii) are optimized based on a training set of patients. Again, we will describe each step in more detail:

Estimation of control points The preoperative vessel centerline can be described by a sequence of 3D points $V_{3D} = \{v_1, \ldots, v_{nv}\}$ with $v_i \in \mathbb{R}^3$ In this sequence, certain points can be determined as landmarks, namely the aortic bifurcation (AB) v_{AB} and the position at which the stiff wire enters the femoral artery (FA) v_{FA} The first point is automatically determined during segmentation, the latter is estimated using the method described in [10]. Based on these two landmarks, we identify a segment of interest that stretches from FA to 20 cm proximal to the AB landmark with the proximal endpoint v_P Within this segment $[v_{FA}, v_P]$ we determine the most dorsal and most ventral position v_D and v_V of the centerline. In addition, we estimate points that try to capture the straightening caused by the stiff wire. More specifically, we split the sequence into three subsegments $S_1 = [v_{FA}, v_D]$, $S_2 = [v_D, v_{AB}]$, and $S_3 = [v_{AB}, v_P]$ For each segment, we estimate the mean of all points within two overlapping intervals that are defined by the first and the last two thirds of the segments. Lastly, we estimate the mean of all points in the segment $[v_{1/3FAD}, v_{AB}]$ a segment of very strong curvature, and the midpoints between v_D and v_{AB}, v_{AB} and v_P, and $v_{1/3FAD}$ and v_P This results in a list of 16 control points $V_{C_{3D}}$.

Forward-projection of control points As mentioned previously, we assume that the fluoroscopic image for which we want to reconstruct the stiff wire in 3D was acquired at an angulation of approximately 45° RAO for the left and 45° LAO for the right side. The projection can be described by a projection matrix $\mathbb{P} \in \mathbb{R}^{3 \times 4}$ (using homogeneous coordinates). We rotate this projection matrix by 90° LAO (resp. RAO) which corresponds to a 90° rotation around the longitudinal axis, resulting in a projection matrix $\mathbb{P}' \in \mathbb{R}^{3 \times 4}$ The estimated control points $V_{C_{3D}}$ can then be projected forward using the matrix $\mathbb{P}'$, resulting a sequence of 2D points $V'_{C_{2D}} = \{v'_{c1}, \ldots, v'_{c16}\}$ with $v'_{ci} \in \mathbb{R}^2$.

Weighted polynomial fitting At the given angulation, the course of the wire can be described by a polynomial function of degree three to five. We make use of this by fitting a polynomial of degree five to the control points $V'_{C_{2D}}$ using weighted least squares. For each control point, we define a weight w_i to control its influence during fitting. The weights w are optimized based on a training set of six patients by minimizing the mean squared modified Hausdorff distance (mHD) between the estimated course and the 2D ground truth in the respective projection image using random search. The fitted polynomial then provides the estimated virtual 2D course W'_{2D} of the catheter.

2.4 Reconstruction from real and virtual views

For reconstruction, we utilize the method described in [2]. Given the acquisition geometry, all possible correspondences between points along the sequences W_{2D} and W'_{2D} are computed. Based on this, a mapping between W_{2D} and W'_{2D} of optimal correspondences is determined that respects the continuity of the device. These are then used to reconstruct the wire in 3D.

Table 1. 3D reconstruction error for vessels with stiff wire (SW) only, and stiff wire and delivery device (DD) inserted. Reported are mean and standard deviation with respect to Hausdorff distance and modified Hausdorff distance in mm.

	Baseline reconstruction		Proposed method	
	SW only	SW and DD	SW only	SW and DD
Modified Hausdorff distance	0.97±0.14	0.97±0.17	3.82±1.97	4.49±1.61
Hausdorff distance	2.32±0.36	2.17±0.39	7.34±3.47	9.36±3.41

3   Results

From the 32 iliac arteries (left and right), we excluded three that contained only a substantially softer pigtail catheter. All patients used for training were excluded from further analysis. For the remaining 10 patients, we reconstructed the wire in the left and right iliac artery as described above. To assess the baseline error, we additionally reconstructed the stiff wire based on segmentations in two projections (45° LAO/RAO). Errors in this reconstruction may stem from patient breathing and heartbeat during acquisition of the CBCT, or errors in the annotation. The results of the reconstruction can be found in Tab. 1. Additionally, we investigated the stability of the approach in case the projection image is acquired ±20° from the trained 45° projection. The results and examples of estimated virtual projections can be found in Fig. 2.

4   Discussion and conclusion

The error of the proposed method with a mean mHD of 4.1 mm for the left and the right wire lies well below the typical vessel diameter of the iliac artery of approximately 10-17 mm. It is in range with errors reported by preoperative FEM simulation with a mean 3.8 mm mHD between real and simulated wires [7]. We see a slightly higher error when both a stiff wire and a delivery device is inserted likely because the delivery device causes even more straightening of the vessel. The proposed approach is optimized for the region around the iliac bifurcation and angulations around 45° LAO/RAO. Due to the heuristic selection of control points and the restriction we impose by a polynomial fitting, we see a high

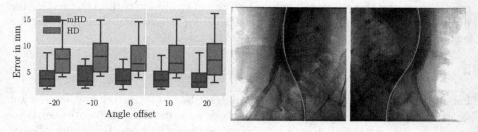

Fig. 2. Left: Error when deviating from a 45° LAO/RAO angulation. Right: Examples for estimated projections (dotted red line), the true wire course is highlighted in green.

deviation outside this field of view. While we see a stable estimation when varying the angles in a reasonable range, the approach has to be adapted for other regions, e.g., around the renal arteries. Furthermore, it requires a preoperative CT segmentation and a registration to the intraoperative images, both generally available in the context of image fusion. It has to be noted that reconstruction accuracy strongly depends on the accuracy of the initial rigid registration.

Within the current workflow for iliac artery deformation correction, these limitations are acceptable, and the accuracy and speed of the method of below 100 ms allows for intraoperative use. In future work, we aim to look into directly reconstructing the device in 3D to be more independent of the anatomical region and integrate tissue properties such as calcifications into the reconstruction.

Disclaimer. The methods and information presented here are based on research and are not commercially available.

References

1. Tacher V, Lin M, Desgranges P, et al. Image guidance for endovascular repair of complex aortic aneurysms: comparison of two-dimensional and three-dimensional angiography and image fusion. J Vasc Interv Radiol. 2013;24(11):1698–1706.
2. Hoffmann M, Brost A, Jakob C, et al. Semi-automatic catheter reconstruction from two views. Proc MICCAI. 2012; p. 584–591.
3. Baert SAM, van de Kraats EB, van Walsum T, et al. Three-dimensional guide-wire reconstruction from biplane image sequences for integrated display in 3-D vasculature. IEEE Trans Med Imaging. 2003;22(10):1252–1258.
4. van Walsum T, Baert SAM, Niessen WJ. Guide wire reconstruction and visualization in 3DRA using monoplane fluoroscopic imaging. IEEE Trans Med Imaging. 2005;24(5):612–623.
5. Petković T, Homan R, Lončarić S. Real-time 3D position reconstruction of guidewire for monoplane X-ray. Comput Med Imaging Graph. 2014;38(3):211–223.
6. Brückner M, Deinzer F, Denzler J. Temporal estimation of the 3d guide-wire position using 2d X-ray images. Proc MICCAI. 2009; p. 386–393.
7. Gindre J, Bel-Brunon A, Rochette M, et al. Patient-specific finite-element simulation of the insertion of guidewire during an EVAR procedure: guidewire position prediction validation on 28 cases. IEEE Trans Biomed Eng. 2017;64(5):1057–1066.
8. Lessard S, Kauffmann C, Pfister M, et al. Automatic detection of selective arterial devices for advanced visualization during abdominal aortic aneurysm endovascular repair. Med Eng Phys. 2015;37(10):979–986.
9. Breininger K, Würfl T, Kurzendorfer T, et al. Multiple device segmentation for fluoroscopic imaging using multi-task learning. Intravascular Imaging Comput Assist Stenting Large-Scale Annotat Biomed Data Expert Label Synth. 2018; p. 19–27.
10. Breininger K, Pfister M, Koutouzi G, et al. Estimation of femoral artery access location for anatomic deformation correction. Proc Conf Image-Guid Interv Fokus Neuroradiol. 2017; p. 23–24.

Regularized Landmark Detection with CAEs for Human Pose Estimation in the Operating Room

Lasse Hansen[1], Jasper Diesel[2], Mattias P. Heinrich[1]

[1]Institute of Medical Informatics, University of Lübeck, Germany
[2]Drägerwerk AG & Co. KGaA, Lübeck, Germany
`hansen@imi.uni-luebeck.de`

Abstract. Robust estimation of the human pose is a critical requirement for the development of context aware assistance and monitoring
systems in clinical settings. Environments like operating rooms or intensive care units pose different visual challenges for the problem of human
pose estimation such as frequent occlusions, clutter and difficult light-
ing conditions. Moreover, privacy concerns play a major role in health
care applications and make it necessary to use unidentifiable data, e.g.
blurred RGB images or depth frames. Since, for this reason, the data
basis is much smaller than for human pose estimation in common scenarios, pose priors could be beneficial for regularization to train robust
estimation models. In this work, we investigate to what extent existing pose estimation methods are suitable for the challenges of clinical
environments and propose a CAE based regularization method to correct estimated poses that are anatomically implausible. We show that
our models trained solely on depth images reach similar results on the
MVOR dataset [1] as RGB based pose estimators while intrinsically being
non-identifiable. In further experiments we prove that our CAE regularization can cope with several pose perturbations, e.g. missing parts or
left-right flips of joints.

1 Introduction

Human pose estimation is a typical computer vision task that has been studied
for decades and is a key component for a variety of higher level applications ranging from motion control in video games or car entertainment systems to video
surveillance and behavioral understanding. The conventional estimation process
is driven by the underlying image data, capturing local appearance, as well as
structured prediction to produce globally plausible poses. Similar to other fields,
purely data driven deep learning methods, in particular convolutional neural
networks (CNNs) yield impressive results on public datasets and have nowadays
replaced hand-crafted features and graphical models. With their success research
shifts to more challenging scenarios. Pose estimation in clinical environments offers great opportunities by providing contextual information about the patient
or staff for assistance and monitoring systems, but also has to cope with strong
occluded and cluttered settings such as the operating room. At the same time

clinical pose estimation datasets are much smaller than large-scale annotated datasets like MPII [2] making it harder to reliably train deep learning models. Explicit regularization of predicted poses is a possibility to recover plausible poses.

1.1 Related work

Early successful methods for human pose estimation relied on hand-crafted image features and sophisticated body part models [3]. DeepPose [4] was the first work that trained a deep neural network to directly regress joint positions. Following the success of CNNs for the image classification task subsequent methods used CNNs in a fully convolutional manner to generate heatmaps of joint locations [5]. In general, predicting heatmaps showed to be more robust than directly regressing pixel positions. Recent state-of-the-art pose estimators often adopt variants of stacked hourglass networks (SHGs) [6] as basic building blocks. SHGs capture both local and global context within multi-scale CNN architectures. Stacking multiple of these hourglasses combined with intermediate supervision further improves the network's final performance.

The most recent methods described above model the human body only implicitly. In this work we aim at explicitly regularizing poses and therefore consider research that uses global priors in neural networks. Convolutional Autoencoders (CAEs) [7] were introduced as unsupervised feature extractors. They reduce the input data with spatial filters and pooling operations into a latent space from which the original input must be reconstructed. The learned features from the encoder can then be reused in a supervised classification task. [8] showed that the CAEs latent space could also be used to regularize segmentation of ultrasound images. Therefore during training, the model predictions are forced to follow the distribution of the learnt low dimensional representations of priors. In the field of human pose estimation [9] trained an autoencoder on 3D joint locations to regress the 3D positions from 2D images via its regularized latent space.

1.2 Contribution

In this work we investigate how SHG, a state-of-the art human pose estimator, performs in a challenging clinical setting. We show that SHG models trained on normalized depth images yield a similar performance on the MVOR dataset [1] as RGB based methods and can therefore conclude that the use of depth images is a suitable image modality to tackle privacy concerns in visual health care applications. Given the small amount of training data (in contrast to non-clinical settings), we observe frequent anatomically implausible pose predictions. We therefore propose a CAE based postprocessing of predicted poses. Our experiments show that this new approach can reliable recover poses from input perturbations such as joints that are missing or symmetrically switched.

2   Materials and methods

Our architecture for regularized pose estimation consists of two independent components – an SHG that predicts heatmaps from raw input data and a CAE to recover plausible poses from the initial joint locations. Fig. 1 for a schematic overview of the two-stage pipeline.

2.1   Pose estimation

Pose estimation of input image data, e.g. RGB or depth, is conducted with SHGs from [8]. The output of the network is a heatmap with N channels, where N is the number of landmarks to detect. The final predictions are given by the maximum activation of the heatmap. Ground truth targets consist of a 2D Gaussian (kernel) centered on the corresponding joint location. One hourglass consists of multiple convolution and pooling layers to process features down to a very low resolution, whereby at each pooling step one further convolution is applied at the current level and added to the corresponding layer on the symmetric bottom-up sequence. Multiple hourglasses with intermediate supervision can be stacked to further improve the performance.

2.2   Pose regularization

For regularization of implausible poses we propose a convolutional autoencoder that is trained with different synthetic perturbations on the input data to enforce the explicit learning of a body pose model. The CAE is composed of two parts, the encoder and the decoder. In the encoding step a heatmap with N channels is transformed into a small-low-dimensional feature map (e.g. 4x4 pixels) by a series of convolution and pooling layers. With every convolution the number of features is doubled. After the last pooling layer the spatial relation is broken and the flattened tensor is fed into a two-layer neural network. The number of output features of the last linear layer specifies the dimension of the latent representation and should be small enough to force the CAE to learn a representative body pose embedding. The decoder reverses the operations of the encoding, whereby

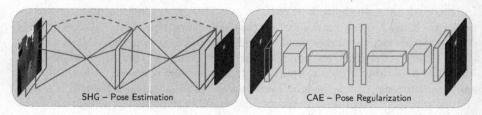

Fig. 1. We propose a two-stage architecture for regularized pose estimation from single depth images. A stacked hourglass network infers heatmaps for human joint locations. In a subsequent step a convolutional autoencoder corrects implausible pose predictions. The two networks are trained separately, whereby the pose regularizer is explicitly forced to learn a body model via perturbations of the input data.

	head	shoulder	elbow	wrist	hip	mean
SHG_{depth}	97.6	90.5	78.2	80.0	71.2	83.5
SHG_{rgb}	97.0	90.5	77.4	79.5	71.7	83.2
$OpenPose_{rgb}$	91.0	88.8	74.5	58.1	56.4	73.8
$AlphaPose_{rgb}$	87.7	88.9	77.8	64.7	61.8	76.2

Table 1. Independent quantitative evaluations for pose estimation.

convolutions and pooling operations are replaced by transposed convolutions and indexed unpooling, respectively. To ensure that the CAE can actually act as a pose regularizer typical pose errors are explicitly incorporated in the training. In this work we propose three different synthetic augmentations: swapping two corresponding joints of the left and right body part, removing a single joint and applying a high random offset to one of the joints. All input channels are randomly scaled and Gaussian noise is added to further reduce the risk of learning an identity mapping.

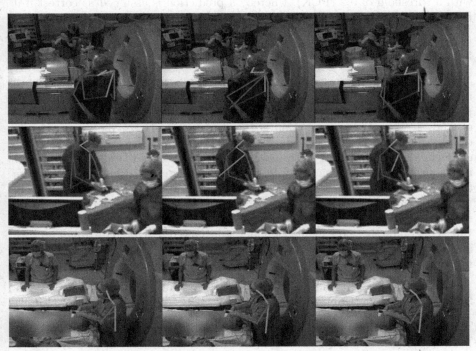

Fig. 2. Qualitative and quantitative results on the MVOR dataset. The example images show ground truth (left), SHG predictions (middle) and CAE regularized joints (right). Body poses were inferred from depth frames and overlayed on rgb images for better visualization.

Table 2. Independent quantitative evaluations for pose regularization.

	w/o reg.	CAE reg.
swap	80.3	97.1
remove	90.0	96.6
offset	90.7	96.5

3   Results

All experiments were conducted on the MVOR dataset [1]. It consists of 732 multi-view frames from three RGB-D cameras providing registered depth and anonymized rgb images synchronized in time. The images were recorded in an operating room at the University Hospital of Strasbourg over a period of four days. Each day was used as one fold in a 4-fold cross validation. For the task of 2D pose estimation the ground truth annotations consist of 2926 bounding boxes and upper-body poses. As evaluation metric we use percentage of correct keypoints with a threshold of 0.2 (PCK), whereby a prediction is assumed as correct if it falls within $0.2 \cdot \max(bbox_h, bbox_w)$ pixels of the ground truth annotation.

3.1   Pose estimation

We first evaluate the pose estimation network on both image modalities, depth and RGB. The SHG with two stacks is implemented in PyTorch. Training was performed for 50 epochs with the Adam optimizer and an initial learning rate of $2.5e-4$. The objective function is the mean squared error between the predicted and ground truth heatmaps. We use random affine transformations to augment the input data. For training with depth images it was crucial to normalize each image independently to correct for different distances of the person to the camera.

Fig. 2 shows the results of the SHG models. Training with the two image modalities gives a similar PCK of approximately 83.5. For comparison, PCK values of two further pose estimation methods, OpenPose[10] and AlphaPose[11], are reported from [1]. We note that both estimators are pretrained on MPII without fine-tuning on MVOR.

3.2   Pose regularization

The general training setting is the same as for our pose estimation network. The CAE encodes body poses in a 16-dimensional latent vector. During training Gaussian noise with a std of 0.05 is added to the input heatmap and one of the three perturbations ('swap', 'remove', 'offset') is applied with a probability of 0.5 each. We evaluate the capability of the CAE to recover plausible poses for each input perturbation independently by applying the corresponding augmentation strategy on all test images. In a last experiment we regularize the predicted heatmaps from the SHG by feeding them directly into the CAE.

The isolated evaluation of our CAE shows improved mean PCK values of 80.3 to 97.1, 90.0 to 96.6 and 90.7 to 96.5 for the swap, remove and offset perturbation, respectively. The subsequent regularization of the SHG predictions on depth images leads to a mean PCK of 84.4. Qualitative results in Fig. 2 visualize the regularization of implausible and incomplete poses (Tabs. 1 and 2).

4   Discussion

We successfully validated a state-of-the-art pose estimator, namely SHG, for upper body pose estimation in a new challenging clinical environment. Thereby, we could show that depth frames as input modality reached a better performance than blurred RGB images, implying that depth information can be a natural choice for computer vision algorithms in health care applications that depend on anonymized input data. Our CAE based regularization can reliable recover plausible poses from a set of input perturbations and as a simple and independent post processing step the CAE leads to a small improvement in mean PCK. To further improve on the results the CAE could be incorporated in an end-to-end training in the pose estimation step, e.g. using the latent space for a regularization loss as in [9]. Finally, we believe our self-supervised regularization method has great potential for future use in landmark detection and foresee further research in different domains, e.g. localisation in CT or MRI volumes.

References

1. Srivastav V, Issenhuth T, Kadkhodamohammadi A, et al.   MVOR: a multi-view RGB-D operating room dataset for 2D and 3D human pose estimation. arXiv:180808180. 2018;.
2. Andriluka M, Pishchulin L, Gehler P, et al.   2D human pose estimation: new benchmark and state of the art analysis. Proc CVPR. 2014; p. 3686–3693.
3. Felzenszwalb P, McAllester D, Ramanan D. A discriminatively trained, multiscale, deformable part model. Proc CVPR. 2008; p. 1–8.
4. Pishchulin L, Andriluka M, Gehler P, et al.   Strong appearance and expressive spatial models for human pose estimation. Proc ICCV. 2013; p. 3487–3494.
5. Toshev A, Szegedy C. Deeppose: human pose estimation via deep neural networks. Proc CVPR. 2014; p. 1653–1660.
6. Wei SE, Ramakrishna V, Kanade T, et al.   Convolutional pose machines. Proc CVPR. 2016; p. 4724–4732.
7. Newell A, Yang K, Deng J. Stacked hourglass networks for human pose estimation. Proc ECCV. 2016; p. 483–499.
8. Masci J, Meier U, Cireşan D, et al. Stacked convolutional auto-encoders for hierarchical feature extraction. Int Conf Artif Neural Netw. 2011; p. 52–59.
9. Oktay O, Ferrante E, Kamnitsas K, et al. Anatomically constrained neural networks (ACNNs): application to cardiac image enhancement and segmentation. IEEE Trans Med Imaging. 2018;37(2):384–395.
10. Tekin B, Katircioglu I, Salzmann M, et al.   Structured prediction of 3D human pose with deep neural networks. arXiv:160505180. 2016;.
11. Cao Z, Simon T, Wei SE, et al. Realtime multi-person 2D pose estimation using part affinity fields. Proc CCVPR. 2017; p. 7291–7299.

Abstract: Does Bone Suppression and Lung Detection Improve Chest Disease Classification?

Ivo M. Baltruschat[1,2,3,4], Leonhard A. Steinmeister[1,3], Harald Ittrich[1], Gerhard Adam[1], Hannes Nickisch[4], Axel Saalbach[4], Jens von Berg[4], Michael Grass[4], Tobias Knopp[1,2]

[1]Department for Diagnostic and Interventional Radiology and Nuclear Medicine, University Medical Center Hamburg-Eppendorf, Germany
[2]Institute for Biomedical Imaging, Hamburg University of Technology, Germany
[3]DAISYLabs, Forschungszentrum Medizintechnik Hamburg, Germany
[4]Philips Research, Hamburg, Germany
i.baltruschat@uke.de

Chest radiography is the most common clinical examination type. To improve the quality of patient care and to reduce workload, researchers started developing methods for automatic pathology classification. In our paper [1], we investigate the effect of advanced image processing techniques – initially developed to support radiologists – on the performance of deep learning techniques.

First, we employ bone suppression, an algorithm to artificially remove the rib cage in chest X-ray images. Secondly, we use automatic lung field detection to crop images to the lung area. Furthermore, we consider the combination of both. For convolutional neural network (CNN) training and evaluation, DICOM images from the Indiana dataset (Open-I [2]), were examined by two expert radiologists and annotated with respect to eight different pathologies. We pretrain our CNN on the largest publicly available X-Ray dataset (ChestX-ray14) and fine-tune it by using the DICOM data.

In a five-times re-sampling scheme, we use receiver operating characteristic (ROC) statistics to evaluate the effect of the pre-processing approaches. Using a convolutional neural network (CNN), optimized for X-ray analysis, we achieve a good performance with respect to all pathologies on average. While, the combination of bone suppression and lung field detection improves slightly the average ROC area from 0.891 ± 0.013 to 0.906 ± 0.012. Contrary, for selected pathologies, a substantial improvement can be reported i.e. for *mass* the area under the ROC curve increased by 9.95%. The ensemble with pre-processed trained models yields the best overall results with 0.912 ± 0.011 AUC on average.

References

1. Baltruschat IM, Steinmeister LA, Ittrich H, et al. When does bone suppression and lung field segmentation improve chest X-ray disease classification? Proc ISBI. 2019;.
2. Demner-Fushman D, Kohli MD, et al. Preparing a collection of radiology examinations for distribution and retrieval. J Am Med Inform Assoc. 2015; p. 304–310.

Towards Automated Reporting and Visualization of Lymph Node Metastases of Lung Cancer

Nico Merten[1,2], Philipp Genseke[3], Bernhard Preim[1,2], Michael C. Kreissl[1,3], Sylvia Saalfeld[1,2]

[1]Research Campus *STIMULATE*
[2]Department of and Graphics, Otto-von-Guericke University
[3]Department of Radiology and Nuclear Medicine, University Hospital Magdeburg
nmerten@isg.cs.uni-magdeburg.de

Abstract. For lung cancer staging, the involvement of lymph nodes in the mediastinum, meaning along the trachea and bronchi, has to be assessed. Depending on the staging results, treatment options include radiation therapy, chemotherapy, or lymph node resection. We present a processing pipeline to automatically generate visualization-supported case reports to simplify reporting and to improve interdisciplinary communication, e.g. between nuclear medicine physicians, radiologists, radiation oncologists, and thoracic surgeons. To evaluate our method, we obtained detailed feedback from the local division of nuclear medicine: Although patient-specific anatomy was not yet considered, the presented approach was deemed to be highly useful from a clinical perspective.

1 Introduction

Worldwide, lung cancer has the highest incidence and mortality rates [1]. Popper [2] reports that depending on the type of lung carcinoma, cancer cells can migrate via blood vessels and cause distant metastases in the brain, bones, and the adrenal glands. Furthermore, they can also migrate via the lymphatic system and cause lymph node metastases.

In addition to the direct assessment of lung carcinomas, e.g. measuring their size and examining their shape, and whether distant metastases are present, the involvement of the mediastinal lymph nodes has to be taken into consideration in order select the right treatment option for the individual patient. Mountain et al. [3] introduced the lymph node map that enables a uniform classification for lung cancer staging by grouping lymph nodes into lymph node stations. Multiple extensions and variations of this classification exist. For example, Rusch et al. [4] decreased the classification granularity by grouping stations into zones.

We present our processing pipeline that automatically generates case reports (Fig. 1). Our approach is related to the tumor therapy manager by Rössling et al. [5], which examines lymph node levels to support treatment planning for cases with head and neck cancer. Additionally, it is also related to the tool of Birr et al. [6], which creates interactive oncology reports for the operation planning of lung tumors. Here, reports are used to document medical findings, and to support

Fig. 1. A detailed overview of the processing pipeline to generate visualization-supported case reports for lymph node metastases for lung cancer staging.

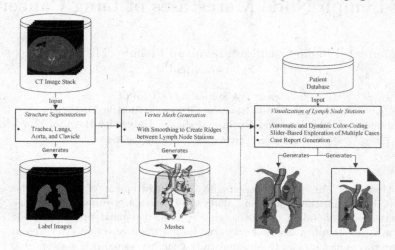

interdisciplinary communication between physicians that make diagnoses and surgeons, e. g. to plan lymph node resections.

2 Materials and methods

The processing pipeline was implemented using MeVisLab 2.8.2 [7] and a detailed overview of the pipeline is depicted in Fig. 1.

2.1 Structure segmentation

For the first step, a computed tomography (CT) scan is used to create initial segmentation masks for important anatomical structures, namely the trachea, both lungs, the aorta, and the clavicle, which are then used to define lymph node

Fig. 2. A focused depiction of the lymph node stations 1L/R, 2L/R, 4L/R, and 5 (Tab. 1).

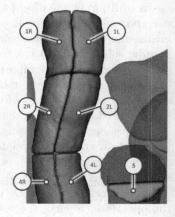

stations. Considered stations, their anatomical location, and how they are geometrically encoded in the resulting visualizations and case reports are compiled in Tab. 1.

To obtain these segmentation masks, a region-growing approach with manual seed point definition was used. This is possible since the radio densities of the aforementioned and nearby structures are different enough to prevent an over-segmentation. However, to create lymph node stations, further processing was necessary (Fig. 1 and 2). For our results, this was done manually: Starting a region-growing in the aortic arch included large parts of the heart, ascending arteries, and the abdominal aorta. Therefore, the aorta's segmentation mask was cut by defining clipping planes to exclude not needed anatomy. Two additional planes were then used to separate station 5 from the aorta.

All other stations are geometrically encoded using the trachea surface mesh. First, to separate the left and right lymph node stations, the segmentation mask was divided in the middle from the top to the carina. This processing step was automated by computing the axis-aligned bounding box for each axial slice and separating the left and right half. The horizontal *cuts* were also done manually using the vertical center of the clavicle (stations 1 and 2) and the upper edge of the aortic arch (stations 2 and 4). In Fig. 2, this is depicted in detail. To separate the stations 10, 11 and 12, the skeletonization method of Selle et al. [8] was used, which is implemented in the DtfSkeletonization module in MeVisLab and resulted in a directed graph with the root node at the top of the trachea. While graph nodes represent airway branching points, graph edges represent the intermediate airways between these points. The airways behind the first bifurcation that divides the trachea into the primary bronchi are assigned to the stations 4L and 4R. Near the hilum, the primary bronchi are divided to separate the stations 4 and 10 from each other. The subsequent edges are assigned to the stations 10 (primary bronchi near hilum to lobar bronchi), stations 11 (lobar bronchi), and stations 12 (subsequent bronchi after lobar bronchi). Finally, to create station 7 at the bifurcation of the trachea, clipping planes were used to create the upside down, saddle-like geometry.

Although no lymph node stations were encoded using the lung parenchyma, it was segmented and visualized to create a visual context for the airways. However, segmenting the lung parenchyma via region-growing results in holes due to a rather high contrast between parenchyma and blood vessels. Therefore, a morphological closing operator was applied to close major holes.

2.2 Vertex mesh generation

For each segmentation mask, a surface mesh is generated using the neighboring cells algorithm of Bade et al. [9], which is implemented in the WEMIsoSurface module in MeVisLab. After mesh generation, the Laplacian mesh smoothing from the WEMSmooth module is applied to all meshes to reduce staircase artifacts and to enhance the visual separation between adjacent lymph node stations by creating ridges along mesh borders.

Table 1. Used lymph node stations, their anatomical location, and how they are geometrically encoded in the visualizations and case reports. The anatomical directions sinistra (left) and dextra (right) are abbreviated with L and R, respectively.

Lymph Node Station	Anatomical Location	Geometric Encoding
1L & 1R	Supraclavicler	Trachea, above clavicler
2L & 2R	Upper Paratracheal	Trachea, above aortic arch
4L & 4R	Lower Paratracheal	Rest of Trachea until Hilum
5	Subaortic	Segment at aortic arch
7	Subcarinal	Trachea, just above carina
10L & 10R	Hilum	Primary bronchi near Hilum
11L & 11R	Interlobar	Near Hilum to lobar bronchi
12L & 12R	Lobar	Subsequent bronchi

3   Results

In the last processing step, the previously created meshes are visualized and color-coded (Fig. 3). To create the color-coding, the user has to import a patient database with one or multiple cases that include the patient name, gender, and the individual metastases findings for each lymph node stations. We used the comma-separated values (CSV) file format, because it can easily be generated and processed. Using the slider at the top right, users can interactively browse through all imported patients and the color-coding is adapted with respect to a patient's individual findings. Additionally, the color-coding for the lymph node stations and anatomic landmarks can be changed. Furthermore, the opacities of the landmarks can be changed interactively. To do that, the order-independent transparencies method of Barta et al. [10] was implemented.

At the bottom right, users can export screenshots of the rendering canvas on the left and automatically generate case reports in the portable document format (PDF) by defining an export path. The internal case report generation pipeline is depicted in Fig. 4: Information about the patient and a screenshot of the currently presented 3D visualization are collected and merged via Python scripting in a LaTeX source file. When all information are present, a PDF case report is generated by invoking a LaTeX program, e. g. `pdflatex`.

4   Discussion

To evaluate our developed method, we received detailed feedback from our local division of nuclear medicine. First, the clinical suitability of the presented geometric encoding of lymph node stations was assessed. On the one hand, it was noted that the current approach introduces a rather high degree of anatomical abstraction, because lymph nodes are separate anatomic structures, but at this moment, they are represented via tracheal mesh geometry (Tab. 1). On the other hand, the current approach was found to be easy to understand as well as to make clinical reports more straightforward to interpret.

Fig. 3. The graphical user interface with the resulting lymph node station visualization. On the right, the color-coding of the stations and anatomic landmarks can be changed. Furthermore, the individual metastases findings are presented in a list. At the bottom right, users can export automatically generated case reports (Fig. 4).

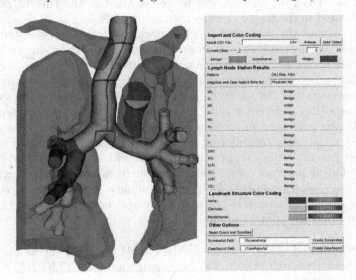

For now, obtaining the initial segmentation masks and separating them into lymph node stations was done manually. Our clinical cooperation partners stated that segmenting patient-specific anatomy for each new case would be too time-consuming in a clinical workflow, however, it was also mentioned that, currently, this was not necessary. Although this is not a favorable condition, it can be argued that always using the already obtained set of segmentation masks and surface meshes can be an advantageous, because the resulting case reports are

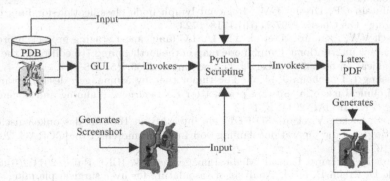

Fig. 4. A detailed overview of the case report generation pipeline. A sreenshot of the 3D visualization is merged with patient information and individual lymph node metastases findings from the patient database (PDB; Fig. 1). All information are collected via Python scripting and are then compiled in a case report via LaTeX.

uniform and comparable to each other. Moreover, this increases the familiarity with visualization-supported reports.

For lung cancer staging, our clinical colleagues use combined PET/CT scans with the F18-FDG radionuclide, which are not used in the current processing pipeline. Related to the tumor therapy manager by Rössling et al. [5], it would be desirable to extend the presented pipeline towards a computer-assisted diagnosis prototype, which enables an automatic derivation of staging suggestions from suspicious metabolic activity of lymph nodes. Currently, users are required to create and maintain an additional database with individual lymph node metastases findings, however, this can easily be done using table processing software. Furthermore, regarding different staging classifications, e. g. by Mountain or Rusch et al. [3, 4], the presented processing pipeline and GUI can easily be adapted, which enables fast software tailoring for different clinical workflows. Finally, we searched for potential clinical applications areas with our cooperation partners: From the clinical point of view, resulting visualization-supported reports are seen as a very helpful addition for interdisciplinary communication scenarios, e. g. tumor board reviews, the planning of lymph node resections, or for the documentation in the context of clinical trials.

Acknowledgement. This work is partly funded by the Federal Ministry of Education and Research within the Forschungscampus *STIMULATE* (Grant Number 13GW0095A).

References

1. Bray F, Ferlay J, et al. Global cancer statistics 2018: GLOBOCAN estimates of incidence and mortality worldwide for 36 cancers in 185 countries. CA Cancer J Clin. 2018;.
2. Popper HH. Progression and metastasis of lung cancer. Cancer Metastasis Rev. 2016;35(1):75–91.
3. Mountain CF, Dresler CM. Regional lymph node classification for lung cancer staging. Dis Chest. 1997;111(6):1718–1723.
4. Rusch VW, Asamura H, et al. The IASLC lung cancer staging project: a proposal for a new international lymph node map in the forthcoming 7th edition of the TNM classification for lung cancer. J Thorac Oncol. 2009;4(5):568–577.
5. Rössling I, Dornheim J, et al. The tumor therapy Mmanager: design, refinement and clinical use of a software product for ENT surgery planning and documentation. Proc IPCAI. 2011; p. 1–12.
6. Birr S, Dicken V, et al. 3D-PDF: ein interaktives Tool für das onkologische Reporting und die Operationsplanung von Lungentumoren. Proc CURAC. 2011; p. 11–16.
7. Ritter F, Boskamp T, et al. Medical image analysis. IEEE Pulse. 2011;2(6):60–70.
8. Selle D, Preim B, et al. Analysis of vasculature for liver surgical planning. IEEE Trans Med Imaging. 2002;21(11):1344–1357.
9. Bade R, Konrad O, et al. Reducing artifacts in surface meshes extracted from binary volumes. J WSCG. 2007;15(1-3):67–74.
10. Barta P, Kovács B, et al. Order independent transparency with per-pixel linked lists. Budap Univ Technol Econ. 2011;.

Workflow Phase Detection in Fluoroscopic Images Using Convolutional Neural Networks

Nikolaus Arbogast[1,2], Tanja Kurzendorfer[1,2], Katharina Breininger[1],
Peter Mountney[3], Daniel Toth[4,5], Srinivas A. Narayan[4], Andreas Maier[1]

[1]Pattern Recognition Lab, Department of Computer Science,
Friedrich-Alexander-Universität Erlangen-Nürnberg, Erlangen, Germany
[2]Siemens Healthcare GmbH, Forchheim, Germany
[3]Siemens Healthineers, Medical Imaging Technologies, Princeton, NJ, USA
[4]School of Biomedical Engineering and Imaging Sciences, King's College London,
London, UK
[5]Siemens Healthineers, Frimley, UK
nikolaus.arbogast@fau.de

Abstract. In image guided interventions, the radiation dose to the patient and personnel can be reduced by positioning the blades of a collimator to block off unnecessary X-rays and restrict the irradiated area to a region of interest. In a certain stage of the operation workflow phase detection can define objects of interest to enable automatic collimation. Workflow phase detection can be beneficial for clinical time management or operating rooms of the future. In this work, we propose a learning-based approach for an automatic classification of three surgical workflow phases. Our data consists of 24 congenital cardiac interventions with a total of 2985 fluoroscopic 2D X-ray images. We compare two different convolutional neural network architectures and investigate their performance regarding each phase. Using a residual network, a class-wise averaged accuracy of 86.14 % was achieved. The predictions of the trained models can then be used for context specific collimation.

1 Introduction

With high precision and real-time imaging, C-arm fluoroscopy is the common modality of choice for image guided interventions to enable minimally invasive procedures [1]. However a major problem is the amount of radiation exposure to the patient and personnel during operations like cardiac resynchronization therapy, endovascular aneurysm repair, or congenital cardiac disease treatment [2]. Especially in latter intervention, the majority of the patients are underage and often have to undergo this process several times, thus, the total dose received can have a severe impact on their health [3].

Therefore, the reduction of unnecessary radiation is one of the most essential tasks in image-guided therapies. Collimation is a widespread approach to block and limit X-rays to a certain field of view without losing important information. One way of adjusting the collimator's blades is to do this manually by the physician himself, which leads to interruptions and slows down the clinical workflow.

Hence, a desired method is the automatic detection of a region of interest that will determine the irradiated area in the given context.

Workflow phase detection can be a useful strategy to define an object of interest and reposition the collimator depending on the specific stage of an operation. A state-of-the-art method to classify a cholescystectomy into seven phases by DiPietro et al. [4] includes the analysis of 15 different sensor signals. An algorithm comparison between a support vector machine, conditional random forest, and hidden Markov model showed that the latter performed best with an accuracy of 81.1 % compared to the given ground truth. On the same task, a learning-based method by Yengera et al. [5] uses videos as input for a network, consisting of a convolutional neural network (CNN) and a long short-term memory. This method achieves an accuracy of 89.6 %.

In this work, we investigate a learning-based approach for workflow phase detection of intra-operative fluoroscopic images from congenital cardiac interventions. This has already been investigated in a similar way by Alhrishy et al. [6] using a network consisting of two convolutional layers. In addition to a more powerful network, we extend their work by taking a closer look at the networks performance for each workflow phase. The aim is to automatically identify three different surgical workflow phases. This information can then be used for context specific collimation.

2   Materials and methods

2.1   Data

Our data consists of 2985 grayscale 2D X-ray images from 24 clinical cases of congenital cardiac disease treatments, which are subdivided into three workflow phases:

0. Navigation phase: insertion of guidewires and catheters, Fig. 1 a);
1. Deployment phase: transport and deployment of a therapeutical device (e.g. stent, ballon, valve), Fig. 1 b);

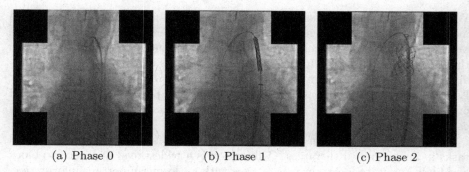

(a) Phase 0   (b) Phase 1   (c) Phase 2

Fig. 1. Example images for the three phases of congenital cardiac treatments. (a) Navigation phase. (b) Pre-deployment phase. (c) Post-deployment phase.

2. Post-deployment phase: inspection of deployed device, Fig. 1 c).

Every frame was labeled manually by a medical expert with two years of experience. The corners of each image are blacked out for anonymization purposes. The aim is to train a network to match its prediction $\hat{y} \in \mathbb{R}^c$ with the ground truth label $y \in \mathbb{R}^c$ for a given image $X \in \mathbb{R}^{h \times w}$, where c corresponds to the number of classes, h to the height and w to the width of an image.

2.2 Preprocessing

Every image goes through several preprocessing steps for data augmentation and more stability during training. Some images showed artifacts in form of white lines caused by the collimator or filter positioning during the intervention. In cases where the lines are located within the irradiated area (Fig. 2 a)), the data is manually excluded from each data set. The remaining artifacts in all sets are cleared with a contour analysis, setting every pixel outside the detected countour of the frame to 0 to prevent the network from learning them as features. An example for this is shown in Fig. 2 b) - d). The training data is then normalized in a range between $[0, 255]$ to prepare it for data augmentation. To stay close to a realistic case of an image guided intervention, only specific kinds of augmentation methods are used: horizontal flip, rotation of $\pm 15°$, translation in x-/y-direction by ± 100 pixels, Gaussian blur, random noise, and random contrast.

After augmentation, the image is again normalized to a range of $[0, 1]$. Due to the memory limitation of the graphics card and time consumption of the training, the images are downscaled from their original resolution of 1024×1024 to 256×256. At this patch size it is still possible for a human to classify every image correctly. It has to be noted that the artifact removal for all sets and the data augmentation of the training set is performed on the original size.

2.3 Data composition

The clinical cases are assigned to training, validation, and testing set such that all sets contain approximately the same relative proportion of each phase. It should

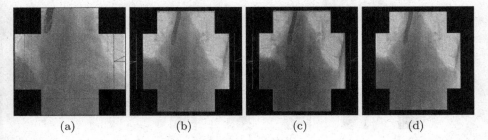

(a)	(b)	(c)	(d)

Fig. 2. Example images with artifacts. (a) Intern: Artifacts inside the irradiated area. (b) Extern: Artifacts outside the irradiated area. (c) Contour analysis: Red contour marking the boundary of the irradiated area. (d) Cleared: Image after artifact removal.

be pointed out that the images from one intervention are not split amongst two or more sets. Without data augmentation of the training set the split between training, validation, and testing is 62.5 %, 16.4 %, and 21.1 %, respectively. The data is highly unbalanced, both with respect to the number of images per intervention and phase. To avoid overfitting, the cases are sampled such that every case is equally represented by the same number of images. Thus, the dependency on interventions with many image sequences is decreased. Furthermore, to tackle the issue of uneven distribution of labels, the training data is also sampled over its classes. This means that during training, we sample images such that all phases are presented to the network with the same frequency.

2.4   CNN architectures

In this paper, two different networks are compared, an adapted AlexNet [7] and a ResNet18 [8]. For both CNNs the 4D input tensor contains grayscale images of the resolution 256×256. All weights of the networks are He initialized as this works best with ReLU activations according to He et al. [9].

The adapted AlexNet differs from its original architecture [7] in respect to the amount of filters applied for convolution, kernel size of the first layer, number of neurons in the fully connected layer, and batch normalization after every convolutional layer instead of local response normalization after first and second layer. The first layer applies $f_{1A} = f_A$ initial filters, with $f_A \in \{8, 16, 32, 64\}$. The number of neurons in the first two fully connected layers are $d_{1/2} = d$, with $d \in \{16, 32, 64\}$, and are regularized with a dropout rate of 50 %. The model for the adapted AlexNet is visualized in Fig. 3.

The structure of the ResNet18 proposed in this work refers to its original architecture introduced by He et al. [8], however, with some minor differences regarding the kernel size of the initial convolution and the strides throughout the network. The adapted ResNet18 applies $f_{1R} = f_R$ filters for the first convolutional layer with kernel size 3×3 and stride of 2, with $f_R \in \{64, 128\}$. The output is max-pooled with a 3×3 kernel and stride of 2 before being processed by the first residual building block. Every block convolves with a stride of 1, with

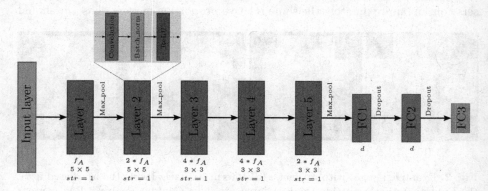

Fig. 3. Architecture of adapted AlexNet.

Table 1. Recall for each phase and balanced accuracy of every set for AlexNet and ResNet18. The model with the best balanced accuracy for validation set is shown.

Network	Set	Phase 0	Phase 1	Phase 2	Bal. acc.
	Training	96.16%	99.95%	99.61%	98.58%
AlexNet	Validation	96.64%	35.29%	65.66%	65.86%
	Testing	86.40%	80.49%	60.90%	75.93%
	Training	95.84%	100.0%	98.80%	98.21%
ResNet18	Validation	89.36%	91.18%	71.72%	84.08%
	Testing	83.77%	92.68%	81.96%	86.14%

the exception of the very first convolution of the initial building block, where the stride is 2. At the end of each block the amount of filters is doubled. The last layer of both networks is a fully connected layer that maps its input to the number of classes and applies a softmax activation, representing the probabilities for every image to belong to the respective phase. Both networks were trained by optimizing the cross entropy function loss using the ADAM optimizer.

3   Results

The training is performed with a grid search over several parameters. For AlexNet, we vary the number of initial filters, the learning rate, the number of fully connected neurons, and the batch size. For each setting, we train the network for 100 epochs. For ResNet18, the parameters are restricted to the number of filters in the first layer and learning rate with 50 epochs for every combination. To take the uneven distribution of phases in validation and test set into account, we evaluate the performance of the networks using balanced accuracy. We select the trained network that achieves the highest balanced accuracy on the validation set. The performance of AlexNet and ResNet18 is summarized in Tab. 1 showing the accuracy for every phase and the overall balanced accuracy, respectively.

4   Discussion

The evaluation shows that ResNet18 achieved better classification results when compared to the adapted AlexNet. However, both networks are overfitting on the training set, and curiously perform less accurate for the validation set than for the testing set. The latter can be explained by fact that the validation set contains several inconclusive images, which the models are not trained for, e.g. double or hardly visible stents. ResNet18 seems to be able to deal with these special images better than AlexNet. AlexNet especially misclassified images depicting stent markers in phase 1, which are frequently represented in the validation, but not in the testing set. In general, the investigated data set is highly diverse which makes workflow phase classification a very challenging task. In addition to high variations in image quality, we see a number of structures in the images that are not directly related to the workflow phase, such as contrast agent injections or transesophageal echoprobes. A larger data set that better represents the variety of possible images will likely help with misclassifications in these cases.

In this work, we compared two CNN architectures to classify congenital cardiac interventions into three workflow phases. Our evaluation showed that ResNet18 performed better than the adapted AlexNet when confronted with the same task. Thus, it can be hypothesized that increasing network depth results in a higher accuracy. We propose that our model for workflow phase detection can be combined with device detection approaches like intraoperative stent segmentation [10] or can be adapted for other image guided interventions to benefit not only automatic collimation, but also clinical time management or operating rooms of the future. This investigation presents promising first steps towards workflow phase classification. To allow for intraoperative use, the robustness of the classification has to be further improved. Further research could examine different CNN architectures with other training data and regularization methods to improve the performance and stability of this strategy.

Disclaimer: The methods and information presented here are based on research and are not commercially available.

References

1. Bicknell C. Occupational radiation exposure and the vascular interventionalist. Eur J Vasc Endovasc Surg. 2013;46(4):431.
2. Giordano BD, Baumhauer JF, Morgan TL, et al. Patient and surgeon radiation exposure: comparison of standard and mini-C-arm fluoroscopy. J Bone Joint Surg Am. 2009;91(2):297–304.
3. Johnson JN, Hornik CP, Li JS, et al. Cumulative radiation exposure and cancer risk estimation in children with heart disease. Circ. 2014;130(2):161–167.
4. DiPietro R, Stauder R, Kayis E, et al. Automated surgical-phase recognition using rapidly-deployable sensors. Proc MICCAI Workshop M2CAI. 2015;.
5. Twinanda AP, Yengera G, Mutter D, et al. RSDNet: learning to predict remaining surgery duration from laparoscopic videos without manual annotations. arXiv:180203243. 2018;.
6. Alhrishy M, Toth D, Narayan SA, et al. A machine learning framework for context specific collimation and workflow phase detection. Comput Methods Biomech Biomed Engin. 2018;.
7. Krizhevsky A, Sutskever I, Hinton GE. ImageNet classification with deep convolutional neural networks. Adv Neural Inf Process Syst. 2012; p. 1097–1105.
8. He K, Zhang X, Ren S, et al. Deep residual learning for image recognition. Proc CVPR. 2016; p. 770–778.
9. He K, Zhang X, Ren S, et al. Delving deep into rectifiers: surpassing human-level performance on imagenet classification. Proc ICCV. 2015; p. 1026–1034.
10. Breininger K, Albarqouni S, Kurzendorfer T, et al. Intraoperative stent segmentation in X-ray fluoroscopy for endovascular aortic repair. Int J Comput Assist Radiol Surg. 2018;13(8).

Abstract: Interpretable Explanations of Black Box Classifiers Applied on Medical Images by Meaningful Perturbations Using Variational Autoencoders

Hristina Uzunova, Jan Ehrhardt, Timo Kepp, Heinz Handels

Institut für Medizinische Informatik, Universität zu Lübeck
uzunova@imi.uni-luebeck.de

The growing popularity of black box machine learning methods for medical image analysis makes their interpretability to a crucial task. To make a system, e.g. a trained neural network, trustworthy for a clinician, it needs to be able to explain its decisions and predictions. In our work we tackle the problem of explaining the predictions of medical image classifiers, trained to differentiate between different types of pathologies and healthy tissue [1].

There is a variety of neural network explanation methods, such as gradCAMs and guided backpropagation that directly use the learned network weights to deduct the most important image features. However, such methods are based on heuristics and depend on the network architecture. Another intuitive solution to determine which regions of an image influence the trained classifier is to find out whether the classifier changes its prediction when those regions are deleted. This idea is model-agnostic and can be formulated as an explicit minimization problem and thus efficiently implemented on the GPU. However, the meaning of "deletion"of image regions, in our case pathologies in medical images, is not defined. Usually, deleting image regions would be based on image perturbations, but intuitive solutions like replacing the values by zeros or blurring regions, may not have the desired effect for medical applications.

We contribute by defining the deletion of suspicious regions, as the replacement by their healthy looking equivalent generated using a variational autoencoder (VAE). We train the VAE on healthy images only and thus expect it to only be able to reconstruct healthy looking images in test phase even if the input contains pathologies. This healthy reconstruction is then used to perturb the pathological regions. In our tests on retinal OCTs with age-related macular degeneration and brain MRI images with lesions, we show that this perturbation method outperforms other perturbation techniques and shows more robust results compared to heuristic methods.

References

1. Uzunova H, Ehrhardt J, Kepp T, et al. Interpretable explanations of black box classifiers applied on medical images by meaningful perturbations using variational autoencoders. Proc SPIE. 2019;Accepted.

Abstract: Deep Transfer Learning for Aortic Root Dilation Identification in 3D Ultrasound Images

Jannis Hagenah[1], Mattias Heinrich[2], Floris Ernst[1]

[1]Institut für Robotik und Kognitive Systeme, Universität zu Lübeck
[2]Institut für Medizinische Informatik, Universität zu Lübeck
hagenah@rob.uni-luebeck.de

Valve-sparing aortic root reconstruction presents an alternative to valve replacement. However, choosing the optimal prosthesis size for the individual patient is a critical task during surgery. To assist the surgeons in their decision making, a pre-operative surgery planning tool based on 3D ultrasound data has been proposed. One step in the workflow is the automatic discrimination of healthy and pathologically dilated aortic roots. Up to date, hand-crafted features were extracted from the images for this purpose of training a classifier. A study showed the limited classification accuracy of this method, indicating that feature learning would present a promising alternative. However, training deep neural networks requires large datasets.

In this work, we propose transfer learning to use image features derived by deep neural networks on the available very small data sets [1]. For this purpose, we used the pretrained deep neural network VGG16. We used the activation of the last convolutional layer as extracted features of the input image.

To simplify the problem, we manually identified two prominent horizontal slices through the ultrasound volume: The coaptation plane and the commissure plane. We propagated both images through the network and stitched the resulting features together to describe one aortic root sample. We did this for the whole data set of 48 images (24 healthy, 24 dilated). On the resulting dataset, we trained a Random Forest classifier (400 trees) and evaluated the classification accuracy using 10-fold cross validation.

Using the transferred deep features we could reach a classification accuracy of 84 %, which clearly outperformed the hand-crafted features (71 % accuracy). Adding the hand-crafted features to the transferred ones did not increase the accuracy (83 %) Hence, all of the information contained in the hand-crafted features can be provided using transfer learning. Even though the VGG16 network was trained on RGB photos and different classification tasks, the learned feaures are still relevant for ultrasound image analysis of aortic root pathology identification. Hence, transfer learning makes deep learning possible even on very small ultrasound data sets.

References

1. Hagenah J, Mattias H, Floris E. Deep transfer learning for aortic root dilation identification in 3D ultrasound images. Curr Dir Biomed Eng. 2018;4.1:71–74.

Abstract: Leveraging Web Data for Skin Lesion Classification

Fernando Navarro[1], Sailesh Conjeti[2], Federico Tombari[1], Nassir Navab[1,3]

[1]Computer Aided Medical Procedures, Technische Universität München, Germany
[2] Deutsches Zentrum für Neurodegenerative Erkrankungen (DZNE), Bonn, Germany
[3]Computer Aided Medical Procedures, Johns Hopkins University, USA
fernando.navarro@tum.de

The success of deep learning is mainly based on the assumption that for the given application, there is access to a large amount of annotated data. In medical imaging applications, having access to a big-well-annotated data-set is restrictive, time-consuming and costly to obtain. Although diverse techniques as data augmentation can be leveraged to increase the size and variability within the data-set, the representativeness of the training set is still limited by the number of available samples. Furthermore, a small-size and well-annotated data-set can not guarantee the generalizability to unseen samples.

As a consequence for the aforementioned problem, we have proposed in [1] to utilize the vast amount of free available data from the web to alleviate the need of a large-well-annotated data-set in the so-called Webly Supervised Learning methodology presented in [2]. Harvesting images from the web presents the opportunity to increase the variability and heterogeneity of the training set at the cost of label noise. These label noises include cross-domain: retrieved images opposite to the dermatology domain and cross-category: retrieved images visually similar to the query image yet belonging to a different class. To overcome the first type of noise we have proposed a search by image technique to increase the search specificity and retrieve only images visually similar to the query. The second type of noise is reduced by modeling the noise in the data-set with a class-transition matrix, estimated from the web-retrieved images as proposed in [3]. To the best of our knowledge, our work has been the first applying webly supervised learning in medical imaging. To validate our methodology, we have tested our system in the context of ten-class fine-grained skin lesion classification. Our results show that the proposed methodology increase the overall classification accuracy from 71.25 % to 80.53 % due to the web-supervision.

References

1. Navarro F, Conjeti S, Tombari F, et al. Webly supervised learning for skin lesion classification. Proc MICCAI. 2018; p. 398–406.
2. Chen X, Gupta A. Webly supervised learning of convolutional networks. Proc CVPR. 2015; p. 1431–1439.
3. Patrini G, Rozza A, Menon AK, et al. Making deep neural networks robust to label noise: a loss correction approach. Proc CVPR. 2017; p. 2233–2241.

Machbarkeitsstudie zur CNN-basierten Identifikation und TICI-Klassifizierung zerebraler ischämischer Infarkte in DSA-Daten

Maximilian Nielsen[1], Moritz Waldmann[2], Andreas Frölich[2], Jens Fiehler[2], René Werner[1]

[1]Institut für Computational Neuroscience, Universitätsklinikum Hamburg-Eppendorf
[2]Klinik und Poliklinik für Neuroradiologische Diagnostik und Intervention, Universitätsklinikum Hamburg-Eppendorf
maximilian.nielsen@tuhh.de

Kurzfassung. Ziel der vorliegenden Machbarkeitsstudie ist es, zu prüfen, ob eine bildbasierte TICI-Klassifikation von ischämischen Infarkten mittels aktueller Machine Learning-Methoden automatisiert werden kann. Der TICI-Score (Thrombolysis in Cerebral Infarction) beschreibt den lokalen Befund am Infarktort und nachgeschaltete Hirndurchblutung nach endovaskulärer Behandlung. Die zugrunde liegenden Bilddaten sind (2D+t)-Bildserien aus zwei orthogonalen Ansichten (lateral und anterior-posterior), die mittels digitaler Subtraktionsangiographie (DSA) aufgenommen wurden. Basierend auf 698 Bildsequenzen wurde untersucht, inwieweit mittels CNN (Convolutional Neural Network) anhand von entweder aus den Zeitserien abgeleiteten Minimum Intensity Projection-Daten oder unter expliziter Berücksichtigung der Zeitserieninformation eine korrekte Klassifikation erfolgt. Im Zuge dessen wurden im Hinblick auf die zu erwartende Komplexität verschiedene Konfigurationen/Kombinationen von Verschlussort und TICI-Score definiert und analysiert. Die Ergebnisse zeigen, dass es möglich ist, TICI-Score und Verschlussort von ischämischen Infarkten zumindest bei stark unterschiedlichen TICI-Scores verlässlich automatisiert zu bestimmen; die Machbarkeit wird belegt.

1 Einleitung

Digitale Subtraktionsangiographie (DSA) ist derzeit die klinisch etablierte Bildmodalität zur Diagnose von zerebralen ischämischen Schlaganfällen. Bei den resultierenden Datensätzen handelt es sich um 2D-Bilddaten in zeitlicher Abfolge, d.h. (2D+t)-Bilddaten. Die Diagnose selbst erfolgt über sowie die Bestimmung des Schweregrads des Infarkts. Typische Verschlusslokalisationen finden sich im Bereich des Carotis-T (T-Infarkt) und der Arteria cerebri media (M1-Infarkt). Der Schweregrad des Infarkts resultiert aus der residuellen Menge des durch den Verschluss strömenden Blutes bzw. der Durchblutung nachgeschalteter Hirnregionen. Das Ergebnis nach endovaskulärer Behandlung wird gemäß TICI-Score (Thrombolysis in Cerebral Infarction) beurteilt [1]. Der Score reicht von 0 bis 3, wobei Grad 2 weiter in 2a und 2b unterteilt wird. Ein TICI-Score 0 bedeutet, dass keine stattfindet; Grad 3 beschreibt eine vollständige (Abb. 1; TICI-Grad 1: kaum Perfusion, Grad 2a: teilweise Perfusion; Grad 2b: komplette bei jedoch unvollständigem Stromgebiet).

Aktuell erfolgt die TICI-Klassifizierung der Infarkte durch den behandelnden Radiologen. Die visuelle Einschätzung unterliegt jedoch einer starken Observervariabilität [2] und ist insbesondere im Hinblick auf größere Studien mit einem nicht vertretbaren Zeitaufwand verbunden. Folglich zielt die vorliegende Arbeit mittelfristig auf die Automatisierung von Identifikation, Lokalisierung und TICI-Klassifizierung von zerebralen ischämischen Infarkten ab. Verwandte Arbeiten beschäftigen sich momentan im Wesentlichen mit der Vorhersage des Outcomes für den Patienten [3] oder der Bestimmung des Infarktvolumens [4]. Die automatisierte Bestimmung des TICI-Scores, insbesondere unter Verwendung von klinischen DSA-Bilddaten, ist unseres Wissens nach bislang nicht näher betrachtet worden; die vorliegende Arbeit repräsentiert entsprechend einen ersten diesbezüglichen Ansatz. Aufgrund des großen Erfolgs von Convolutional Neural Networks (CNNs) zur Klassifikation von Bilddaten wird auf eine (einfache) CNN-Architektur zur TICI-Klassifizierung zurückgegriffen.

2 Material und Methoden

2.1 Verwendete Bilddaten

Für jeden Patienten lagen je ein prä- und ein postinterventionell aufgezeichneter Datensatz mit jeweils simultan aufgezeichneten DSA-Datensätzen in lateraler und anterior-posteriorer Ansicht vor (isotrope räumliche 0,19 mm; zeitliche 0,33 s; je Sequenz zwischen 6 und 24 Frames). Visuelle Lokalisierung und TICI-Klassifizierung erfolgte durch einen klinischen Experten; jeweilige Angaben dienten als Ground Truth. Die Verteilung der verfügbaren Daten gemäß Infarktlokalisierung und TICI-Score ist Tab. 1 zu entnehmen.

2.2 Bilddatenvorverarbeitung

Als erster Schritt der DSA-Datenvorverarbeitung wurden die aufgabenspezifisch relevanten Strukturen (d.h. kontrastmitteltragende Stukturen) schwellwertbasiert vorverarbeitet: Intensitätswerte oberhalb des Schwellwerts wurden mittels

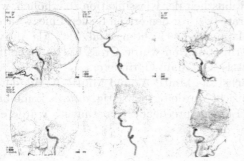

Abb. 1. Beispieldaten (obere Reihe: laterale Ansicht; untere Reihe = anterior-posteriore Ansicht) für einen T-Verschluss mit TICI-Score 0 (links), einen M1-Verschluss mit Score 0 (Mitte) sowie einen Datensatz mit Score 3 (rechts). Bei den Bildern handelt es sich um Minimum Intensity Projecions (minIP) entlang der Zeitachse.

Tabelle 1. Datensatzübersicht, aufgeschlüsselt nach Ort des Infarktes und korrespondierendem TICI-Score. Werte in Klammern bedeuten, dass die korrespondierenden Klassen aufgrund der geringen Fallzahl nicht weiter betrachtet wurden.

Ort	TICI 0	TICI 1	TICI 2a	TICI 2b	TICI 3	gesamt
M1	256	46	101	113	–	525
T	58	(6)	(13)	(18)	–	58
gesamt	323	46	101	113	115	698

des Schwellwertes überschrieben und der resultierende Dynamikbereich auf das Intervall [0;1] skaliert. Der Schwellwert wurde anhand ausgewählter Datensätze heuristisch optimiert und auf alle anderen Daten übertragen. Hierdurch wurde z.B. der Einfluss von Bildartefakten reduziert.

Zur effizienteren Verarbeitung der Daten mittels CNN wurden aus jeder der resultierenden (2D+t)-Bildserien drei Datensätze abgeleitet: eine Minimum Intensity Projection (MinIP) entlang der zeitlichen Achse, die sämtliche verfügbaren Frames des Patienten umfasst (MinIP-A); eine zeitliche MinIP, die auf Basis von lediglich den neun Frames berechnet wurde, die den Zeitpunkt umschließen, der die geringste Intensität aufweist (MinIP-9F; integriert über den gesamten Bildbereich); ein (2D+t)-Datensatz, der vorgenannte neun Frames enthält (3DC-9F). Für den Fall, dass eine Serie weniger als 9 Bilder enthält, wurden erster und letzter Frame repliziert. Eine zeitliche MinIP hat den Effekt, dass für jedes Voxel der Intensitätswert zum Zeitpunkt der lokal maximalen Durchblutung (bzw. der maximalen Kontrastmittelkonzentration) abgebildet wird und somit der Infarktbereich bzw. nicht- oder schlechter durchblutete Bereiche hell im Bild erscheinen. Die vorgenannte Einschränkung auf neun Frames (siehe MinIP-9F und 3DC-9F) soll Unsicherheiten z.B. durch retrograde reduzieren.

Jeweilige Bilddaten wurden von einer ursprünglichen Größe von 1024 × 1024 Pixel auf eine Größe von 512 × 512 Pixel reduziert.

2.3   CNN-Architektur und Datenverarbeitung

Die Architektur des zur Klassifikation verwendeten CNNs orientierte sich an erfolgreichen Designs des ResNets [5]. Das verwendete Netzwerk bestand aus neun 2D-Convolutional- und fünf 2D-Maxpooling-Schichten; zur Klassifikation dienten drei weitere Linear-Layer. Um die Robustheit der Klassifikation zu erhöhen, wurden zudem Dropoutlayer (Dropoutrate 0,5) vor den ersten beiden Linear-Layern und Batchnormalisierung vor den Maxpooling-Schichten genutzt [6]. Als Aktivierungsfunktion diente ReLU; als Verlustfunktion wurde Cross Entropy genutzt; Parameteroptimierung erfolgte mittels des Adam-Optimierers.

Als CNN-Eingabe dienten zunächst die MinIP-A- und MinIP-9F-Bilddaten. Laterale und anterior-posteriore Ansicht wurden gleichzeitig, d.h. als kombinierte zweikanalige Eingabe, genutzt. Für entsprechende Experimente wurde eine Lernrate von 0,001 genutzt.

Zur Verarbeitung der 3DC-9F wurde ebenfalls das genannte CNN-Design verwendet (Lernrate 0,0025); dem 2D-CNN wurde jedoch eine 3D-Convolution- und eine Maxpooling-Schicht vorgeschaltet.

2.4 Experimente und Auswertestrategie

Um die Machbarkeit der CNN-basierten TICI-Score-Bestimmung zu untersuchen und Herausforderungen zu identifizieren, wurden Experimente zu verschiedenen Kombinationen von Infarkt-Schweregrad und - durchgeführt.

Paarweise Differenzierung von TICI-Scores Beginnend mit der visuell einfachen Unterscheidung von TICI 0- und TICI 3-Daten wurde die Schwierigkeit sukzessive erhöht und insbesondere die Differenzierung „benachbarter" TICI-Scores als individuelle 2-Klassenprobleme betrachtet (TICI 0 vs. TICI 1, TICI 1 vs. TICI 2a, etc.). Diese Substudie wurde unter Verwendung der Bilddaten mit M1-Verschluss durchgeführt.

Differenzierung aller TICI-Scores Basierend auf den M1-Verschlussdaten wurde in der nächsten Substudie die Differenzierung sämtlicher TICI-Scores anhand der vorgenannten M1-Verschlussbilddaten evaluiert.

Differenzierung nach Infarktlokalisation Abschließend wurde die Differenzierung von M1-TICI 0- und T-TICI 0-Verschlussdaten (2-Klassenproblem) sowie von M1-TICI 0-, T-TICI 0- und TICI 3-Daten (3-Klassenproblem) untersucht. Auf eine Betrachtung der weiteren T-Verschlussdaten wurde aufgrund der geringen Anzahl verfügbarer Daten verzichtet.

Alle Experimente wurden jeweils auf Basis der MinIP-A-, MinIP-9F- und 3DC-9F-Daten und als 5-fache Keuzvalidierung durchgeführt; die Gößte der Klassifizierung wurde mittels Korrektklassifikationsrate quantifiziert. Um eine balancierte Klassenverteilung während des Trainings zu gewährleisten, erfolgte ein Oversampling der unterrepäsentierten Klassen.

3 Ergebnisse

Die Ergebnisse sind für die betrachteten Kombinationen von Infarktort und TICI-Score in Tab. 2 zusammengefasst; die verwendeten Testdatensätze waren hinsichtlich der Klassenbesetzung balanciert.

3.1 Paarweise Differenzierung von TICI-Scores

Die Unterscheidung von M1-TICI 0-Infarkten und infarktfreien (TICI 3) Bildern zeigen erwartungsgemäß mit im Schnitt 89% und weitestgehend unabhängig von dem betrachteten Bildformat (MinIP-A, MinIP-F9, 3DC-9F) die höchsten

Tabelle 2. Korrektklassifikationsraten der durchgeführten Experimente zur paarweisen Differenzierung von TICI-Scores für M1-Verschlussdaten. (Angabe: Mittelwert [minimale; maximale Rate] der verschiedenen Durchläufe der Kreuzvalidierung).

Betrachtete Scores	MinIP-A	MinIP-9F	3DC-9F
TICI 0 vs. TICI T3	0,89 [0,87; 0,92]	0,89 [0,82; 0,92]	0,89 [0,88; 0,90]
TICI 0 vs. TICI 1	0,73 [0,69; 0,82]	0,79 [0,69; 0,84]	0,81 [0,74; 0,88]
TICI 1 vs. TICI 2a	0,61 [0,36; 0,73]	0,68 [0,55; 0,77]	0,73 [0,65; 0,75]
TICI 2a vs. TICI 2b	0,66 [0,52; 0,88]	0,69 [0,56; 0,84]	0,74 [0,72; 0,78]
TICI 2b vs. TICI 3	0,50 [0,43; 0,56]	0,51 [0,45; 0,58]	0,50 [0,39; 0,60]
Alle	0,55 [0,45; 0,60]	0,56 [0,51; 0,61]	0,55 [0,49; 0,58]

Tabelle 3. Ergebnisse der Experimente zur gleichzeitigen Differenzierung aller TICI-Scores, basierend auf M1-Infarkten (Darstellung: Mittelwert sowie minimale und maximale Korrektklassifikationsraten der Durchläufe der Kreuzvalidierung).

	TICI 0	TICI 1	TICI 2a	TICI 2b	TICI 3
A	0,71 [0,57;0,87]	0,50 [0,19;0,77]	0,59 [0,40;0,79]	0,49 [0,35;0,71]	0,45 [0,38;0,52]
B	0,77 [0,67; 0,84]	0,49 [0,34;0,58]	0,57 [0,42;0,65]	0,50 [0,37;0,61]	0,49 [0,33;0,66]
C	0,65 [0,50;0,73]	0,59 [0,42;0,67]	0,56 [0,48;0,71]	0,49 [0,44;0,56]	0,44 [0,40;0,53]

Korrektheitsraten. Die Differenzierung von M1-Infarkten mit den TICI-Scores 0/1, 1/2a, 2a/2b, zeigen niedrigere Korrektheitswerte, die jeweils jedoch deutlich oberhalb einer zufallsbasierten Klassifikation liegen. Letzteres gilt nicht mehr für die Differenzierung von TICI-Scores 2b und 3.

3.2 Differenzierung aller TICI-Scores

Alle getesteten CNN-Ansätze führten zu einer Gesamtkorrektklassifikationsrate von etwa 55%. Jeweilige Raten für die einzelnen Klassen sind in Tab. 3 aufgeführt. Wie aufgrund o.g. Resultate zu erwarten, ist auch bei gleichzeitiger Betrachtung aller Klassen die Klassifikation von TICI 0-Infarkten am verlässlichsten. Bei detaillierten Betrachtung der Ergebnisse ist festzustellen, dass ein Großteil der Fehlklassifikation der TICI 1-Infarkte auf TICI-Scores 0 und 2a entfallen. Gleiches gilt im Wesentlichen für die anderen TICI-Scores; insgesamt werden > 90% der Daten entweder dem korrekten oder einem direkt „benachbarten" Score zugeordnet.

3.3 Differenzierung nach Infarktlokalisation

Die Unterscheidung von T- und M1-Infarkten mit TICI-Score 0 gelingt mit vergleichsweise hoher Genauigkeit (Korrektheitsraten > 85% für alle Bildformate). Das korrespondierende Dreiklassenproblem führt zu ähnlichen Werten (Korrektklassifikationsraten von im Schnitt etwa 85% für alle Bildformate).

4   Diskussion

Ziel der vorliegenden Arbeit war es, zu beurteilen, ob es möglich ist, Ort und Schweregrad von zerebralen ischämischen Infarkten automatisiert anhand von DSA-Daten mittels Convolutional Neural Networks (CNNs) zu bestimmen.

Die Resultate zeigen, dass Fälle mit niedrigem TICI-Score und verschiedener Infarktlokalisation vergleichsweise gut von TICI 3-Daten differenziert werden können. Insbesondere die Differenzierung von TICI 2b und TICI 3 stellt hingegen eine Herausforderung dar (Korrektheitsraten bei 2-Klassenproblem nicht von Zufallszuordnung zu unterscheiden). Bei Interpretation der genannten Korrektklassifikationsraten sollte jedoch auf das grundlegende Problem einer in Teilen subjektiven, literaturübergreifend nicht einheitlichen Definition von TICI-Scores berücksichtigt werden [7]. Neben weiterer methodischer Entwicklung wird entsprechend in Fortführung der begonnenen Arbeiten eine systematische Evaluation von Intra- und Interratervariabilitäten bei TICI-Scorezuweisung erfolgen.

Der Vergleich der Resultate für MinIP-A, MinIP-9F und 3DC-9F zeigt im Schnitt leicht bessere Korrektheitsraten für 3DC-9F. Diese gehen jedoch aufgrund der Verwendung der 3D-Convolution-Schicht einher mit einem deutlich erhöhten Zeitaufwand für das Training des Netzwerks.

Insgesamt ist das Gesamtergebnis dieser ersten Studie zur automatisierten TICI-Klassifizierung in klinischen DSA-Daten als ermutigend zu beurteilen; die prinzipielle Machbarkeit der automatisierten Bestimmung des TICI-Scores und des Ortes von ischämischen zerebralen Infarktes wurde in großen Teilen belegt und motiviert weitergehende Untersuchungen.

Danksagung. Gefördert durch das Forschungszentrum Medizintechnik Hamburg (02fmthh2017).

Literaturverzeichnis

1. Higashida RT, Furlan AJ, et al. Trial design and reporting standards for intra-arterial cerebral thrombolysis for acute ischemic stroke. Stroke. 2003;34:e109–37.
2. Drewer-Gutland F, Kemmling A, Ligges S, et al. CTP-based tissue outcome: promising tool to prove the beneficial effect of mechanical recanalization in acute ischemic stroke. RoFo. 2015;187:459–66.
3. Asadi H, Dowling R, Yan B, et al. Machine learning for outcome prediction of acute ischemic stroke post intra-arterial therapy. PLoS ONE. 2014;9:e88225.
4. McKinley R, Häni L, Gralla J, et al. Fully automated stroke tissue estimation using random forest classifiers (FASTER). J Cereb Blood Flow Metab. 2016;37:2728–41.
5. He K, Zhang X, Ren S, et al. Deep residual learning for image recognition. Proc CVPR. 2016; p. 770–778.
6. Hinton GE, Srivastava N, Krizhevsky A, et al. Improving neural networks by preventing co-adaptation of feature detectors. CoRR. 2012;abs/1207.0580. Available from: http://arxiv.org/abs/1207.0580.
7. Fugate JE, Klunder AM, Kallmes DF. What is meant by "TICI"? AJNR Am J Neuroradiol. 2013;34:1792–7.

Image-Based Detection of MRI Hardware Failures

Bhavya Jain[1], Nadine Kuhnert[1,2], André deOliveira[1], Andreas Maier[2]

[1]Siemens Healthineers, Erlangen
[2]Fakultät für Pattern Recognition, FAU Erlangen-Nürnberg
bhavya.jain@fau.de

Abstract. Currently in Magnetic Resonance Imaging (MRI) systems, most hardware failures are only detected after a component has stopped functioning properly. In many cases, this results in a downtime of the system. Moreover, sometimes defective parts are not identified correctly, which may result in more parts than necessary being replaced, causing extra costs. Often in MRI systems, hardware related problems have an impact on image quality. Given an imaging protocol and a well-functioning MRI system, certain image quality metrics have a normal range in a given patient population. Thus, such metrics will present a measurable behavior change in case of a hardware problem. We identified such simple and powerful metrics for signal-to-noise ratio, noise variance and symmetry in images for hardware failures related to Shimming and Local RF coils in this work. To be able to calculate these metrics with every MRI image during the clinical workflow, another constraint is the computation time. With the performance of quality metrics on machine learning algorithms and computation time, we are able to identify the failing MRI components with an accuracy of up to 0.96 AUROC.

1 Introduction

In Magnetic Resonance Imaging (MRI) systems, several factors can cause failures such as, installation environment and equipment usage. If the failure cause is misidentified, the downtime is prolonged causing further inconvenience. Currently, the failure causes are investigated manually by the customer service engineer on site which requires time, leading to further unavailability for measurements. In literature, Kuhnert et al. [1] demonstrate that meta information from MRI log files is already sufficient to estimate imaged body part without looking at the image. Lorch et al. in, [2] present a method to detect motion artifact in MRI data based on image-derived features. Peltonen et al. in, [3] propose to use the patient 3D FLAIR volumes to assess the image quality as a replacement of specialized phantom Quality Assessment (QA) procedures. While the need of QA procedures in medical equipment is highly emphasized, much less investigation on detecting the concrete hardware failures with image quality is carried out. In this work, we present a method to detect failing hardware components with the help of image quality metrics.

1.1   Hardware failures

Inhomogeneous magnetic field To acquire the distortion-free images that also correctly represent the imaged body part, the homogeneity in static magnetic field B_0 is of crucial importance. There are many reasons such as objects in MRI system's immediate environment and the patient himself, can have an impact on the magnetic field's homogeneity. Shimming is the technique used to correct such inhomogeneities in the magnetic field. Using ferromagnetic pellets inside of the magnet bore, static homogeneity can be achieved. This technique is known as passive shimming. To correct for the patient specific inhomogeneity in B_0, specialized shimming coils are used. Through these shimming coils current is passed to generate a corrective magnetic field. This technique is known as active shimming. The current that needs to pass through the shimming coil in each direction is calculated using the spherical harmonic (SH) function. If there is a defect in the shimming coil, the homogeneity in the magnetic field could be disturbed due to incorrect shimming. The images generated in such inhomogeneous magnetic fields may contain artifacts and distortions reducing its diagnostic value. We look into symmetry as an image quality metric for detecting failures related to shimming coil.

Defective RF coils Wear and tear is a very common failure mode of the local RF coils. Over the time, due to usage or the intensity of the measurement protocols, the failure modes such as failing noise amplifiers, frequency side bands or fuses can occur, allowing more noise in the received signal and thus in the reconstructed image. Such a gradual change in image quality is difficult to detect unless certain quality analysis measures are being taken at regular interval of time. In this work, we present a method to constantly analyze the quality metrics such as noise and signal-to-noise ratio to detect failures before they can cause an unavailability of the MRI system.

2   Materials and methods

In this section, we present the mathematical models used for calculating image quality metrics related to the hardware failures and the methods used to evaluate these image quality metrics for its correlation with the hardware failures and computation time.

2.1   Image quality metrics

We implemented mathematical models ranging from low to high in their complexity to test if high complexity also leads to higher correlation with hardware failure and thus higher rate of failure detection.

The human body has an extrinsic bilateral symmetry in most cases. The brain however also has an intrinsic left-right bilateral symmetry. If the magnetic filed homogeneity is disturbed, the inherent structural or morphological symmetry

Table 1. The abbreviations and explanation of all the mathematical models implemented to calculate image quality metrics.

Abrv.	Implemented quality metric
Symmetry	
CLR	Cross-correlation between left and right half
CAB	Cross-correlation between upper and lower half
PLR	Phase only correlation between left and right half
PAB	Phase only correlation between upper and lower half
MLR	Mutual information between left and right half
MAB	Mutual information between upper and lower half
GRM	Mean of the gradient magnitude calculated using sobel operators
Noise	
SHM	A 3×3 high-pass filter with MAD
HLH	A 2×2 high-pass filter with MAD
HLM	HH sub-band of the Haar wavelet transform with MAD
HWS	HH sub-band of the Haar wavelet transform with SD
DWS	HH sub-band of the Daubechies wavelet transform with SD
LAP	A fast noise variance method using Laplacian as presented in [4]
Signal-to-noise Ratio	
SSR	Average of intensity value on whole image and noise variance using HLH
RSR	Average of intensity value on a central ROI and noise variance using HLH
SRS	Signal on the segmented (intensity > 10) image and noise using HLH
SSS	Signal on the segmented ROI and noise on ROI using HLH
SHD	Haar DWT, SD of LL-subband as a signal, SD of HH subband as noise
SDW	Daubechies DWT, SD of LL-subband as a signal, SD of HH subband as noise

of the brain may no longer be present in the image. For this image quality metric, we used reference methods as we as a no-reference method: GRM. For noise variance the methods were based on Standard Deviation (SD) and Median Absolute Deviation (MAD). The SNR was calculated on a ROI, whole image as well as segmented image using various methods including Discrete Wavelet Transform (DWT). The brief description is presented in Tab. 1.

2.2 Evaluation methods

Data To study the image features, brain MRI images of 29 volunteers on a 1.5 T system using clinically validated diagnostic protocols [5] were acquired, using 3 defective and 1 normal 20 channel head/neck RF coil. The image data for inhomogeneous magnetic field was acquired with normal coil by modifying the 1st and 2nd order SH functions on echo planner diffusion sequences. We use the mathematical models discussed in Section 2.1 to extract the features from the DICOM images. For symmetry, the failure mode only had an influence on images acquired with echo planner diffusion sequences and only on the middle slides.

Thus, limiting our dataset for symmetry analysis to 1,077 images. Whereas, the final dataset for noise and SNR contained 18,835 images.

Evaluation criteria We used the machine learning (ML) methods to find the predictive performance as well as the correlation of mathematical models discussed in Section 2.1 with the hardware failure. Each of the image quality metric related to hardware failures was evaluated individually, making it a binary classification problem. The classification methods used are: Decision Tree, Support Vector Machine and Logistic Regression with 5-fold cross-validation on a balanced data with 60% training and 40% test partition with the values calculated using mathematical models as input features. The ML algorithms were used with the optimal parameters to ensure the validity of the results in python's sklearn package. We compared the performance of single feature as well as combination of features as an Average of Area under the Receiver Operating Characteristic curve (Avg. AUROC) on the three selected ML algorithms.

The performance of each feature is also evaluated for the time it takes for feature computation on a given machine. The machine we use here is 64 bit system with 4 logical cores and 2.93 GHz of clock speed.

Energy function To come to a final conclusion about which features or combination of features should be chosen, we introduce an Energy function. This Energy function is calculated with Avg. AUROC and Time per image in ms by each feature or combinations of features. An improvement in Avg. AUROC, allows a longer computation time up to a certain limit. The formula is:

$$\text{Energy} = \frac{\text{Average of AUROC}}{\text{Time per image in ms}} \tag{1}$$

3 Results

In the following, the performance of ML algorithms applied on features and feature combinations are presented along with the results of the energy function. As shown in Fig. 1, all the compared symmetry features have an Avg. AUROC of 0.75 and above while the computation time varies between 4 ms for CLR to 300 ms for ALL features on a single image. For noise variance, the computation time of features is in the same range from 20 ms to 40 ms. Due to this, the Energy function values also vary but in a smaller range, as seen in Fig. 2. All the features here however have a value of above 0.8 on Avg. AUROC. Most features as well as combination of SNR calculation have value of above 0.8 on Avg. AUROC except wavelet based features SDW and SHW. As seen in Fig. 3, the energy function values vary highly due to varying computation time of the features.

Fig. 1. Symmetry: results evaluation.

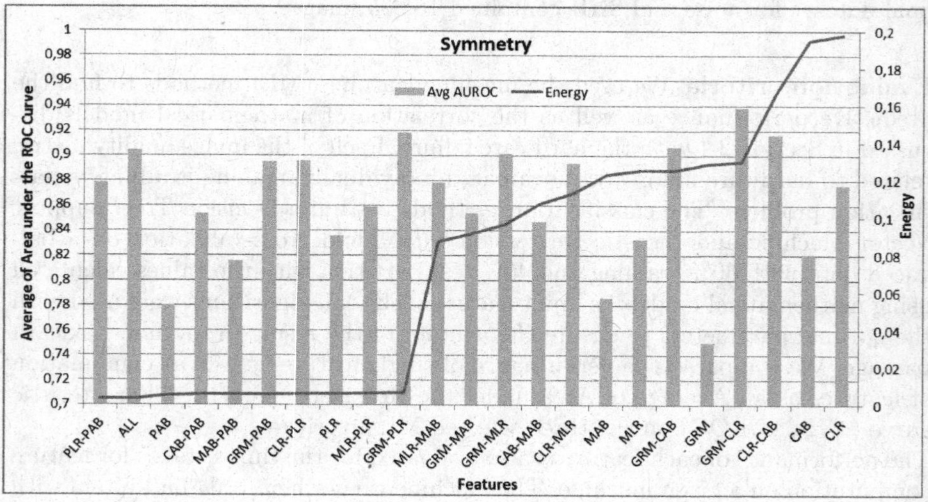

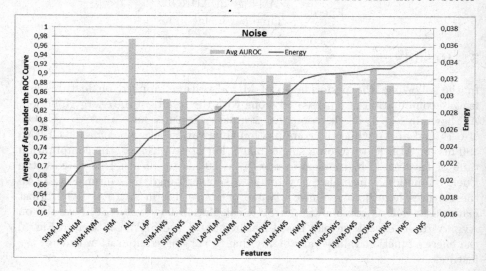

4   Discussion

As observed in the Section 3, the single features such as CLR in symmetry, DWS in noise and SRS in SNR, have higher value on Energy function. Because of lower computation time and with Avg. AUROC of 0.8 and above, single features are a better compromise between the two most important criteria. Although single feature may be sufficient to detect the failing hardware component, the combinations of features GRM-CLR, LAP-HWS and RSR-SRS have a better

Fig. 2. Noise: results evaluation.

Fig. 3. SNR: results evaluation.

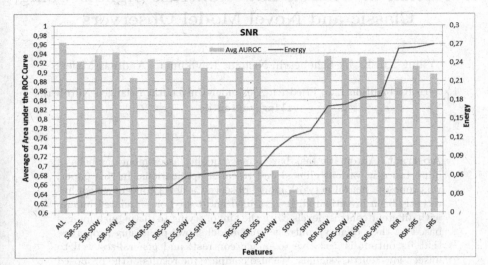

performance on ML algorithms with Avg. AUROC above 0.9, suggesting higher correlation with the respective hardware failure and better modeling of the underlying variability in data due to varying sequences and measured population. With these results we conclude that, the image quality metrics investigated in this thesis, are capable of classifying the images generated with normal vs defective MRI hardware component on ML algorithms. As a next step, more such image quality metrics will be implemented for range of hardware components to improve the services and availability of the MRI system.

References

1. Kuhnert N, Lindenmayr O, Maier A. Classification of body regions based on MRI log files. Proc CORES. 2017; p. 102–109.
2. Lorch B, Vaillant G, Baumgartner C, et al. Automated detection of motion artefacts in MR imaging using decision forests. J Med Eng. 2017;2017(4501647):1–9.
3. Peltonen JI, Mäkelä T, Salli E. MRI quality assurance based on 3D FLAIR brain images. Magn Reson Mater Phys Biol Med. 2018;.
4. Immerkaer J.   Fast noise variance estimation.   Comput Vis Image Underst. 1996;64(2):300 – 302.
5. Mehan WA, González RG, Buchbinder BR, et al. Optimal brain MRI protocol for new neurological complaint. PLoS ONE. 2014;9(10):e110803.

Detection of Unseen Low-Contrast Signals Using Classic and Novel Model Observers

Yiling Xu, Frank Schebesch, Nishant Ravikumar, Andreas Maier

Pattern Recognition Lab, Friedrich-Alexander-Universität Erlangen-Nürnberg
yiling.xu@fau.de

Abstract. Automatic task-based image quality assessment has been of importance in various clinical and research applications. In this paper, we propose a neural network model observer, a novel concept which has recently been investigated. It is trained and tested on simulated images with different contrast levels, with the aim of trying to distinguish images based on their quality/contrast. Our model shows promising properties that its output is sensitive to image contrast, and generalizes well to unseen low-contrast signals. We also compare the results of the proposed approach with those of a channelized hotelling observer (CHO), on the same simulated dataset.

1 Introduction

Medical image analysis techniques have been largely applied to clinical diagnosis in a variety of imaging modalities, including mammography. An important auxiliary task for any such application is to evaluate the image quality. Human observers are the ideal reference, but too costly for frequent studies and in many cases unavailable.

As a surrogate, mathematical model observers are popular among task-based image quality assessment since 90s [1]. In a detection task, model observers are trained to distinguish between signal-present and signal-absent images, and its performance is used to assess image quality. However, a mathematical model observer requires prior knowledge about the signal, which is challenging when dealing with low-contrast images [2].

While classic model observers follow the concepts given by Barrett et al. [1], in recent years there have been attempts to use other algorithmic concepts [3]. With the advent of wide-spread use of deep neural networks, Alnowami et al. [4] proposed a deep learning-based model observer and highlighted its promising performance on both clinical and simulated mammography images. However, the model in this paper contains 5 convolutional layers and more than 570 kernels, requiring significant computational resources, more training data and a long training time. This motivates us to employ emerging deep learning techniques to design a more compact model, with fewer trainable parameters. Our goal is to train a network with affordable cost that generalizes well, and is able to identify the presence or absence of signals in unseen lower contrast images.

2   Materials and methods

2.1   Data set

To train, validate and test the different designs of model observers we used a synthetic database generated using an image creation pipeline from the Conrad framework [5]. The simulation is a re-implementation of parts of a toolbox that has been suggested previously for studies of model observers [6]. Here, a Gaussian shaped signal is modeled by

$$s(x, y; A, s) = A\, e^{-\frac{x^2+y^2}{2s^2}}$$

and its contrast and size are parameterized by A and s, respectively. For a noisy background two separate random image components are drawn from a normal distribution. Noise structure is simulated for both components by convolution of each with a cone-filter, represented as

$$c(x, y) = \begin{cases} 0 & \text{if } |x| < 3\Delta x \wedge |y| < 3\Delta y \\ \frac{1}{\sqrt{x^2+y^2}} & \text{otherwise} \end{cases}$$

where, $\Delta x \times \Delta y$ denotes the pixel dimensions. One of the components is considered the background structure as it would appear as tissue in clinical images. The other serves as noise that would originate from an image acquisition process. Both components are weighted with constant factors and merged to background images b_i, $i = 1, ..., N$ such that signal-present and signal-absent images $I_i^{(p)}$ and $I_i^{(a)}$, respectively, can be created as

$$I_i^{(p)} = s_i + b_i, \qquad I_i^{(a)} = b_i$$

All images are of size 200×200 pixels. We simulate 5 groups of images, each group comprising 240 signal-present images and 240 signal-absent images. Signal intensity of the signal-present images is controlled to span 5 different levels such that images in group 1 are of the highest contrast, while images in group 5 are of the lowest contrast. Signals in group 5 are hardly visible to the human eye (Fig. 1). All signal-absent images contain only background information and are statistically similar. In order to prevent the neural network from learning only mean or variance features, we normalize each image in a pre-processing step, so that they all have the same mean and variance. We evenly assign one-sixth of the data set to a testing set, and the rest are further employed as the training and validation pool.

2.2   Classic model observer

A frequently studied task for model observers is the detection task which in its basic form involves the detection of a known signal at a known location. Based on the performance of a model observer on a selected data set a certain degree of image quality can be assessed [7]. The channelized hotelling observer (CHO) is a group of observers that produce its decision metric from a feature description of the image data. The well-known Laguerre-Gauss channels [8] produce a set of rotationally-invariant features. Thus well applicable for Gaussian signal shapes [9], we compute scores for all tested contrast levels using such a classic model observer, namely, a CHO with 10 Laguerre-Gauss channels. The width parameter that controls the area which is effectively taken into account for the feature computation is selected as $4s$, where s is the size parameter of the signal.

The detectability index SNR_λ is associated with a model observer via its test statistic λ [7]. It is a figure of merit of how separable the two groups are w.r.t. λ and is defined as

$$\text{SNR}_\lambda = \frac{E(\lambda|\text{signal}) - E(\lambda|\text{no signal})}{\sqrt{0.5\,(\text{Var}(\lambda|\text{signal}) + \text{Var}(\lambda|\text{no signal}))}}$$

We choose this model observer and its figure of merit for comparison with the proposed approach using a neural network.

2.3   Neural network architecture and training strategy

In this paper, we propose a convolutional neural network with 2 convolutional layers. The first convolutional layer has 6 kernels of size 11×11, followed by a rectified linear unit (ReLu) activation, batch normalization and an 8×8 max-pooling with 2×2 stride. The second convolutional layer has 3 kernels of size 5×5, followed by ReLu activation, batch normalization and a 2×2 max-pooling with 2×2 stride. The output is then passed to two fully connected layers to reduce the dimension to 2 corresponding to the number of classes. A softmax layer is employed as the final classification layer, with a cross entropy loss function (Fig. 2). This neural network serves as a model observer and predicts a score

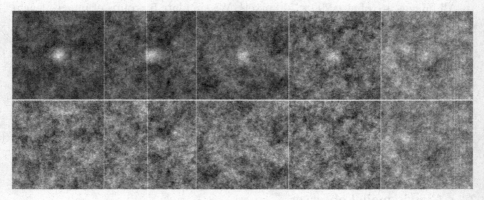

Fig. 1. From left to right: Examples images from highest to lowest contrast (groups 1-5) with signal present (first row), and signal absent (second row). The images shown above are aimed for better visualization, while the actual data are normalized as described in the text.

between 0 to 1.0 as to how likely the image contains a signal. In validation a classification is achieved based on a probability threshold of 0.5.

In order to train the network, we employ the Adam optimizer, with the learning rate set to $1e^{-5}$. The neural network is trained to a maximum of 300 epochs, and after 100 epochs, an early stopping criterion is called if the validation loss has not improved in the preceding 20 epochs. To evaluate the robustness of the neural network and to detect signals in unseen lower contrast images, we always leave out group 5 from the training and validation data sets. A 5-fold cross validation is carried out and consequently, five different sets of weights are trained for our network. We employ these as five individual models in the test phase, using samples from group 5 in the test set.

Besides the probability output from the network itself as a measure of detection confidence, these outputs were also considered as decision scores. By this analogy, SNR_λ can be evaluated for the neural network as well, which allows to qualitatively compare both methods for different contrast levels.

3   Results

We test both classic and neural network based model observers on the test data samples which are separated randomly before the training takes place. As we do 5-fold cross validation in training, we further combine the results from 5 different weight sets by averaging the softmax scores sample-wise. In (Tab. 1) we show its classification accuracy on the test data with adjusted threshold. The accuracy and sensitivity show very good performance in the first 3 groups and decrease as contrast levels go lower. (Fig. 3) shows typical training curves in our experiments, where in this case early stopping criterion was called at epoch 140.

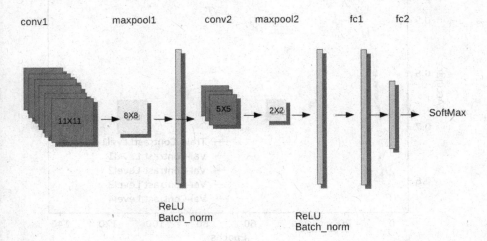

Fig. 2. Illustration of the neural network structure.

Table 1. Performance of the combined neural network model on test data.

Contrast Level	Accuracy	Accuracy(CMO)	Sensitivity	Specificity
1 (highest)	1.0	1.0	1.0	1.0
2	1.0	1.0	1.0	1.0
3	1.0	1.0	1.0	1.0
4	0.975	1.0	0.975	0.975
5 (lowest)	0.9	0.95	0.9	0.9

(Tab. 2) shows SNR_λ values for both classic model observer and our proposed neural network. It can be seen that both models have high SNR_λ on higher contrast levels, and lower SNR_λ on contrast level 4 and 5. Our proposed neural network's ability to distinguish signal-present images from signal-absent images shows a comparable decreasing trend to the classic model observer. Furthermore, The result of our novel model observer suggests the presence of a significant difference between level 1-3, and the two lowest contrast levels, than within level 1-3, which can be seen as alternative reference to human performance (Fig. 1).

4   Discussion

In this paper, we propose a neural network as a model observer. The network is trained with simulated images of four different contrast levels and tested on

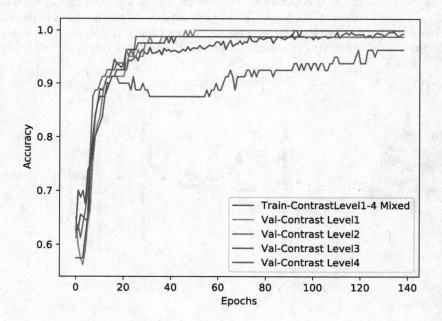

Fig. 3. Train and validation accuracy along training epochs.

Table 2. SNR_λ on test results from both model observers.

Contrast Level	Classic Model Observer	Proposed Neural Network
1 (highest)	10.7	10.5
2	8.0	10.3
3	6.5	9.4
4	5.0	6.1
5 (lowest)	3.4	2.0

images with similar contrast, as well as an unseen lower contrast. The results highlight the model's potential for predicting human performance qualitatively as its classification performance declines with the image contrast, while still being able to detect signals in some of the very low-contrast images. Furthermore, the performance is comparable to a classic model observer. Compared with other techniques, our model requires little knowledge about the signal and demands only reasonable training time. We believe our proposed model observer can also be applicable to clinical data, to assess image quality, among other tasks. For instance, training a network on simulated high- and low-contrast images and then evaluating it on real mammography images, to distinguish between high and low contrast samples, may provide a means for automatically detecting lesions and microcalcifications, which will be a topic of future work.

References

1. Barrett HH, Yao J, Rolland JP, et al. Model observers for assessment of image quality. PNAS. 1993;90:9758–9765.
2. Damien R, Alexandre B, Julien O, et al. Objective assessment of low contrast detectability in computed tomography with channelized hotelling observer. Phys Med. 2016;32:76–83.
3. Kalayeh MM, Marin T, Brankov JG. Generalization evaluation of machine learning numerical observers for image quality assessment. IEEE Trans Nucl Sci. 2013;60(3):1609–1618.
4. Alnowami MR, Mills G, Awis M, et al. A deep learning model observer for use in alterative forced choice virtual clinical trials. Proc SPIE. 2018;.
5. Maier A, Hofmann H, Berger M, et al. CONRAD: a software framework for cone-beam imaging in radiology. Med Phys. 2013;40(11):111914–1–8.
6. Wunderlich A. IQmodelo; 2016. [Online; accessed 28-October-2018]. https://github.com/DIDSR/IQmodelo.
7. He X, Park S. Model observers in medical imaging research. Theranostics. 2013;3(10):774–786.
8. Gallas BD, Barrett HH. Validating the use of channels to estimate the ideal linear observer. JOSA A: Opt, Image Sci, Vis. 2003;20(9):1725–1738.
9. Schebesch F, Maier A. Towards optimal channels for a detection channelized hotelling observer. 3rd Conf Proc Image-Guid Interv Fokus Neuroradiol. 2017; p. 12–13.

Abstract: Imitating Human Soft Tissue with Dual-Daterial 3D Printing

Johannes Maier[1], Maximilian Weiherer[1], Michaela Huber[2], Christoph Palm[1,3]

[1]Regensburg Medical Image Computing (ReMIC), Ostbayerische Technische Hochschule Regensburg (OTH Regensburg), Germany
[2]Department of Trauma Surgery & Emergency Department, University Hospital Regensburg, Germany
[3]Regensburg Center of Biomedical Engineering (RCBE), OTH Regensburg and Regensburg University, Germany
christoph.palm@oth-regensburg.de

Currently, it is common practice to use three-dimensional (3D) printers not only for rapid prototyping in the industry, but also in the medical area to create medical applications for training inexperienced surgeons. In a clinical training simulator for minimally invasive bone drilling to fix hand fractures with Kirschner-wires (K-wires), a 3D printed hand phantom must not only be geometrically but also haptically correct. Due to a limited view during an operation, surgeons need to perfectly localize underlying risk structures only by feeling of specific bony protrusions of the human hand.

The goal of this experiment is to imitate human soft tissue with its haptic and elasticity for a realistic hand phantom fabrication, using only a dual-material 3D printer and support-material-filled metamaterial between skin and bone. We present our workflow to generate lattice structures between hard bone and soft skin with iterative cube edge (CE) or cube face (CF) unit cells. Cuboid and finger shaped sample prints with and without inner hard bone in different lattice thickness are constructed and 3D printed.

The most elastic available rubber-like material is too firm to imitate soft tissue. By reducing the amount of rubber in the inner volume through support material (SUP), objects become significantly softer. This was confirmed by an expert surgeon evaluation. Subjects adjudged 3D printed finger samples in CF design as realistic compared to the haptic of human tissue with a good palpable bone structure. Blowy SUP is trapped within a lattice structure to soften rubber-like 3D print material, which makes it possible to reproduce a realistic replica of human hand soft tissue [1].

References

1. Maier J, Weiherer M, Huber M, et al. Imitating human suft tissue on basis of a dual-material 3D print using a support-filled metamaterial to provide bimanual haptic for a hand surgery training system. Quant Imaging Med Surg. 2018;in press.

A Mixed Reality Simulation for Robotic Systems

Martin Leipert[1,2], Jenny Sadowski[2], Michèle Kießling[2],
Emeric Kwemou Ngandeu[2], Andreas Maier[1]

[1]Chair of Pattern Recognition, FAU Erlangen-Nürnberg
[2]Siemens Healthineers
martin.leipert@fau.de

Abstract. In interventional angiography, kinematic simulation of robotic system prototypes in early development phases facilitates the detection of design errors. In this work, a game engine visualization with output is developed for such a robotic simulation. The goal of this is a better perception of the prototype by more realistic visualization. The achieved realism is evaluated in a user study. Additionally, the inclusion of real rooms' walls into the simulation's collision model is tested and evaluated, to verify smartglasses as a tool for interactive room planning. The walls are reconstructed from point clouds using a mean shift segmentation and RANSAC. Afterwards, the obtained wall estimates are ordered using a simple neighborhood graph.

1 Introduction

This work is based on a kinematic robot simulation, developed for the purpose of risk detection at interventional angiography system prototypes. It uses models directly exported from computer-aided design (CAD) software. The main functionalities are collision detection and angulation testing. Graphical output, with Visualization Toolkit (VTK), is plain, functional and therefore sufficient for the purposes of most engineers. Despite this, for a better understanding of those prototypes and realistic demonstrations, it would be helpful to use the software for more realistic visualization in AR and VR. One possibility to boost the visual quality and to use both – AR and VR – is an implementation with a game engine. These provide low-cost solutions for superior visualization. Furthermore, they offer portability to multiple platforms, AR and VR.

Today's game engines are capable to cover a large variety of use cases. Also in scientific visualization, where the variety of usage fields is large and includes military simulations, virtual museums or archaeological site reconstruction. In science – according to Cowan and Kapralos – the most popular are the multipurpose Unity and Unreal engines [1]. For an evaluation of different operation schemes in robotics, Andaluz et. al. used Unity3D for the simulation of robotic arms in combination with Matlab [2]. To improve the remote comprehension of assembly lines and industrial robots by service technicians, Aschenbrenner et. al. used a visualization of remote robots' poses in Unity, both for a desktop computer and in AR [3]. In the evaluation, participants demonstrated a superior comprehension of the setup in AR, compared to video based visualization. For room capture from data obtained by depth cameras, common plane extraction approaches include region growing and Hough Transform. With the latter, Oesau et al. reached an accuracy of 2.3 cm in spatial reconstruction [4, 5].

In this work, the feasibility of a realistic simulation of prototypes' behavior in AR is evaluated. This is desired for a better understanding of arbitrary workflows – by superior visualization. Also, by an in-situ simulation of different room setups, a better understanding of those is desired. In Mixed Reality (MR) depth sensors offer the possibility of interactive room planing, which is the second aspect examined. The potential benefit is to demonstrate a setting in-situ and to identify difficulties due to collisions.

A suitable game engine was investigated for visualization of the simulation. With the found engine a desktop and an output for the Microsoft HoloLens was designed, including interactive registration of the simulations' basic coordinate system into reality. All visualizations – desktop computer and AR – were evaluated with a user study. A in-situ room capture with the depth camera of the HoloLens is evaluated with a simple room segmentation approach. From the provided depth data, walls are extracted and integrated into the collision model. Primarily, depth data belonging to a wall are distinguished from other objects with mean shift segmentation. From the segmented point clouds, wall models are generated with the Random Sample Consensus (RANSAC) algorithm and out of those the room is reconstructed. The quality of the result is measured by the size deviation to the real rooms.

2   Materials and methods

The game engine of choice was Unity as it is the simplest to develop with – because of C# scripting – offering both good graphics quality and AR support. Of the examined engines, Unity has the best and widest compatibility with AR platforms. A notable consideration was Unreal which offers similar potentials regarding graphics and platforms. Also, the open source engine Godot, with advanced 3D effects, although yet lacking AR support.

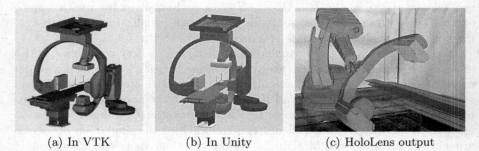

(a) In VTK   (b) In Unity   (c) HoloLens output

Fig. 1. Visualization of a robotic angiography system in VTK, Unity and the Hologram in Augmented Reality on HoloLens.

2.1   Desktop and augmented reality visualization

A reusable implementation based on IPC was required for both desktop and AR. The Remote Procedural Calling (RPC) toolkit gRPC was chosen – because of its good performance and simplicity. A layered architecture was developed around the offered interface, where each layer applies a common design pattern. The visualization backend is made flexible and exchangeable, as objects are generated by an *AbstractFactory* in the simulation. Objects in the Unity process are represented by *Proxies* in the simulation. Access to Unity is simplified by a *Facade* mapping the calls to Unity using object ids. For performance reasons, frequent calls were sent batched, triggered by a timer. The object implementations in Unity use the *Adapter* pattern to map calls to Unity's *GameObjects*. For thread safety, a *Queue* is used to access Unity's *GameObjects*.

To obtain an estimate of improvements in a user study, both outputs – VTK in Fig. 1(a) and Unity in Fig. 1(b) – were demonstrated to the users under supervision, at the same PC and in a randomized order. They had to rate these in terms of rendering fluency, intuitiveness, graphical quality and visualization effectiveness on a scale of 1 (bad) to 5 (excellent). For the study, an excerpt of potential, sporadic and frequent simulation users – from different interested areas – were invited to participate. Of those, 18 participated in the study.

Due to the usage of Transmission Control Protocol (TCP) for IPC, the interface could be reused for an AR visualization – demonstrated in Fig. 1(c). Via a plugin implementing the *Observer* pattern, changes of the *Proxy* objects are mapped to their reflections in AR, resulting in AR objects behaving equal those on desktop. With the Vuforia toolkit – which uses natural feature detection – a marker printed on an A4 sheet of paper, was used to register the coordinate system of the simulation into the real world. Also placement intuitiveness and the perceived realism of AR content, were evaluated in the user study.

2.2   Room capture

With the HoloLens' depth camera, the room is captured. This consists of a two steps procedure. The first is the recording of single wall planes, each time triggered by the user via gesture input. After the user stops the recording, in the second step, the walls are ordered by a wall-neighborhood graph to a room. The Unity class *SurfaceObserver* provides depth-data as 3D point meshes, which are used to estimate the real-world measures. The points within the user's field of view (FoV) are used to sample the wall. As consequence, only a partial sector of the wall is used for plane estimation. Additionally, the surface normals are calculated from the meshes. The feature dimensionality is reduced by a feature transform of the i-th point $\boldsymbol{x}_i^{3\times1} \in \mathbb{R}^{3\times1}$ of the point cloud dataset and the components of its normal $\boldsymbol{n}_i^{3\times1} = \left(n_i^x\ n_i^y\ n_i^z\right)^\top$ Therefore, the feature vector initially consists of surface points and their normals $\boldsymbol{f}_i = \left(x_i^x\ x_i^y\ x_i^z\ n_i^x\ n_i^y\ n_i^z\right)^\top$ From these features, the distance of the point to the camera and the normal direction are obtained as a reduced feature vector $\boldsymbol{f}_i$:

$$f_i = \left(\sin n_i^x \cos n_i^y \; \boldsymbol{n}_i^{3\times1\,\top} \cdot \boldsymbol{x}_i^{3\times1} \right)^\top \tag{1}$$

The transformed data are clustered using mean shift. This does not require a fixed cluster number and works well for a low number of features. Additionally, the only required parameter – the kernel width – can be estimated based on real-world observations [6] (for example the depth measure of cabinets). From the clustered data – which still contain outliers – the wall planes are estimated by the outlier-insensitive RANSAC algorithm. To order the obtained wall planes $W = \{a, b\}$ via a graph to a room of rectangular walls, the neighborhood probability is used as weight w_{ab} of walls $a \in W$ and $b \in W$. It is calculated from the wall's normal $\boldsymbol{n}_W^{3\times1}$ and the camera (and user's) C's position $\boldsymbol{x}_{C,W}^{3\times1}$ at the time of the recording of a and b. Far away walls are considered as less probable neighbors. The parameter β weights the inter-wall angle. Only (close-to) rectangular walls are regarded as possible neighbors.

$$w_{ab} = \left(\boldsymbol{n}_a^{3\times1\,\top} \cdot \boldsymbol{n}_b^{3\times1} + \beta \right) \cdot \left(||\boldsymbol{x}_{C,a}^{3\times1} - -\boldsymbol{x}_{C,b}^{3\times1}||_2 \right) \tag{2}$$

In the graph the neighbors are obtained by selecting the edges with the lowest weight between two walls (which do not have 2 neighbors yet). This works for rectangular rooms. However, it fails if a room has a small cove and the positions of the camera trajectory are close together for adjacent walls of the cove. The possible principal accuracy of the HoloLens' depth camera was tested by estimating the plane of a white wall. The points of the wall, obtained by the depth camera, represent a plane estimated by Singular Value Decomposition (SVD). The 3rd singular value σ_3 of the SVD was taken as an estimate for the standard deviation or measurement noise. The standard deviation of the normal direction was estimated from the singular values σ_2 and σ_3 of the normal array, as the normals point in one main direction, which is covered by σ_1. The evaluation of the approach itself was conducted by taking different room sizes (small: 5653 mm x 4039 mm, medium: 6161 mm x 5654 mm and large: 8050 mm x 5743 mm). Additionally, the medium sized room was cluttered with tables, chairs and packing foil, resulting in a no, medium and maximum clutter setup (Fig. 2(b)). Those setups serve the purpose of planning in rooms, where a previous system is still installed or which are not yet empty. The used evaluation measure was the deviation of the side-lengths of the estimated room towards the ground truth. As accuracy requirement 5 cm was derived from the IEC 60601-1 norm, taking 10 % of the smallest gap of the squeezing safety distance.

3   Results

In the user study, Unity visualization was rated superior to VTK on desktop. Using a paired t-test, a significant improvement could be concluded for rendering performance, visual impression, surface quality and realism. For the visualizations' effectiveness, distracting effects and detail quality no significant improvement was observed. In the AR evaluation, the size of the robot, movements and

Table 1. User study results for the AR visualization.

Property	Mean	Std. Dev.	Median	Percentiles 25%	75 %	Acceptance
Realistic Movements	3.17	1.04	3	3	4	4
Realistic Graphics	3.17	1.15	3.5	2.25	4	3
Realistic Dimensions	3.94	0.87	4	3.25	4.75	3
HoloLens' FoV	1.5	0.62	1	1	2	3
Intuitive Placement	3.11	1.45	3.5	2	4	4

graphics were rated as rather realistic by the majority of participants (Tab. 1). Users perceived sometimes stuttering movements resulting in less realism. As the used marker pattern for registration was small (on a A4 sheet) and used natural feature detection, the robot was often in a skewed position. Also, users considered the HoloLens' FoV of 35° as too small for the visualization a life-sized robot. They had to step back several meters from the marker to see the entire

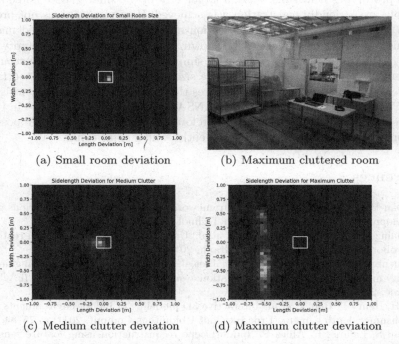

(a) Small room deviation

(b) Maximum cluttered room

(c) Medium clutter deviation

(d) Maximum clutter deviation

Fig. 2. Deviation in different room setups. The small room could be measured relatively precise (a). The room was initially empty. To reach the clutter setups, tables and other furniture were used for medium clutter. Additional packaging foil was used for the maximum clutter setup (b). The obtained estimates showed large relative deviations (c, d) and an additional absolute deviation (d) in the clutter setup.

system and perceived this as a large inconvenience. The principal method of registering the coordinate systems with printed marker was rated as easy, however not as intuitive. For the principal accuracy of the HoloLens' depth camera, the value σ_3 was 24 mm. The singular values of the normals σ_2 and σ_3 were 0.159 and 0.138. Which results in an angular standard deviation of 9.03° and 7.85°. For the empty rooms, the size estimation results were in a range of around 10 cm for the small and the large room (Fig. 2(a)). Contrarily in the clutter setups, the quality of the measurement deteriorated, such that large deviations from the desired accuracy occurred (Fig. 2(c) & 2(d)).

4   Discussion

With a rather simple architecture and small efforts compared to VTK, an improvement of the visualization quality was reached with Unity. Further visual improvement is possible with low effort, as the Unity visualization is yet unpolished. In AR it can be concluded, that with some optimizations (optimized models, fluent movements) a perception of realism, sufficient for the visualization of prototypes is feasible. Also, a larger FoV of the smartglasses is required. A simple, user-friendly registration was achieved. However, this was not precise due to Vuforia's natural feature detection approach. Fiducial, squared marker patterns may solve this. It could be shown, that the integration of empty real rooms in the simulation is possible with simple methods. However, the accuracy requirement was failed to achieve as the size estimation error is still too large. However, the noise measurement indicates that the accuracy requirement is feasible. Using small wall patches with RANSAC resulted in tilted planes in room capture. Another drawback of the therefore insufficient approach. A possible solution is the use of constraints or the entire wall's point cloud.

References

1. Cowan B, Kapralos B. A survey of frameworks and game engines for serious game development. Proc IEEE Adv Learn Technol. 2014; p. 662–664.
2. Andaluz H, Chicaiza F, Gallardo C, et al. Unity3D-MatLab simulator in real time for robotics applications. Comput Graph. 2016; p. 246–263.
3. Aschenbrenner D, Maltry N, Kimmel J, et al. ARTab: using virtual and augmented reality methods for an improved situation awareness for telemaintenance. IFAC Pap Online. 2016;49(30):204–209.
4. Du H, Henry P, Ren X, et al. Interactive 3D modeling of indoor environments with a consumer depth camera. Proc Int Conf Ubiquitous Comput. 2011; p. 75–84.
5. Oesau S, Lafarge F, Alliez P. Indoor scene reconstruction using feature sensitive primitive extraction and graph-cut. J Photogramm Remote Sens. 2014;90:68–82.
6. Comaniciu D, Meer P. Mean shift: a robust approach toward feature space analysis. IEEE Trans Pattern Anal Mach Intell. 2002;24(5):603–619.

Image Quality Assessments

Medha Juneja[1], Mechthild Bode-Hofmann[2], Khay Sun Haong[3],
Steffen Meißner[5], Viola Merkel[4], Johannes Vogt[1], Nobert Wilke[3], Anja Wolff[1],
Thomas Hartkens[1]

[1]Technology Lab, medneo GmbH, Berlin
[2]Ernst von Bergmann Poliklinik Potsdam
[3]Radiologisches Zentrum Höchstadt / Nürnberg / Fürth
[4]Radiologische Praxis Merkel
[5]Sana Gesundheitszentren Berlin-Brandenburg GmbH
medha.juneja@medneo.com

Abstract. Deep learning with Convolutional Neural Networks (CNN) requires large number of training and test data sets which involves usually time-consuming visual inspection of medical image data. Recently, crowdsourcing methods have been proposed to gain such large training sets from untrained observers. In this paper, we propose to establish a lightweight method within the daily routine of radiologists in order to collect simple image quality annotations on a large scale. In multiple diagnostic centres, we analyse the acceptance rate of the radiologists and whether a substantial total number of professional annotations can be acquired to be used for deep learning later. Using a simple control panel with three buttons, 6 radiologists in 5 imaging centres assessed the image quality within their daily routine. Altogether, 1527 DICOM image studies (MR, CT, and X-ray) have been subjectively assessed in the first 70 days which demonstrates that a considerable number of training data sets can be collected with such a method in short time. The acceptance rate of the radiologists indicates that more data sets could be acquired if corresponding incentives are introduced as discussed in the paper. Since the proposed method is incorporated in the daily routine of radiologists, it can be easily scaled to even more number of professional observers.

1 Introduction

Quality control of radiological images has been an intense field of research in the last 25 years [1], because it is essential for excluding problematic acquisitions and avoiding bias in subsequent reading of the images. Also, many image processing and analysis techniques rely on a constant image quality and can result in erroneous conclusion if the image quality is not sufficient.

Automatic image quality control enables technicians at the modality to verify the image quality directly after acquisition and makes it possible to repeat the acquisition while the patient is still in the scanner. *Quantitative* image quality measurements have been proposed to facilitate such automatic control [2, 3]. Image quality is not necessarily objective but might be subjectively judged by radiologists based on their personal preferences: an "optimized" image quality for one radiologist might not be satisfying for another. Furthermore, it is not clear if the proposed specific quantitative measurements capture all aspects of image quality. Thus, a quality-controlled acquisition based on purely quantitative measurements might not differentiate images sufficiently and is preferably combined with subjective annotations based on visual inspection.

Recently, it has been proposed to train CNN using visual ratings by radiologists in order to incorporate subjective aspects in automatic image quality control. For example, Esses et al. [4] use a CNN for automated classifying T2-weighted liver acquisitions in either diagnostic or non-diagnostic quality and compare this automated approach with evaluation by two radiologists. A similar approach was suggested in [5] for brain images. Typically, training such CNNs requires a large number of annotated data sets assessed by experts. In order to overcome the time-consuming visual inspection of the image data, the authors in [5] and [6] propose crowdsourcing methods as a means to involve large number of individuals to rate the large number of training and test image data. With such an approach it is not clear if all observers are qualified to make such an assessment and might introduce label noise. In this paper, we propose to incorporate a lightweight subjective assessment of the image quality in the daily routine of radiologists and to use such assessments for a CNN later. We analyse whether the proposed method is accepted by the radiologist and if the specified evaluation criteria allows sufficient differentiation of image quality.

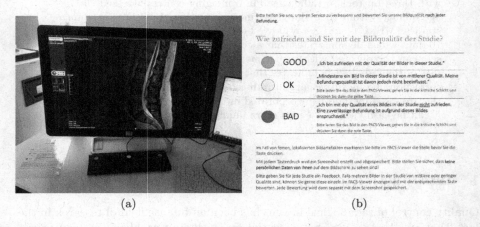

(a)   (b)

Fig. 1. (a) The assessment control panel placed in front of the radiologists work station. (b) Written instructions handed to the radiologists.

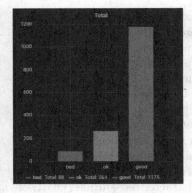

Fig. 2. Total number of assessments by radiologists. Within the first 70 days, in total 1527 annotated DICOM studies (MR, CT and X-ray) have been collected with 1175 good, 264 ok and 88 bad rated studies.

2   Materials and methods

A control panel with 3 buttons is set up at the diagnostic station as shown in Fig. 1(a). The radiologist assesses the image quality of the entire DICOM study by pressing one of the buttons (green = "good", yellow = "ok", red = "bad") at any time during the reading process. Besides the assessment of radiologist, a screenshot of the Picture Archiving and Communication System (PACS) viewer is captured and anonymised according to General Data Protection Regulation

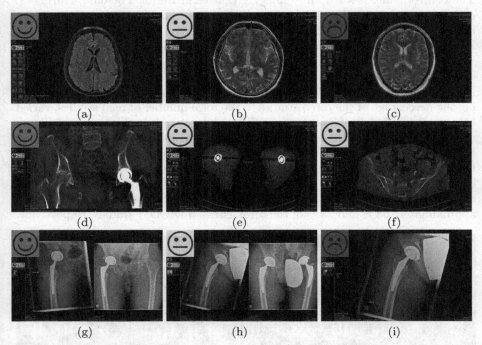

Fig. 3. Example (a)-(c) MR images of the head region, (d)-(f) CT images of pelvis region and (g)-(i) X-ray images of hip region annotated as good (green), ok (yellow) and bad (red).

(GDPR) to identify which type of sequence the radiologist looked at during the assessment. It is part of the standard operating procedure (SOP) of all centres, that patients sign a consent form for improving image quality.

After a brief personal introduction, written instructions on how to provide subjective assessment of image quality using the control panel as stated in Fig. 1(b) are handed to the radiologist. In order to minimize the overhead for radiologists, they are asked to rate the image quality of the entire DICOM study of the patient instead of rating individual sequences. If he considers an individual image slice as "ok" or "bad", then the entire sequence is rated as "ok" or "bad". The radiologist enlarges the image sequence in the PACS viewer before submitting his assessment. The acquired screenshot enables the automatic identification of the individual sequence image through optical character recognition (OCR) of the PACS text overlays. The radiologist is instructed to rate the DICOM study with "ok" if at least one of the images in the study is of average quality, but the diagnostic quality is not affected. The study is rated as "bad", if the radiologist *feels uncomfortable* performing diagnosis based on these images.

3   Results

The control panel is set up in 5 imaging centres in Berlin, Potsdam, Nürnberg, and Fürth and 6 radiologists were enrolled who read magnetic resonance (MR), computed tomography (CT) and X-ray studies.

Total collected assessments is shown in Fig. 2 with number of feedbacks varying from day to day as shown in Fig. 4 whereby the actual image quality depends on each modality as seen in Fig. 5. An example of anonymised annotated screenshots of rated images is shown in Fig. 3. The acceptance rate of radiologists, i.e. the percentage of the rated studies to the total number of read studies, varied between 2.1 % and 100 % as shown in Tab. 1 suggesting that even more training data sets could be acquired if corresponding incentives are introduced. It turned out, that Radiologist #1 uses a different workstation for reading studies and hence, rated only 2 studies with the feedback tool. Radiologist #2 rated all the studies, but he reads only a small number of patients. The largest number of assessments were received from Radiologist #3 and Radiologist #4 who rated approximately 68 % and 23 % of the total assessed DICOM studies, respectively.

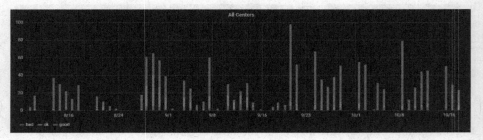

Fig. 4. Number of image quality assessments by radiologists per day.

Fig. 5. Percentage of assessments based on modalities.

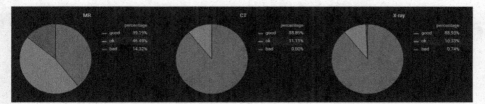

All 6 radiologists reported that the proposed method does not interfere in their daily work. The control panel itself was also judged to be user-friendly.

Fig. 6 illustrates the effect of change in the parameters of an MR protocol on the assessment of quality at a specific time point.

4 Discussion

We demonstrated that the proposed lightweight method to collect subjective assessment of image quality from radiologists in their daily routine results in a considerable number of annotated images in a short amount of time. Within 70 days 1527 DICOM studies have been rated by 6 enrolled radiologists.

The method has several drawbacks. Firstly, it is not compulsory for the radiologists to provide an assessment for each DICOM study. That means only a fraction of the diagnosed images are actually assessed. Secondly, even though most images are rated as "good quality" in our study, radiologist might pay more attention to images of bad quality in general, and, therefore, rate bad quality images more often than good quality images. Thirdly, the radiologists rate a large spectrum of images, i.e. different modalities like MR, CT, and X-ray images and even different types within each modality. It needs to be seen, if CNNs can be trained on a sub-group of those varieties. Fourthly, the control panel for the assessment may not be installable at all reading stations because of technical constraints.

Our initial results suggest that the method could be improved by providing an incentive to the radiologists such as establishing a process to identify critical acquisition protocols based on the assessments and adjust their parameters as shown in Fig. 6. Furthermore, in order to enable assessments on third party or

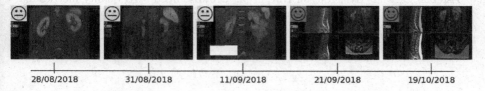

| 28/08/2018 | 31/08/2018 | 11/09/2018 | 21/09/2018 | 19/10/2018 |

Fig. 6. Effect of change of MR protocol on the assessment of quality. Radiologist repeatedly rated the same protocol as average. After adjusting the parameters of the protocol on 13/09/2018, the protocol was rated "good" subsequently.

Table 1. Assessments of each radiologist and their corresponding acceptance rate.

Radiologist	Total ratings	GOOD	OK	BAD	Unrated	Acceptance rate
#1	93	0	0	2	91	2.1 %
#2	19	16	3	0	0	100 %
#3	2346	975	58	2	1258	44.1 %
#4	1198	165	169	24	838	29.9 %
#5	408	10	2	18	378	7.3 %
#6	675	9	32	42	590	12.3 %

remote workstation, a web browser-based widget could be used which would not require an installation of software on the reading station.

The strength of the proposed method is based on its lightweight approach which can be incorporated in the daily routine of the radiologist: In contrast to [4] we were able to enrol more radiologists (6 instead of just 2) and establish the method at multiple centres, which indicates an easy scale up to even more radiologists and centres. The approach does not rely on untrained observers like [5] and [6].

Furthermore, if large number of radiologists participate, there is the prospect to train CNNs for specific sub-groups of radiologists who would then benefit from a "personalized" automatic image quality control at the modality.

References

1. Gardner EA, Ellis JH, Hyde RJ, et al. Detection of degradation of magnetic resonance (MR) images: comparison of an automated MR image-quality analysis system with trained human observers. Acad Radiol. 1995;2(4):277–281.
2. Rao TVN, Govardhan A. Assessment of diverse quality metrics for medical images including mammography. Int J Comput Appl. 2013;83(4).
3. Esteban O, Birman D, Schaer M, et al. MRIQC: Advancing the automatic prediction of image quality in MRI from unseen sites. PloS one. 2017;12(9):e0184661.
4. Esses SJ, Lu X, Zhao T, et al. Automated image quality evaluation of T2-weighted liver MRI utilizing deep learning architecture. J Magn Reson Imaging. 2018;47(3):723–728.
5. Keshavan A, Yeatman J, Rokem A. Combining citizen science and deep learning to amplify expertise in neuroimaging. bioRxiv. 2018; p. 363382.
6. Esteban O, Blair RW, Nielson DM, et al. Crowdsourced MRI quality metrics and expert quality annotations for training of humans and machines. bioRxiv. 2018; p. 420984.

Abstract: HoloLens
Streaming of 3D Data from Ultrasound Systems to Augmented Reality Glasses

Felix von Haxthausen[1], Floris Ernst[1], Ralf Bruder[1], Mark Kaschwich[2]
Verónica García-Vázquez[1]

[1]Institut für Robotik und Kognitive Systeme, Universität zu Lübeck
[2]Division of Vascular- and Endovascular Surgery, Department of Surgery,
University Hospital Schleswig-Holstein, Campus Lübeck
vonhaxthausen@rob.uni-luebeck.de

Two-dimensional ultrasound (US) imaging is one of the most common tools for diagnostic procedures. However, this imaging modality requires highly experienced and skilled operators to mentally reconstruct three-dimensional (3D) anatomy from these images. Additionally, the physician's gaze is focused on the screen of the US system instead of the probe and patient. In order to overcome these problems, we propose real-time 3D US in combination with augmented reality (AR) glasses (specifically Microsoft HoloLens) to render the volume relative to the US probe [1]. Raw data access to the US system was provided by an in-house modification and volumes were sent from the US system (GE Vivid 7) to a computer via Ethernet. On the computer, the data was first converted from spherical to Cartesian coordinates and then the zeros (mainly presented outside the pyramid-shaped US volume) were compressed using run-length encoding. A multi-language remote procedure call (gRPC) was used to transmit the encoded data from the computer to HoloLens via Wi-Fi. The AR marker attached to the US probe, which allows the placement of the virtual volume next to the probe, was tracked using HoloLensARTToolkit. This approach was evaluated regarding the rate of displayed volumes on HoloLens and the end-to-end latency. US volumes (depth of 15 cm, matrix size in spherical coordinates of 495 x 72 x 26) were acquired at a frame rate of 13.8 Hz. On HoloLens, the volumes had a matrix size in Cartesian coordinates of 103 x 74 x 134. Our results show that the volumetric data was rendered with a time interval of 72 ± 55 ms and an end-to-end latency of 259 ± 85 ms. The loss-less data encoding allowed a decrease of 63 % in data size. There is a growing interest in using real-time 3D US for clinical applications and HoloLens gives the possibility of a more intuitive visualization of volumetric data than using a standard screen. Future work will evaluate the AR marker tracking and other transmissions paths in order to lower the end-to-end latency.

References

1. von Haxthausen F, Ernst F, Bruder R, et al. Streaming of 3D data from ultrasound systems to augmented reality glasses (HoloLens). Proc CURAC. 2018; p. 2–3.

Open-Source Tracked Ultrasound with Anser Electromagnetic Tracking

Alfred Michael Franz[1,4], Herman Alexander Jaeger[2], Alexander Seitel[4],
Pádraig Cantillon-Murphy[2,3], Lena Maier-Hein[4]

[1]Institute for Computer Science, Ulm University of Applied Sciences, Ulm, Germany
[2]University College Cork, Cork, Ireland
[3]Tyndall National Institute, Dyke Parade, Cork, Ireland
[4]Division of Computer Assisted Medical Interventions, German Cancer Research
Center (DKFZ), Heidelberg, Germany
franz@hs-ulm.de

Abstract. Image-guided interventions (IGT) have shown a huge potential to improve medical procedures or even allow for new treatment options. Most ultrasound(US)-based IGT systems use electromagnetic (EM) tracking for localizing US probes and instruments. However, EM tracking is not always reliable in clinical settings because the EM field can be disturbed by medical equipment. So far, most researchers used and studied commercial EM trackers with their IGT systems which in turn limited the possibilities to customize the trackers in order minimize distortions and make the systems robust for clinical use. In light of current good scientific practice initiatives that increasingly request research to publish the source code corresponding to a paper, the aim of this work was to test the feasibility of using the open-source EM tracker (Anser EMT) for localizing US probes in a clinical US suite for the first time. The standardized protocol of Hummel et al. yielded a jitter of $0.1 \pm 0.1\,\text{mm}$ and a position error of $1.1 \pm 0.7\,\text{mm}$, which is comparable to $0.1\,\text{mm}$ and $1.0\,\text{mm}$ of a commercial NDI Aurora system. The rotation error of Anser EMT was $0.15 \pm 0.16°$, which is lower than at least $0.4°$ for the commercial tracker. We consider tracked US as feasible with Anser EMT if an accuracy of 1–$2\,\text{mm}$ is sufficient for a specific application.

1 Introduction

Promising contributions in the area of Image-guided interventions (IGT) [1] have shown a huge potential to improve medical outcome of existing procedures or allow for new treatment options by enhancing the information available during the intervention. If, for example, the pose of an ultrasound (US) probe can be determined accurately, conventional US images can be enhanced in different ways: (1) preoperative data can be visualized together with US images [2, 3], (2) instruments can be shown in relation to the US image [2], and (3) 2D US machines can record 3D images by combing 2D scans from different viewing angles [4]. If localization data is used to train neural networks, 3D US is later possible without a tracker [5].

Key component of many IGT systems is a tracking device, most frequently used for determining the pose of medical devices. Optical tracking allows for accurate localization [1], but requires a free line-of-sight (LoS) from a camera to optical markers which is cumbersome during freehand motion of a US probe. Electromagnetic (EM) trackers can localize small EM sensors in relation to a field generator (FG) without LoS [3]. Hence, most US-based IGT systems use EM tracking for localizing US probes (e.g., [2]). However, meanwhile it is apparent that EM tracking is not always reliable in clinical settings because the EM field can be disturbed, e.g. by medical devices or the patient stretcher [3]. To study these distortions, standardized assessment protocols for testing EM trackers in specific clinical environments with a maximum of comparability have been published [3, 6]. So far, most researchers used and studied commercial EM trackers with their IGT systems which in turn limited the possibilities to customize the trackers in order minimize distortions and make the systems robust for clinical use.

In parallel, recent discussions in the scientific community yielded the request to publish all source code of scientific results [7]. In the special case of IGT prototypes, this should at best include the source code for the tracking algorithms. In this regard, a welcome development is that open-source EM tracking systems have been published recently [8, 9] and enable researchers to develop IGT systems with open soft- and hardware. However, these systems have not been tested in a tracked US context so far and it remains unclear if tracking is accurate and robust in related clinical environments. In this study, we assess the feasibility of using the open-source EM tracker (Anser EMT) [9] for localizing US probes in a clinical US suite for the first time.

2 Materials and methods

2.1 Tracked ultrasound setup

Anser EMT is a open-source EM tracking platform for IGT [9]. Full system design schematics, instructions, and code can be accessed online[1]. The flat FG of Anser EMT creates a magnetic field in a working volume of 25 x 25 x 25 cm^3 and is capable of tracking up to 16 EM sensors in the latest version. In this study, a NDI 5-DOF sensor (Northern Digital, Waterloo, Canada, Model no. 610099) was used. It was fixed to a linear US probe (type L14-5w) of a Zonare ZS3 Ultrasound System (ZONARE Medical Systems, Mountain View, California) as shown in Fig. 1.

Anser EMT supports the OpenIGTLink [10] protocol for connection to open-source IGT toolkits. For this study, the Medical Imaging Interaction Toolkit (MITK) was connected to the system and the plugin Hummel Protocol Measurements[2] was used for further processing and evaluation of the data. All software

---

[1] http://openemt.org
[2] org.mitk.gui.qt.igt.app.hummelprotocolmeasurements

used for this project is available open-source under the link mentioned earlier and in the MITK repository[3].

2.2   Standardized assessment of tracked ultrasound

We used a standardized assessment protocol proposed by Hummel et al. [6] to assess our tracked US setup. 5 x 5 = 25 positional measurements were performed on a polycarbonate board (Hummel Board) in a known grid with 5 cm distances as shown in Fig. 1. Orientational measurements were done in 31 steps of 11.25° for a 360° rotation the middle of the board. For all positions, 150 measurement samples were recorded over 10 s at an update rate of 15 Hz.

The jitter error at one position was defined as the root mean square error of 150 samples. To determine positional accuracy, the Euclidean distances between two adjacent measured sensor locations, each averaged over 150 samples, were computed. The deviation to the reference of 5 cm was defined as distance error and determined for all 16 distance measurements (4 horizontal x 4 vertical) of the 5 x 5 grid. As another measure for positional accuracy, a grid matching error was determined. This error represents the fiducial registration error (FRE) obtained when matching the measured grid positions (n=25) to the grid of known reference positions with the optimal rigid transformation in a least square sense [11]. The angle differences between pairs of measured orientations and the known relative sensor rotation of 11.25° were determined to get the orientational errors.

The assessment of the tracked US with Anser EMT was performed in a clinical US suite of the German Cancer Research Center (DKFZ), as shown in Fig. 1. The Hummel Board was placed at a height of 11 cm above the FG on the patient stretcher. The FG was aligned in the middle of the covered volume.

---

[3] https://phabricator.mitk.org/source/mitk/

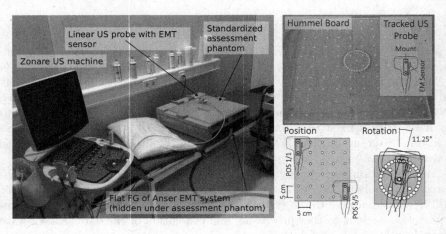

Fig. 1. Experimental setup in the US suite. A linear US probe is equipped with an EMT sensor and fixed on a special mount. The mount can be moved to known positions on the standardized assessment phantom (Hummel Board).

Table 1. Comparison to the NDI Aurora tracker in the US suite [12]. A subset of 4 x 3 = 12 positions and 180° of rotation measurements of the Anser EMT data was evaluated for this table to be comparable. Note, that the configuration of the field generator (FG) in [12] was different. We took the results from the bottom level of [12] which had a similar distance to patient stretcher and FG as in this study.

System	Setup	Field Generator	Prec.[mm]	Acc.[mm]	Rot_1[°]
Anser EMT	Tracked US	Flat FG (below)	0.07	1.11	0.1
Anser EMT	US Suite	Flat FG (below)	0.18	1.65	\<na\>
NDI Aurora	US Suite	Compact FG with US probe (above) [13]	0.09	1.03	0.4

For comparison, the position measurements were repeated in the same setup on the patient stretcher but without a US probe (US suite). In addition, reference data of comparable experiments (position and rotation) in a distortion-free lab environment (Lab ref) is available from a previous study [9].

3   Results

The precision (jitter error) was 0.1 ± 0.1 mm (Lab and Tracked US) and 0.2 ± 0.1 mm (US Suite) on average ($\mu \pm \sigma$, n=25 grid points) with a maximum error of 0.7 mm. The positional errors of the 5 cm distance measurements on the board in all setups are shown as boxplots in Fig. 2 and usually stay below 2 mm. The grid matching error was 1.5 mm (Lab), 2.2 mm (US suite) and 2.9 mm (Tracked US). The average sensor locations in the tracked US setup are visualized in Fig. 3. Orientation measurements yielded an error of $0.15 \pm 0.16°$ (n=31) in the tracked US setup which was increased by around 0.1° compared to reference measurement ($0.04 \pm 0.02°$ [9]). All measurements taken in this study are provided open data in the Open Science Framework[4] together with comparative data sets of other trackers.

4   Discussion

The jitter error of 0.1 ± 0.1 mm and the position error of 1.1 ± 0.7 mm is comparable to 0.1 mm jitter and 1.0 mm position error of a commercial tracker (NDI Aurora) in the same environment [12] as shown in Tab. 1. As for the measurements in a laboratory environment in an earlier study [9], the rotational errors of

---

[4] https://osf.io/aphzv/

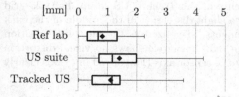

Fig. 2. Relative position errors of 4 x 4 = 16 measured 5 cm distances illustrated as box-whiskers plots. The diamonds show the mean values, the whiskers the minimum and maximum values.

Anser EMT are also small, below 0.3° in our measurements, which is better than published results of other trackers (e.g., at least 0.4° [12], but up to 3° [13] for a NDI Aurora system). When looking at the grid matching error, we see a slight drop in accuracy between US suite (2.2 mm) and Tracked US (2.9 mm). This is not reflected by the 5 cm distance evaluation, where the median error is similar in both setups (1.2 mm). If only distances between pairs of points are evaluated, slight field distortions as we see in the back row of the position measurements (Fig. 3) can have little effect on the metric, but matching the whole grid can reveal these distortions. Therefore, we propose to always have a look at both metrics, and also at the raw data points, when interpreting Hummel protocol results.

Most errors are relatively small, which is good for the system, but raises the question if manual measurements are accurate enough to determine its limits in accuracy. In an earlier study a reference measurement was repeated three times to analyze reproducibility [13]. The average 5 cm distance error measured was in the range of 0.3-0.5 mm. In case of this study, the difference between the average errors in the US suite (1.4 mm) and Tracked US (1.1 mm) setup, as shown in Fig. 2, might be caused by the natural variation of manual measurements. However, the results still show, that the errors stay below 1 to 2 mm in most of the cases and demonstrate a high accuracy for the tracked US setup.

We used a 5 DoF sensor for our experiments. Depending on the application, 6 DoF of the probe are required. In this case either a second 5 DoF sensor or a slightly bigger 6 DoF sensor can be used. According to our experience with EM trackers, it is unlikely that a second or different sensor would affect tracking accuracy or robustness except for slight manufacturing tolerances.

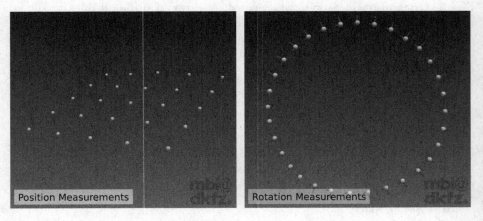

Fig. 3. 3D visualization of the measurements in the Tracked US setup. Left: 25 grid points of the position measurements. Only a slight distortion in the middle of the back row is visible. Right: 32 rotation measurements, visualized as the measured position together with the sensor coordinate axes in red. The circle shows no visual distortion of the measurements. Please note that only the sensor axis (longer red line) was clearly defined because a 5 DoF sensor was used.

All in all, although the positional error is slightly increased when tracking the US probe in the US suite, we consider tracked US as feasible with the Anser EMT system if an accuracy of 1-2 mm is sufficient for a specific application.

Acknowledgement. This work was supported by the European Union through the ERC starting Grant COMBIOSCOPY (ERC-2015-StG-37960) and by the Irish Health Research Board (POR/2012/31), Science Foundation Ireland (15/TIDA/2846). We acknowledge the German Cancer Research Center (DKFZ), Heidelberg, and the Institute of Image-Guided Surgery (IHU), Strasbourg for supporting this work.

References

1. Cleary K, Peters TM. Image-guided interventions: technology review and clinical applications. Annu Rev Biomed Eng. 2010;12:119–142.
2. Tomonari A, Tsuji K, Yamazaki H, et al. Feasibility of the virtual needle tracking system for percutaneous radiofrequency ablation of hepatocellular carcinoma. Hepatol Res. 2013;43(12):1352–1355.
3. Franz AM, Haidegger T, Birkfellner W, et al. Electromagnetic tracking in medicine: a review of technology, validation and applications. IEEE Trans Med Imaging. 2014;33(8):1702–1725.
4. Mercier L, Langø T, Lindseth F, et al. A review of calibration techniques for freehand 3-D ultrasound systems. Ultrasound Med Biol. 2005;31(4):449–471.
5. Prevost R, Salehi M, Sprung J, et al. Deep learning for sensorless 3D freehand ultrasound imaging. Proc MICCAI. 2017; p. 628–636.
6. Hummel JB, Bax MR, Figl ML, et al. Design and application of an assessment protocol for electromagnetic tracking systems. Med Phys. 2005;32(7):2371–2379.
7. Ince DC, Hatton L, Graham-Cumming J. The case for open computer programs. Nature. 2012;482:482–485.
8. Li M, Bien T, Rose G. Construction of a conductive distortion reduced electromagnetic tracking system for computer assisted image-guided interventions. Med Eng Phys. 2014;36(11):1496–1501.
9. Jaeger HA, Franz AM, O'Donoghue K, et al. Anser EMT: the first open-source electromagnetic tracking platform for image-guided interventions. Int J Comput Assist Radiol Surg. 2017;12(6):1059–1067.
10. Tokuda J, Fischer GS, Papademetris X, et al. OpenIGTLink: an open network protocol for image-guided therapy environment. Int J Med Robot. 2009;5(4):423–434.
11. Horn BKP. Closed-form solution of absolute orientation using unit quaternions. J Opt Soc Am A. 1987;4(4):629–642.
12. Franz AM, Marz K, Seitel A, et al. Combined modality for ultrasound imaging and electromagnetic tracking. Biomed Tech (Berl). 2013;.
13. Franz AM, Marz K, Hummel J, et al. Electromagnetic tracking for US-guided interventions: standardized assessment of a new compact field generator. Int J Comput Assist Radiol Surg. 2012;7(6):813–818.

Navigierte Interventionen im Kopf- und Halsbereich
Standardisiertes Assessment eines neuen, handlichen Feldgenerators

Benjamin J. Mittmann[1,3], Alexander Seitel[3], Lena Maier-Hein[3], Alfred M. Franz[2,3]

[1] Institut für Medizintechnik und Mechatronik, Hochschule Ulm
[2] Institut für Informatik, Hochschule Ulm
[3] Abteilung Computer-assistierte Medizinische Interventionen, DKFZ Heidelberg
mittmann@mail.hs-ulm.de

Kurzfassung. Elektromagnetische (EM) Trackingsysteme verwenden zur von OP-Instrumenten am Eingriffsort ein EM Feld, das von einem Feldgenerator (FG) erzeugt wird. Üblicherweise sind die FG umso größer, je höher die Reichweite ihres Trackingvolumens ist. Der kürzlich von der Firma NDI (Northern Digital Inc., Waterloo, ON, Canada) vorgestellte Planar 10-11 FG vereint erstmals eine kompakte Bauweise und ein dazu verhältnismäßig großes Trackingvolumen. Mit einem standardisierten Messprotokoll wurde der FG auf seine Robustheit gegenüber externen Störquellen und seine Genauigkeit geprüft. Die mittlere Positionsgenauigkeit beträgt 0,59 mm (Standard-Setup) bei einem mittleren Jitter von 0,26 mm. Der mittlere Orientierungsfehler fällt mit 0,10° sehr gering aus. Der höchste durch ein Metall verursachte Positionsfehler (4,82 mm) wird von Stahl SST 303 hervorgerufen. Bei Stahl SST 416 ist der Positionsfehler (0,10 mm) am geringsten. Im Vergleich zu zwei anderen FG von NDI erreicht der Planar 10-11 FG tendenziell bessere Genauigkeitsergebnisse. Wegen seiner Kompaktheit und der damit verbundenen mobilen Einsatzfähigkeit könnte der FG daher dazu beitragen, den Gebrauch von EM Trackingsystemen in der Klinik zu steigern.

1 Einleitung

Bei medizinischen Interventionen spielt die Beachtung angrenzender Risikostrukturen allgemein eine bedeutende Rolle. Durch den Einsatz sogenannter intraoperativer Trackingsysteme (IOT) kann die Wahrscheinlichkeit, eine Risikostruktur ungewollt zu verletzen, minimiert werden. Sie ermöglichen eine genaue von OP-Instrumenten am Eingriffsort und bieten dem Operateur visuelle Hilfestellungen durch Augmented-Reality-Darstellungen. In der Neurochirurgie, einem Gebiet, das besondere Präzision vom Operateur verlangt, kommen IOT standardmäßig zum Einsatz [1]. In vielen anderen Fachbereichen hingegen hat sich der Routineeinsatz von IOT im Klinikalltag bislang nicht durchgesetzt.

Wie Studien der vergangenen Jahre belegen, könnten insbesondere minimalinvasive Eingriffe im Hals- und Kopfbereich künftig von IOT profitieren. Beispiele hierfür sind perkutane Punktionen wie die Punktion von Knoten innerhalb der Schilddrüse [2], endoskopische Interventionen wie die Endoskop-geführte Nasennebenhöhlenchirurgie [3] oder Kathetereingriffe wie die Thrombektomie zur Behandlung eines akuten Schlaganfalls. In der aktuellen Forschung zur Thrombektomie wird darauf verwiesen, dass ein des Katheters helfen könnte, die Reperfusion der Arterien früher zu ermöglichen [4].

Die zur von OP-Instrumenten notwendige Positionsbestimmung der Instrumente erfolgt in der Regel durch ein optisches System (Optisches Tracking) oder durch ein elektromagnetisches (EM) System [5]. Optische Tra-ckingsysteme bieten den Vorteil hoher Positionsgenauigkeit. Allerdings ist zur Positionsbestimmung eine durchgängige Sichtlinie (Line-Of-Sight) des optischen Trackers zum getrackten Objekt notwendig. EM Trackingsysteme benötigen keine Line-Of-Sight und können daher potentiell bei perkutanen oder endoskopischen Eingriffen eingesetzt werden. Sie weisen allerdings eine schlechtere Posi-tionsgenauigkeit auf verglichen mit den optischen Systemen [6]. Für elektromagnetische Trackingsysteme wird ein Feldgenerator (FG) benötigt, der im Raum ein EM Feld erzeugt, in dem EM Sensoren lokalisiert werden können. Das Raumvolumen, in dem die von EM Sensoren möglich ist, bezeichnet man als Trackingvolumen. Üblicherweise nehmen die Größenabmessungen der FG mit der Größe und Reichweite des Trackingvolumens zu. Je größer der FG ist, umso höher ist der Installationsaufwand in der Klinik und umso höher sind die Installationskosten. Dieser Sachverhalt stellt hinsichtlich der praktischen Anwendbarkeit von EM Trackingsystemen im Klinikalltag bis heute ein Problem dar. Ein anderes bekanntes Problem von EM Trackingsystemen ist die mangelnde Robustheit gegenüber externen Störquellen, die das EM Feld des FG verzerren. Eine nahe Platzierung des FG am Zielbereich kann aber die Robustheit des Systems steigern [7]. Solch eine nahe Platzierung ist häufig jedoch nur mit FG kompakter Bauweise realisierbar.

Kürzlich stellte die Firma NDI den neuen Planar 10-11 FG vor. Er vereint erstmals eine kompakte Bauweise (112 mm x 97 mm x 31 mm) und ein dazu verhältnismäßig großes, zylinderförmiges Trackingvolumen (Durchmesser: 340 mm, Höhe: 340 mm). Durch die damit verbundene mobile Einsatzfähigkeit könnte der FG neue Bereiche im klinischen Einsatzgebiet der EM Trackingtechnologie eröffnen. Wie in Abb. 1 skizziert ist, ließe sich der FG z.B. in ein Vakuumkissen integrieren, auf das der Patient seinen Kopf oder seinen Nacken legt. Durch den geringen Abstand des FG zum Kopf befindet sich der gesamte Kopf des Patienten im Trackingvolumen des FG.

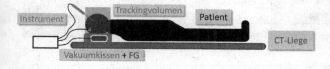

Abb. 1. Einfaches klinisches Setup für Interventionen im Kopf- und Halsbereich: Der FG ist in ein Vakuumkissen integriert und unterhalb des Patientenkopfes positioniert.

Es soll nun untersucht werden, ob der Planar 10-11 FG trotz seines relativ großen Trackingvolumens eine vergleichbar hohe Trackinggenauigkeit aufweist, wie andere FG mit ähnlich großen Trackingvolumina. Von Interesse ist dabei auch die Robustheit des FG in Bezug auf Metalle medizinischer Instrumente, da sie die Messgenauigkeit negativ beeinflussen können.

2   Methoden

Zur messtechnischen Bewertung des Planar 10-11 FG wurde das standardisierte Messprotokoll von Hummel et al. [8] verwendet. Um die Vergleichbarkeit der Messergebnisse mit früheren Messungen anderer FG zu gewährleisten, orientierten wir uns an den in [7] geschilderten Versuchsaufbauten – dem Standard-Setup, bei dem der FG seitlich von der Hummel-Messplatte befestigt ist, und dem Mobile-Setup, bei dem der FG mittig über der Messplatte platziert wird (Abb. 2). In beiden Setups erfolgten sowohl Positions- als auch Rotationsmessungen. Hierzu wurde der 6DOF Cable Tool; 2,5 mm x 11 mm von NDI an definierten Positionen auf der Messplatte platziert wie in Abb. 3 veranschaulicht. Für jede Messposition wurden 150 Messwerte innerhalb von 10 Sekunden mit einer Updaterate von 15 Hz aufgezeichnet. Die Wurzel aus den mittleren quadratischen Abweichungen (RMSE) der 150 Messwerte wurde als Jitter definiert. Die Positionsgenauigkeit ermittelten wir mit Hilfe des Mittelwerts der betragsmäßigen Differenzen zwischen den berechneten mittleren euklidischen Distanzen und der real vorliegenden Distanz (5 cm) direkt benachbarter Sensorpositionen innerhalb des (3 × 4)-Gitters beim Mobile-Setup bzw. des (5 × 6)-Gitters beim Standard-Setup. Die Wahl der Gittergröße erfolgte beim Standard-Setup entsprechend der Größe des Trackingvolumens. Beim Mobile-Setup orientierten wir uns an der Gittergröße vorheriger Studien zum Compact FG von NDI [7]. Die Positionsmessungen erfolgten für beide Setups auf drei verschiedenen Ebenen (unten, mitte, oben; Ebenenabstand: 5 cm). Den Orientierungsfehler berechneten wir anhand der Winkeldifferenz zwischen Paaren von 32 gemessenen Orientierungen und der bekannten relativen Sensorrotation in Höhe von 11,25°. Im Mobile-Setup erfolgten in gleicher Weise wie in [8] Metallmessungen mit vier

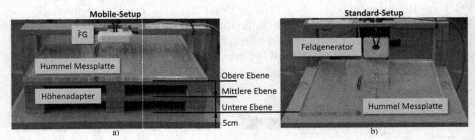

Abb. 2. a) Versuchsaufbau beim Mobile-Setup für Messungen der oberen Ebene. Der FG ist mittig über der Messplatte montiert. b) Versuchsaufbau beim Standard-Setup für Messungen der unteren Ebene. Der FG ist seitlich von der Messplatte befestigt.

verschiedenen Metallen: Stahl SST 303, Stahl SST 416, Bronze und Aluminium. Dabei wurden die Metalle nacheinander in fünf definierten Höhen H1 – H5 im EM Feld des FG platziert und die Position des fixierten EM Sensors bestimmt (Abb. 3c). Anhand der Abweichung zur Referenzposition des Sensors konnte dann der Einfluss des Metalls auf die Messgenauigkeit bestimmt werden.

Zur Untersuchung eines sehr kleinen Mikrosensors, der in Instrumente wie Nadeln integriert werden kann, erfolgten mit dem Micro 6DOF Sensor (0,8 mm × 9,0 mm) von NDI zum Vergleich auf der mittleren Ebene im Standard-Setup Positions- und Rotationsmessungen entsprechend Abb. 3.

3   Ergebnisse

Die Ergebnisse zu den Positions- und Metallmessungen mit dem Cable Tool sind in Abb. 4 dargestellt. Der mittlere Jitter beträgt im Mobile-Setup 0,03 mm und im Standard-Setup 0,26 mm. Im Mobile-Setup beträgt die mittlere Positionsgenauigkeit 0,16 mm und im Standard-Setup 0,59 mm. Der durch ein Metall verursachte Positionsfehler ist tendenziell umso größer, je näher das Metall am FG platziert ist. Die größte Abweichung von der Referenzposition wird durch Stahl SST 303 hervorgerufen (4,82 mm). Bei Stahl SST 416 hingegen fällt die Abweichung am geringsten aus (0,10 mm).

Die Orientierungsfehler betragen im Mobile-Setup 0,04° | 0,05° | 0,22° für ROT_1 | ROT_2 | ROT_3 und im Standard-Setup 0,15° | 0,08° | 0,06°.

Die Ergebnisse der Vergleichsmessungen mit dem Mikrosensor fallen in allen Kategorien schlechter aus. Im Standard-Setup (mittlere Ebene) liegt der Jitter

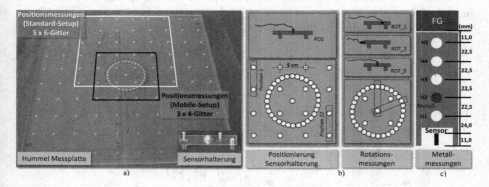

Abb. 3. a) Messplatte nach Hummel et al. [8]. Eingezeichnet sind die zwei Bereiche, in denen der EM Sensor mit Hilfe der Sensorhalterung für die Positionsmessungen platziert wurde im Abstand von je 5 cm. Für die Rotationsmessungen im Standard-Setup wurde der FG seitlich am oberen Rand des (3 × 4)–Gitters platziert. b) Sensormontage an der Sensorhalterung für die Positions- und Rotationsmessungen. Der abgebildete Kreis umfasst 32 Messpositionen mit einem Winkelabstand von je 11,25°. c) Mit Hilfe einer hölzernen Halterung werden 4 verschiedene Metalle nacheinander in den Höhen H1 – H5 im EM Feld des FG platziert und die Position des Sensors ermittelt.

bei 0,35 mm und der Positionsfehler bei 0,90 mm. Der mittlere Orientierungsfehler von ROT_1, ROT_2 und ROT_3 beläuft sich im Standard-Setup auf $0,57°$.

Die Rohdaten aller Messungen und die verwendete Software zur Auswertung der Messdaten sind frei zugänglich [1].

4   Diskussion

Der Planar 10-11 FG wurde mit einem standardisierten Messprotokoll auf seine Genauigkeit und Robustheit geprüft. Die Auswertungsergebnisse belegen, dass der FG trotz des relativ großen Trackingvolumens in störungsfreier Umgebung EM mit Submillimeter-Genauigkeit ermöglicht.

Im Gegensatz zum Mobile-Setup reichen im Standard-Setup die Messpositionen bis an den Rand des Trackingvolumens. Da im Standard-Setu sowohl der Jitter als auch der Positionsfehler höher ausfallen als im Mobile-Setup, ist davon auszugehen, dass die Messgenauigkeit des FG zum Rand des Trackingvolumens hin abnimmt. Dieses Verhalten konnten wir besonders rechts unten an der Eckposition des (5×6)-Gitters feststellen (Abb. 3). Hier detektierten wir auf der oberen Ebene einen einzelnen Ausreißer mit einem Positionsfehler von 7,16 mm.

Aus früheren Studien [7, 8, 9] ist bekannt, dass EM Trackingsysteme anfällig gegenüber externen Störquellen sind. Auch beim Planar 10-11 FG wird der Messfehler durch metallische Störquellen erhöht. Ein quadratischer Zusammenhang zwischen der Entfernung des Metalls zum FG und dem Positionsfehler kann angenommen werden (Abb. 4c).

Mit dem Mikrosensor erhielten wir ungenauere Messergebnisse im Vergleich zum Cable Tool-Sensor. Das betraf besonders die Rotationsmessungen, bei denen einzelne Orientierungsfehler von bis zu $8°$ registriert werden konnten. Die Messgenauigkeit hängt daher nicht allein vom FG und externen Störquellen ab. Sie

---

[1] https://osf.io/aphzv/

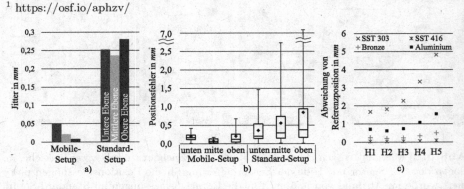

Abb. 4. Ergebnisse zum 6DOF Cable Tool-Sensor: a) Mittlere Jitter im Mobile- und Standard-Setup. b) Positionsfehler dargestellt als Box-Plots. Die Rauten zeigen den Mittelwert, die Whisker den min. bzw. max. Fehlerwert. Der Positionsfehler ist definiert als Mittelwert der n Differenzen zwischen den gemessenen Distanzen und der bekannten 5 cm Referenzdistanz mit n = 17 (Mobile-Setup) bzw. n = 49 (Standard-Setup). c) Positionsfehler durch metallische Zylinder zwischen FG und EM Sensor.

wird auch vom verwendeten EM beeinflusst. Obwohl immer kleinere Mikrosensoren im Submillimeterbereich (0,3 mm) hergestellt werden können [9], sollte es daher bei der Planung navigierter medizinischer Interventionen stets zu einer Abwägung kommen zwischen den vielfältigeren Einsatzmöglichkeiten der Mikrosensoren und der für den Eingriff erforderlichen Trackinggenauigkeit.

Vergleichbare Messungen von Maier-Hein et al. [7] mit dem Planar FG, im Folgenden als Standard FG bezeichnet, und dem Compact FG von NDI ergaben tendenziell schlechtere Genauigkeitsergebnisse. Unter Laborbedingungen beträgt der mittlere Jitter des Compact FG 0,05 mm. Er ist damit etwa doppelt so groß wie der Vergleichswert des Planar 10-11 FG. Der mittlere Jitter des Standard FG fällt mit 0,2 mm etwas kleiner aus als der Jitter des Planar 10-11 FG. Sowohl der Positionsfehler als auch der Orientierungsfehler des Planar 10-11 FG sind verglichen mit den beiden anderen FG deutlich kleiner (z.B. Positionsfehler im Mobile-Setup: Faktor 3,13 kleiner).

Das in Abb. 1 vorgestellte einfache Setup erleichtert die praktische Anwendbarkeit von EM Trackingsystemen im Klinikalltag. In Kombination mit seiner guten Trackinggenauigkeit könnte der Planar 10-11 FG daher aus unserer Sicht dazu beitragen, den Einsatz von IOT in der Klinik zu steigern.

Danksagung. Das Projekt wurde vom Deutschen Zentrum für Luft- und Raumfahrt (DLR) finanziert (Projekt OP 4.1). Herzlichen Dank an die NDI Europe GmbH (Radolfzell, Deutschland) für die Bereitstellung des Feldgenerators.

Literaturverzeichnis

1. Chartrain AG, Kellner CP, Fargen KM, et al. A review and comparison of three neuronavigation systems for minimally invasive intracerebral hemorrhage evacuation. J Neurointerv Surg. 2018;10(1):66–74.
2. Turtulici G, Orlandi D, Corazza A, et al. Percutaneous radiofrequency ablation of benign thyroid nodules assisted by a virtual needle tracking system. Ultrasound Med Biol. 2014;40(7):1447–1452.
3. Irugu DVK, Stammberger HR. A note on the technical aspects and evaluation of the role of navigation system in endoscopic endonasal surgeries. Indian J Otolaryngol Head Neck Surg. 2014 Jan;66(1):307–313.
4. Yoo AJ, Tommy A. Thrombectomy in acute ischemic stroke: challenges to procedural success. J Stroke. 2017;19(2):121–130.
5. Peters T, editor. Image-Guided Interventions. Springer–Verlag, Berlin; 2008.
6. Franz AM, Haidegger T, Birkfellner W, et al. Electromagnetic tracking in medicine: a review of technology, validation, and applications. IEEE Trans Med Imaging. 2014 Aug;33(8):1702–1725.
7. Maier-Hein L, Franz AM, Birkfellner W, et al. Standardized assessment of new electromagnetic field generators in an interventional radiology setting. Med Phys. 2012;39(6):3424–3434.
8. Hummel JB, Bax MR, Figl ML, et al. Design and application of an assessment protocol for electromagnetic tracking systems. Med Phys. 2005;32(7):2371–2379.
9. Yaniv Z, Wilson E, Lindisch D, et al. Electromagnetic tracking in the clinical environment. Med Phys. 2009;36:876–892.

Abstract: Multispectral Imaging Enables Visualization of Spreading Depolarizations in Gyrencephalic Brain

Leonardo Ayala[1,2,3], SJ Wirkert[1], MA Herrera[3], Adrián Hernández-Aguilera[3], AS Vermuri[1], E Santos[3], L Maier-Hein[1,2]

[1]Division of Computer Assisted Medical Interventions, German Cancer Research Center, Heidelberg, Germany.
[2]Medical Faculty, University of Heidelberg, Heidelberg, Germany.
[3]Department of Neurosurgery, Heidelberg University Hospital, Heidelberg, Germany.
l.menjivar@dkfz-heidelberg.de

Spreading Depolarization (SD) is a phenomenon in the brain related to the abrupt depolarization of neurons in gray matter which results from a break-down of ion gradients across the neuron membrane and propagates like a wave of ischemia. While modulating the hemodynamic response of the SDs is a therapeutic target, the lack of imaging methods that allow for monitoring SDs with high spatiotemporal resolution hinder progress in the field. In this work, we address this bottleneck with a new method for brain imaging based on multispectral imaging (MSI). Our approach to visualizing SDs uses a machine learning-based algorithm for estimation of tissue oxygenation using MSI data acquired from the brain. Due to the lack of a gold standard method for measuring oxygen saturation in tissue, training a machine learning-based algorithm is not straightforward in this scenario. The proposed method tackles this problem with *in silico* training data, with the generated spectral reflectances covering a wide range of spectra that can be observed in vivo [1]. To validate our methodology in an initial feasibility study, we used a swine model of SD. A craniotomy exposed the parietal cortex, and SDs were induced using 2-5 μL KCl drops placed in regions selected by visual inspection in the parietal cortex. SDs were continuously monitored with two ECoG recording strips that were placed on the lateral margins of the craniotomy. Our new approach to oxygenation estimation based on MSI was successfully applied to visualize the SDs in the gyrencephalic brain. As it has the potential to monitor SDs with high spatio-temporal resolution without a complex hardware setup, this tool could be used in studies of new treatment strategies and development of drugs that can target the hemodynamic response of the SDs.

References

1. Wirkert SJ, Vemuri AS, Kenngott HG, et al. Physiological parameter estimation from multispectral images unleashed. Proc MICCAI. 2017;1:134–141.

Combining Ultrasound and X-Ray Imaging for Mammography
A Prototype Design

Qiuting Li[1,2], Christoph Luckner[1,2], Madeleine Hertel[2], Marcus Radicke[2], Andreas Maier[1]

[1]Pattern Recognition Lab, Friedrich-Alexander-Universität Erlangen-Nürnberg, Germany
[2]Siemens Healthcare GmbH, Forchheim, Germany
qiutingli.deu@gmail.com

Abstract. This study aims at the combination of 3D breast ultrasound and 2D mammography images to improve the accuracy of diagnosis of breast cancer. It was shown that ultrasound breast imaging has advantages for differentiating cysts and solid masses which are not visible in an X-ray image. Moreover, the specificity in X-ray imaging decreases with an increasing breast thickness, so that ultrasound is usually used as an adjunct to X-ray breast imaging. A fully automatic system to obtain both 2D mammography and 3D ultrasound images is used. The alignment of a 2D mammography image in the cone-beam coordinate system and 3D ultrasound image in a Cartesian coordinate system is the essential task in this study. We have shown that deviations up to 23 mm caused by the cone-beam system can be calculated and corrected utilizing the geometry information of the hardware. The multimodal image reading tool is presented in a GUI for clinical diagnosis. The presented setup might lead to a distinct improvement in efficiency and add diagnostic value to the acquisition.

1 Introduction

Breast cancer is the most common cancer of women and accounts for 25% of all cancers worldwide. In 2012, about 1.7 million women were diagnosed with breast cancer and about half a million women died because of it [1]. X-ray imaging, including mammography, plays an essential role for breast lesion detection and is currently the only medical modality for screening purposes [2]. If a woman has a very dense breast it is difficult to detect malignant masses even in high-quality mammograms. However, it has already been shown that breast ultrasound can detect most solid masses which are non-palpable and invisible in mammography [3]. In this work, we present an image reading tool for a hardware prototype, introduced in [4] and [5], which aims at improving the accuracy and efficiency of breast screening diagnosis and the detection of lesions.

2   Methods and materials

2.1   Hardware prototype

As can be seen in the schematic drawing in Fig. 1 an ultrasound transducer is mounted on top of the compression paddle. The mammography unit is a MAM-MOMAT Inspiration (SIEMENS Healthcare GmbH). To allow the penetration of the ultrasound lotion, a special kind of gauze is used instead of the original compression plate. The X-ray acquisition is performed first, followed by an automatically executed ultrasound scan. This workflow has the advantage that patients do not have to be transferred to a different location in order to receive an additional ultrasound acquisition. Furthermore, as the patient does not move between the two subsequent scans, the multimodal images (X-ray and US) are acquired in the same real-world coordinate system. This information will also be used for the geometric mapping between the different coordinate systems which is analyzed in section 2.3.

2.2   Software prototype

Fig. 2 illustrates the dedicated graphical user interface (GUI) which was designed to display the acquired images in an aggregated manner. In the top left corner, a 2D mammogram of a phantom is shown. On the right side, the xy-plane (top) and the xz-plane (bottom) of the 3D ultrasound volume of the same phantom is displayed. The 3D ultrasound image has the size of 722 * 691 * 443 in x, y, z-axis with the pixel spacing as 0.52/ 0.21/ 0.10 respectively. The red crosshairs indicate the currently selected location. After selecting a location in one of the images, the cursor automatically moves to the corresponding position in the other two images, taking also the cone-beam projection geometry of the X-ray image into account.

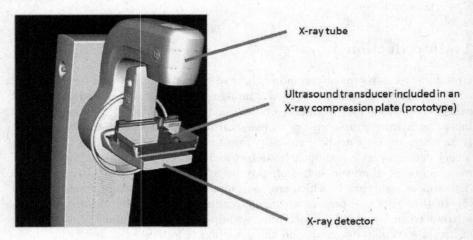

X-ray tube

Ultrasound transducer included in an X-ray compression plate (prototype)

X-ray detector

Fig. 1. Image of the hardware prototype [5] .

However, as the X-ray projection image contains only two-dimensional information the depth information is non-existent. This yields that the position in the xy-plane is correct, whereas the depth has to be obtained manually. This is usually done by scrolling through the US volume to find the correct slice which contains the lesion. To address this problem, a 2D resliced ultrasound image is created in order to connect the 2D X-ray image to the 3D ultrasound volume. Therefore, the beam path for the ray which corresponds to a clicked pixel using the underlying geometry information is computed. Then, a 2D plane coplanar withthe beam path is created and the US volume is resliced accordingly. Note that due to the reslicing process, the 2D ultrasound slice has a different pixel spacing than the original 3D ultrasound image. For the interpolation between adjacent voxels, a linear interpolation scheme is applied. In Fig. 3 an exemplary case is shown. The selected lesion is marked by a red cross and the corresponding resliced 2D plane is shown below. As can be seen in the lower image, the red line indicating the path of the X-ray beam intersects with the marked lesion which is highlighted by the yellow rectangle. Thus, this view enables to select the correct slice with just one additional click.

2.3   Geometric mapping

In a first step, the ultrasound image is aligned to mammogram geometrically, using the center lines of both images. This is sufficient since the ultrasound transducer is attached to the compression paddle, and thus the center line of both images (3D US and 2D mammogram) are at the same position, regardless of the projection geometry. In the subsequent step, we calculate the deviation between

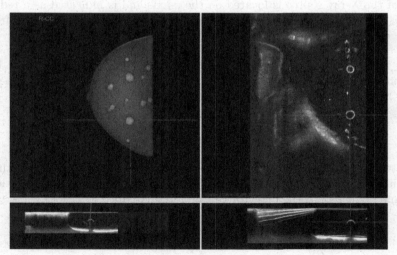

Fig. 2. Dedicated GUI, top left: 2D mammography image of a phantom, top right: 3D US image (xy-plane), bottom left: 2D resliced US intersection, and bottom right: 3D US image (xz-plane).

Fig. 3. 2D mammogram (top) and 2D resliced ultrasound image (bottom). The red cross indicates the selected lesion and the red line in the lower image the path of the X-ray beam. The yellow rectangle highlights the location of the lesion.

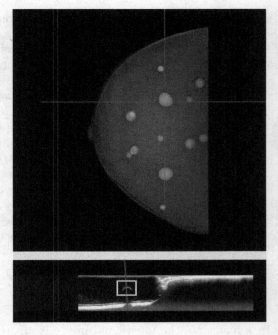

the parallel-beam projection of the US transducer and the cone-beam projection of the X-ray system. In Fig. 4 a schematic drawing representing the geometry of the presented prototype in the xz-plane is shown. For the sake of simplicity, we omit the y-coordinate for the derivation of the formulas in this paper. The focal point of the X-ray source is located on the z-axis and is indicated as a red dot. The distance between source and detector is denoted as SID. The cone-angle α can be computed as

$$\tan \alpha = \frac{x'}{z'} \tag{1}$$

Assuming that the detector lies within the plane $z = 0$, a ray intersecting a point $p(x', z')$ inside the breast is projected onto the detector at

$$\hat{p}_{\text{Xray}} = \begin{pmatrix} \tan \alpha \cdot \text{SID} \\ 0 \end{pmatrix} \tag{2}$$

In contrast to the cone-beam projection geometry of the X-ray system, the ultrasound device has a parallel-beam projection geometry, thus the projection of the same point p onto the detector can be formulated as

$$\hat{p}_{\text{US}} = \begin{pmatrix} x' \\ 0 \end{pmatrix} \tag{3}$$

It follows immediately, that there is a deviation Δx between the two projected points which can be evaluated with respect to the cone-angle α and point p

$$\Delta x = |\tan \alpha \cdot \text{SID} - x'| \tag{4}$$

Please note that we do not consider the impact of magnification as the distance between the object and detector is neglectable small compared to the SID.

3   Results

The value of the deviation caused by the cone-beam is affected by the distance between the point p and the vertical beam from the X-ray source (SID) as well as the height from point p to the X-ray detector. Tab. 1 shows the values of deviation for different cases. The SID of the prototype is 650 mm. In total, three different distance to center x' and two different local heights of the breast in equidistant spacing have been chosen to test according to the width of the test images and the height of the compressed breast phantom. Based on Fig. 4 it becomes clear that the deviation increases with bigger angles, higher local heights and longer distances to the center.

4   Conclusion

In this paper, we present a customized reading solution for a hardware prototype combining ultrasound and X-ray imaging which might be capable of accelerating the workflow speed and improving the diagnostic accuracy. A 2D X-ray image

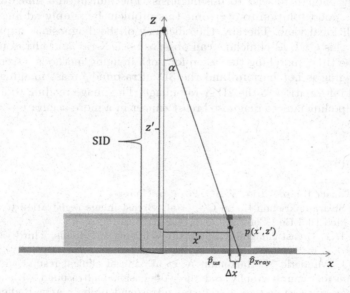

Fig. 4. Graphical representation of the cone-beam geometry. The compressed breast is indicated by the orange rectangle. The ultrasound transducer is shown as a small gray rectangle. Δx depicts the geometric deviation between a point p at the location that is projected onto the detector using a cone-beam projection geometry (mammogram) and a parallel-beam projection geometry (US).

Table 1. Overview about the deviation for various distances, angles and heights for a fixed SID = 650 mm and breast height = 100 mm. If not specified differently, the units in this table are given in mm.

Distance to center x'	Cone-angle α [°]	Local height SID$-z'$	Deviation Δx
50	4.4	50	3.8
100	8.7	50	7.7
150	13	50	11.5
50	5.1	100	7.7
100	10.2	100	15.4
150	15.1	100	23.1

acquired in cone-beam geometry should be linked to a Cartesian 3D-ultrasound volume. Therefore, the center lines of 3D US images and 2D X-ray images are aligned using prior knowledge about the hardware geometry. In the next step, the cone-beam deviation was calculated with given geometry information such that a pixel in the 3D ultrasound image can be matched correctly to the 2D cone-beam X-ray image.

In order to avoid scrolling through many slices an additional view is introduced. Deviations up to 23 mm and a slice thickness of 0.5 mm of the ultrasound images result in about 46 possible slices for the location of the lesion which is already big enough to lead to misdiagnosis. The multimodal image alignment is hereby a good solution to overcome this problem by simply adding one click in the additional view. Thereby, the efficiency of the diagnosis is improved distinctly by this GUI, as clinicians can observe both X-ray and ultrasound image at the same time, matching the lesion for both imaging methods. Overall, ultrasound imaging is not harmful and the 3D ultrasound breast imaging provides additional information to the 2D X-ray image. The image reading tool might be able to help clinicians to diagnose breast cancer in a more accurate and efficient way.

References

1. World Cancer Report 2014. WHO. 2014; p. Chapter 1.1.
2. Guo Y, Sivaramakrishna R, Lu CC, et al. Breast image registration techniques: a survey. Med Biol Eng Comput. 2006;44(1-2):15–26.
3. Kopans DB. Breast Imaging. Lippincott Williams & Wilkins, Third Ed. 2007; p. 555.
4. Emons J, Wunderle M, Hartmann A, et al. Initial clinical results with a fusion prototype for mammography and three-dimensional ultrasound with a standard mammography system and a standard ultrasound probe. Acta Radiol. 2018; p. 0284185118762249.
5. Schaefgen B, Heil J, Barr RG, et al. Initial results of the FUSION-X-US prototype combining 3D automated breast ultrasound and digital breast tomosynthesis. Eur Radiol. 2018;28(6):2499–2506.

Towards In-Vivo X-Ray Nanoscopy
Acquisition Parameters vs. Image Quality

Leonid Mill[1,6], Lasse Kling[2,5], Anika Grüneboom[3], Georg Schett[3],
Silke Christiansen[4,5], Andreas Maier[1]

[1]Pattern Recognition Lab, Friedrich-Alexander-University
Erlangen-Nuremberg, Erlangen
[2]Max Planck Institute for the Science of Light, Erlangen
[3]Department of Internal Medicine 3 and Institute for Clinical Immunology,
Friedrich-Alexander-University Erlangen-Nuremberg and University Hospital
Erlangen, Erlangen
[4]Freie Universität Berlin, Berlin
[5]Helmholtz Zentrum Berlin für Materialien und Energie, Berlin
[6]Institute of Optics, Information and Photonics, Friedrich-Alexander-University
Erlangen-Nuremberg, Erlangen
leonid.mill@fau.de

Abstract. X-ray microscopy is a powerful imaging technique that permits the investigation of specimen on nanoscale with resolution of up to 700 nm in 3-D. In the context of bio-medical research this is a promising technology that allows to study the microstructure of biological tissues. However, X-ray microscopy (XRM) systems are not designed for in-vivo applications and are mainly used in the field of material sciences in which dose is irrelevant. High resolution scans may take up to 10 hours. Our long-term goal is to utilize this modality to study the effects of disease dynamics and treatment in-vivo on mice bones. Therefore, a first step towards this ambitious goal is to evaluate the current state-of-the-art to determine the required system parameters. In this work, we investigate the impact of different XRM settings on the image quality. By changing various acquisition parameters such as exposure time, voltage, current and number of projections, we simulate the outcome of XRM scans, while reducing the X-ray energy. We base our simulations on a high resolution ex-vivo scan of a mouse tibia. The resulting reconstructions are evaluated qualitatively as well as quantitatively by calculating the contrast-to-noise ratio (CNR). We demonstrate that we can reach comparable image quality while reducing the total X-ray energy which forms a foundation towards the upcoming experiments.

1 Introduction

X-ray microscopy (XRM) is as a modality that is currently used mostly in the field of material sciences to study materials and and their composition such as alloys, batteries or integrated circuits [1]. The submicron resolution of up to 700 nm makes this technology also attractive for medical applications as the investigation of biological tissues such as bones. Yet, XRM systems are, in comparison to conventional computed tomography (CT) systems, not designed for in-vivo imaging. The small source-to-object distance, which produces a high energetic throughput, in combination with long acquisition times exceeds the bearable amount of dose for living animals as mice [2]. Stochastic effects would already emerge at a total body dose of 10 Gy [3]. Still, the high potential of these methods to monitor medication implied changes of tiny bone microstructures, makes in-vivo application of XRM systems worth investigating. Hence, methods that allow the reduction of the X-ray dose are essential.

Therefore, we first of all have to evaluate the suitability of such a system to perform long-term in-vivo studies and the hardware updates that are required to guarantee the survival of the animal. As Mill et al. [4] demonstrated using an in-vivo motion pattern, hardware modifications are needed in order to compensate for breathing motion and muscle relaxation. In this work, we investigate, how the XRM system parameters influence the reconstructed image quality, while reducing the emitted X-ray energy. Therefore, we conduct multiple simulations with various exposure times, voltages, currents, and number of projections, while the source-to-object distance remains constant. Subsequently, we evaluate the reconstruction results qualitatively as well as quantitatively using the CNR.

2   Materials and methods

2.1   X-ray physics and photon energy considerations

To simulate the image quality for different XRM parameter settings, we have to consider the underlying X-ray physics of such a system in order to determine the total energy and thus, the total number of photons that hit the detector. The total energy E_{total} that reaches the detector is [5, 6, 7]

$$E_{\text{total}} = \xi \cdot \overbrace{\underbrace{k \cdot U_A \cdot Z}_{\eta} \cdot \underbrace{I_A \cdot U_A}_{J_0}}^{J_{\text{source}}} \cdot t \cdot n \cdot e^{-x \cdot \mu} \tag{1}$$

where ξ describes the energy loss caused by the system including geometric properties and quantum efficiency of the scintillator and detector, η is the efficiency of the X-ray source with the constant $k = 1 \cdot 10^{-9} \ V^{-1}$, Z the atomic number of the anode material, J_0 the electrical power at the X-ray source consisting of the current I_A and voltage U_A, t the exposure time for a single projection, n the number of projections and $e^{-x \cdot \mu}$ the attenuation that is caused by the transmission X-ray source with target thickness x and linear attenuation μ. Thus, knowing the average kinetic energy E_{kin} of all X-ray photons, we can compute the number of photons N that enter the surface area of the detector

$$N = \frac{E_{\text{total}}}{E_{\text{kin}}} \tag{2}$$

2.2   Compressive sensing

Iterative regularized reconstruction is a common technique in medical imaging and allows for reduction of acquisition time, dose, and projections. The main idea, is to augment the reconstruction process by additional prior knowledge that is introduced using regularization techniques. A typical reconstruction is obtained by minimizing an energy function that is composed of a raw data error $||\boldsymbol{Ax} - \boldsymbol{p}||_2$ and a regularization term $R(\boldsymbol{x})$

$$\frac{1}{2}||\boldsymbol{Ax} - \boldsymbol{p}||_2^2 + \lambda R(\boldsymbol{x}) \tag{3}$$

where $\boldsymbol{x}$ is the reconstruction volume, $\boldsymbol{A}$ the projection operator, and $\boldsymbol{p}$ the projection data. In our experiments, we used a bilateral filter in every third iteration to approximate the effect of total variation regularization following the approach in [8].

2.3   Experimental setup

The base volume for the noise simulation is a high resolution reconstruction of a mouse tibia. The scan was performed ex-vivo using a Zeiss Xradia Versa 520 XRM with 2000 projections, a exposure time of 4 s per projection, and an angular increment of $0.18°$. The isotropic voxel size of the volume is 1.35 μm.

As Eq. 1 is just a coarse approximation of the system behavior, we adjusted the detection efficiency of the acquisition system such that the noise level of the simulated scan was matched to the noise level of the ex-vivo scan. The field of view (FOV) of all scans was 1 mm^3, the isotropic resolution of a voxel in the reconstructed volume was 1 μm. The source-to-object distance was kept constant with 11 mm. We used the open source reconstruction framework CONRAD [9] for all simulations. Noise simulation was performed assuming monochromatic X-rays as described in [10].

3   Results

Fig. 1 shows the simulation results for different settings of the XRM system with the ground truth (GT) (Fig. 1a) showing a detailed reconstruction of a mouse tibia. The associated simulation parameters are listed in Tab. 1. Changing the system parameters towards a faster acquisition time introduces noise and artifacts, which go along with a considerable decrease of the image quality (Fig. 1b). As a result, the microstructure of the bone disappears completely. However, in comparison to Fig. 1b, a considerable improvement of the image quality can be achieved while still reducing the total X-ray energy (Fig. 1c). This is a result of a decrease of the voltage U_A while subsequently increasing the current I_A. As a consequence, the total X-ray power remains nearly constant, while the faster acquisition time reduces the total X-ray energy. Furthermore, Compressive Sensing as reconstruction algorithm can lead to a even better image quality as shown in

(Fig. 1d) while using the same acquisition parameters as for the scan in Fig. 1c. Besides the qualitative evaluation, the images are compared using the CNR for a region of interest (ROI). It is calculated as follows

$$\text{CNR} = \frac{\mu}{\sigma} \qquad (4)$$

where μ is the mean value of the ROI and σ the standard deviation. Tab. 1 shows the acquisition parameters and the calculated CNR for each image. We obtain a CNR of 6.71 for the GT reference image compared to a CNR of 2.33 for Fig. 1b. As a result of the system parameter optimization, we achieve a CNR of 3.83 for Fig. 1c. Using Compressive Sensing as reconstruction algorithm results in a CNR value of 6.96 for Fig. 1d, which is comparable to the GT image quality.

4   Discussion

In this work, we evaluate the impact of different XRM system settings on the reconstructed image quality. Depending the chosen parameters, we compute the

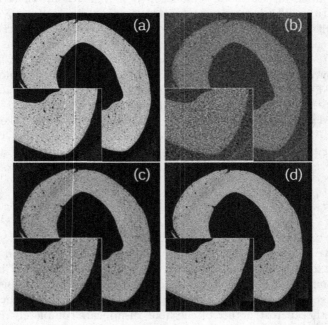

Fig. 1. Simulation results for different XRM parameter settings. The GT (a) image shows a detailed reconstruction of a mouse bone. A change of the system parameters towards a faster acquisition time introduces noise and artifacts that goes along with a decrease of the image quality (b). An optimized XRM setting leads to a considerable improvement of the image quality, while still remaining a lower X-ray energy (c). The reconstruction (d) shows a further reduction of noise using compressive sensing.

Table 1. Acquisition parameters and the CNR values for the associated reconstructions that are shown in Fig. 1.

Image	t [s]	I_A [μ A]	U_A [kV]	E_{kin} [keV]	n	E_{total} [mJ]	CNR
Fig. 1a	4	87	80	40	2000	429.48	6.71
Fig. 1b	0.4	87	80	40	1000	21.474	2.33
Fig. 1c	0.05	172	40	20	1000	2.523	3.83
Fig. 1d	0.05	172	40	20	1000	2.523	6.96

number of photons that reach the detector and by using the CONRAD software framework, we simulate the outcome of XRM scans while reducing the total X-ray energy. The simulations are performed such that the exposure time, voltage, current and number of projections are kept variable while parameters such as the source-to-object distance or the voxel size remain constant. The result of the simulation shows that a reduction of the acquisition time alone, introduces artifacts combined with a strong noise pattern which both result in a low image quality and a loss of the information about the bone's microstructure. Yet, an improved image quality can be achieved by optimizing the system parameters towards a higher CNR while still reducing the acquisition time and therefore the X-ray energy. This can be attained by decreasing the operating voltage U_A while subsequently increasing the current I_A. Although the total X-ray power J_{source} of the source remain nearly constant, a decrease of U_A also goes along with a decrease of the average kinetic energy E_{kin} of the photons. Since the linear attenuation coefficient μ of the object highly depends on the photon energy [7], a lower E_{kin} increases the attenuation of the object. As a consequence, on the one hand, more photons are absorbed by the object itself. Yet on the other hand, the proportion between absorbed and detected photons increases. Subsequently, this leads to a higher CNR while the further reduction of the exposure time goes along with a significant reduction of the total X-ray energy from 429.48 mJ for the GT scan to 2.523 mJ for the scan in Fig 1c. Additionally, by using Compressive Sensing as reconstruction algorithm, a resulting image quality with a CNR value of 6.96 can be achieved which is comparable to the image quality of the GT with a CNR value of 6.71.

In the context of in-vivo imaging using an XRM, where acquisition time and dose are crucial factors, the results presented in this work indicate that a sufficient image quality can be achieved by using optimized scanning parameters while reducing dose and time. However, the simulation in this work uses a coarse approximation of the system behavior by introducing a factor ξ in Eq. 1, which describes the energy loss caused by the system itself including the properties of the scintillator and detector. This factor was estimated by comparing the noise levels of the simulated reconstruction to the noise level of the ex-vivo scan. In addition, to determine optimal parameters that allow for in-vivo imaging, dose and its effects on the tissue has to be considered. Thus, dose computation and Monte-Carlo-Simulations will be subjects of our future work.

References

1. Englisch S, Wirth J, Schrenker N, et al. Mechanical failure of transparent flexible silver nanowire networks for solar cells using 3D X-ray nano tomography and electron microscopy. Microsc Microanal. 2018;24(S2):558–559.
2. Broerse JJ. Dose-mortality studies for mice irradiated with X-rays, gamma-rays and 15 MeV neutrons. Int J Radiat Biol Relat Stud Phys, Chem Med. 1969;15(2):115–124. Available from: https://doi.org/10.1080/09553006914550201.
3. Baker JE, Fish BL, Su J, et al. 10 Gy total body irradiation increases risk of coronary sclerosis, degeneration of heart structure and function in a rat model. Int J Radiat Biol. 2009;85(12):1089–1100.
4. Mill L, Bier B, Syben C, et al. Towards in-vivo X-ray nanoscopy. Proc BVM. 2018; p. 115–120.
5. Maier A, Steidl S, Christlein V, et al. Medical Imaging Systems: An Introductory Guide. Heidelberg, Berlin: Springer; 2018.
6. Dössel O. Bildgebende Verfahren in der Medizin. Heidelberg, Berlin: Springer; 2016.
7. Hubbell JH, Seltzer SM. Tables of X-ray mass attenuation coefficients and mass energy-absorption coefficients 1 keV to 20 MeV for elements Z= 1 to 92 and 48 additional substances of dosimetric interest. National Inst. of Standards and Technology-PL, Gaithersburg, MD (United States). Ionizing Radiation Div.; 1995.
8. Manhart M, Aichert A, Struffert T, et al. Denoising and artefact reduction in dynamic flat detector CT perfusion imaging using high speed acquisition: first experimental and clinical results. Phys Med Biol. 2014;59(16):4505–4524.
9. Maier A, Hofmann HG, Berger M, et al. CONRAD: a software framework for cone-beam imaging in radiology. Med Phys. 2013;40(11):111914–1–8.
10. Maier A, Fahrig R. GPU denoising for computed tomography. Graph Process Unit-Based High Perf Comput Radiat Ther. 2015;113.

Abstract: Beamforming Sub-Sampled Raw Ultrasound Data with DeepFormer

Walter Simson[1], Magdalini Paschali[1], Guillaume Zahnd[1], Nassir Navab[1,2]

[1]Computer Aided Medical Procedures, Technische Universität München, Germany
[2]Computer Aided Medical Procedures, Johns Hopkins University, USA
walter.simson@tum.de

Converting reflected sonic signals to an ultrasound image, beaforming, has been traditionally formulated mathematically via the simple process of delay and sum (DAS). Recent research has aimed to improve ultrasound beamforming via advanced mathematical models for increased contrast, resolution and speckle filtering. These formulations, such as minimum variance, add minor improvement over the current real-time, state-of-the-art DAS, while requiring drastically increased computational time and therefore excluding them from wide-spread adoption. Simultaneously, there is a parallel drive to increase ultrasound frame acquisition rates, for applications such as cardiac imaging, where high frame rates are required to accurately capture the complete subject motion.

In order to improve contrast, resolution and accuracy of reconstructed ultrasound images while increasing acquisition speed, a new paradigm, *Deep-Forming* [1], has been developed to leverage the strengths of deep learning for accelerated sub-sampled ultrasound reconstruction. In this novel work, a fully-convolutional neural network [2] trained with a composite loss of L_1 and $L_{\text{MS-SSIM}}$ [3], is utilized to map sub-sampled raw channel data from an ultrasound transducer to a fully sampled beamformed signal. Experiments were conducted on an in-vivo dataset of 19 participants including scans of a variety of anatomies. Results showed that all anatomies were successfully reconstructed by DeepFormer while using both sub- or fully-sampled raw data with a high relative structural similarity, suggesting that the lateral resolution of the reconstructed images can be maintained even with sparsely sampled channel data. The overall similarity between the reconstructed images and the ground truth for fully- and sub-sampled raw data remained similar with an SSIM of 0.5554 and 0.5550 respectively, highlighting the potential of DeepFormer to serve as a step towards arbitrary reconstruction based on sub-sampled raw ultrasound signals.

References

1. Simson W, Paschali M, Navab N, et al. Deep learning beamforming for sub-sampled ultrasound data. IEEE Int Ultrasonics Symp (IUS). 2018;.
2. Roy AG, Conjeti S, Navab N, et al. QuickNAT: segmenting MRI neuroanatomy in 20 seconds. ArXiv e-prints. 2018;ArXiv: 1801.04161.
3. Zhao H, Gallo O, Frosio I, et al. Loss functions for image restoration with neural networks. IEEE Trans Comput Imaging. 2017;3(1):47–57.

Shape Sensing with Fiber Bragg Grating Sensors
A Realistic Model of Curvature Interpolation for Shape Reconstruction

Sonja Jäckle[1], Jan Strehlow[2], Stefan Heldmann[1]

[1]Fraunhofer MEVIS, Lübeck
[2]Fraunhofer MEVIS, Bremen
sonja.jaeckle@mevis.fraunhofer.de

Abstract. Fiber optical sensors such as Fiber Bragg Grating (FBG) are more and more used for shape sensing of medical instruments. Estimating the shape via measured wavelengths is difficult and underlies a long pipeline of calculations with many different sources of errors. In this work we introduce a novel approach for more realistic interpolation of curvature used in subsequently applied reconstruction algorithms. We demonstrate and compare our method to others based on simulation of different types of shapes. Furthermore, we evaluated our approach in a real world experiment with measured FBGs data.

1 Introduction

In recent years, many Fiber Bragg Grating (FBG) based systems for estimating the shape of medical instruments, such as flexible needles, have been introduced [1, 2, 3]. FBGs are reflectors which are constructed as short segments of an optical fiber and are able to reflect a specific range of the incoming light. This property enables to measure mechanical strain and temperature changes [4]. Placing multiple FBGs at the same location allows to estimate curvature and direction angle. Most common systems use three fibers in a triplet configuration [1, 5, 6].

Shape reconstruction of flexible structures is challenging and various approaches have been proposed. The most common method is based on solving Frenet-Serret formulas [5, 7]. In [6] the reconstruction is build on piece-wise connecting circle segments, and in [8] an algorithm based on parallel transport is introduced. In general, reconstruction becomes difficult for bend shapes with high curvature and the accuracy of the reconstructed shape is poor.

All these approaches have the same assumption, that the sensor values are point-wise measurements. Thus, the spatial extent of FBGs is neglected and the curvature and direction angles are modeled as values of the FBG array center. Then the missing values are typically estimated by a linear or cubic interpolation.

For more accurate reconstruction, we present a novel approach that takes the spatial extent of the FBG into account and models the sensor values as averages of the sensor region. In the following, we describe the model of our interpolation approach, present results on simulated and real-world recorded data and compare our method with state-of-the-art cubic interpolation [2, 6].

2   Materials and methods

We consider a fiber system with n arrays of FBGs placed along the instrument. Each of these arrays contains three FBGs in a triplet configuration and a fourth FBG in the center. All FBGs have fixed length ℓ and the FBG arrays are uniformly distributed with center-to-center distance d. An illustration of a flexible instrument with a FBG system is shown in Fig. 1.

2.1   Shape reconstruction

Shape reconstruction is typically performed via the following steps:

1. For each FBG sensor the strain is determined by estimating the wavelength shift of the measured wavelength.
2. Using the strains of all FBGs, the curvature and direction angles can be computed for all arrays.
3. The missing curvatures and direction angles are determined by interpolation.
4. The shape is reconstructed with the obtained curvature and direction angles.

In this paper we focus on the third step. We introduce a novel approach that takes the FBG geometry into account for curvature interpolation. In the shape reconstruction step we follow the method introduced by Roesthuis et al. [5].

2.2   Averaging cubic interpolation

For curvature estimation and the interpolation step, respectively, we take the physical properties of a FBG into account: We assume n sensors with length ℓ

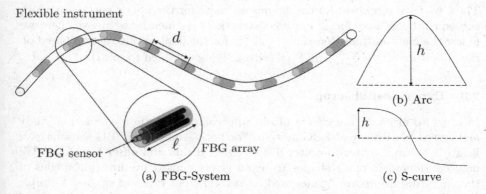

(a) FBG-System   (b) Arc   (c) S-curve

Fig. 1. Image (a) shows a FBG system of medical instrument with center-to-center distance d and sensor length l. Images (b) and (c) show sketches of the simulated shapes dependent on the height h.

that are equidistantly distributed along the fiber of length L with centers $t_i :=$ $t_0 + d \cdot i \in [\frac{\ell}{2}, L - \frac{\ell}{2}]$ $i = 0, \ldots, n-1$ and center-to-center distance $d = |t_{i+1} - t_i|$ Thus, we model the observed value C_i from ith sensor as an average, i.e

$$C_i = \frac{1}{\ell} \int_{t_i - \frac{\ell}{2}}^{t_i + \frac{\ell}{2}} c(t)\, dt \qquad (1)$$

where $c : [0, L] \to \mathbb{R}^+$ denotes the curvature of the fiber parameterized in arc length. Furthermore, we make the modeling assumption that the curvature c can be represented as a b-spline defined on the FBG centers, i.e $c(t) = \sum_{j=0}^{n-1} w_j S_j(t)$ with cubic b-splines $S_j(t) := S\left(\frac{t-t_0}{d} - j + 2\right)$, cubic b-spline basis

$$S(t) := \frac{1}{6} \begin{cases} t^3 & \text{if } t \in [0, 1[\\ -3t^3 + 12t^2 - 12t + 4 & \text{if } t \in [1, 2[\\ 3t^3 - 24t^2 + 60t - 44 & \text{if } t \in [2, 3[\\ (4 - t)^3 & \text{if } t \in [3, 4[\\ 0 & \text{else} \end{cases} \qquad (2)$$

and w_j are the corresponding weights. With (1) we get

$$C_i = \sum_{j=0}^{n-1} w_j I_{ij}, \text{ with } I_{ij} = \frac{1}{\ell} \int_{t_i - \frac{\ell}{2}}^{t_i + \frac{\ell}{2}} S_j(t)\, dt \qquad (3)$$

and the weights can be determined by solving the linear system

$$\begin{pmatrix} I_{00} & I_{01} & \cdots \\ I_{20} & \cdots & I_{n-2n-1} \\ \cdots & I_{n-1n-2} & I_{n-1n-1} \end{pmatrix} \begin{pmatrix} w_0 \\ \cdots \\ w_{n-1} \end{pmatrix} = \begin{pmatrix} C_0 \\ \cdots \\ C_{n-1} \end{pmatrix} \qquad (4)$$

Thus, we have established a continuous estimate for the fiber's curvature which subsequently is used for shape reconstruction. As mentioned above, here we follow the method from Roesthuis et al. [5] for the final reconstruction based on the curvature $c(t) = \sum_{j=0}^{n-1} w_j S_j(t)$ with weights obtained from (4).

2.3   Experimental setup

In order to evaluate the effects of our approach, we made a simulation study and tested it with a real FBG system. For both studies the FBG sensors have length $\ell = 5\,\text{mm}$ center-to-center distance $d = 10\,\text{mm}$ and offset $t_0 = 5\,\text{mm}$ We only considered in-plane shapes to avoid errors caused by direction angles of the curvature. Moreover, we focused on two different types of shapes: a simple arc 1(b) and a s-curve 1(c). For our simulations we generated the shape and then simulated a FBG system with 10 FBG arrays: we calculated the measured values of each FBG array by averaging the curvature over the length of the array and finally adding Gaussian noise. For both shapes we made measurements for different heights h as shown in Fig. 1. In the real experiment we used a fiber system with 3 fibers in a triplet configuration and one fiber at the center. It has 8 FBG arrays equally distributed over 80 mm so every 10 mm segment has one array in the center. We deformed the fiber to an arc and a s-curve, captured and annotated the shape with a camera, and compared the obtained ground truth to the reconstructed shape.

In both settings we compared our method with shape reconstruction using nearest neighbor interpolation, i.e. constant curvature over the 10 mm segments, and with a regular cubic interpolation of the measured curvatures in the

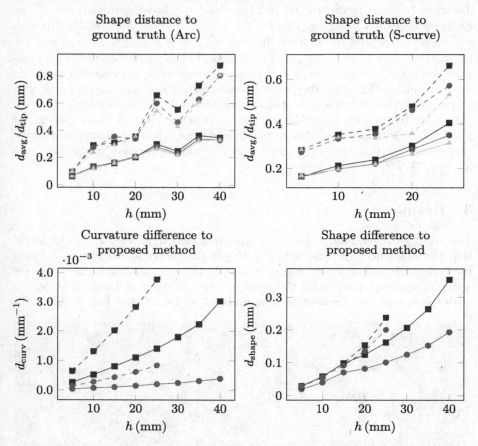

Fig. 2. Results of the simulation study: The figures in the first row show the average (solid) and the tip (dashed) distance of the shape reconstruction to the ground truth using nearest neighbor (■), cubic (●) and averaged cubic (▲) interpolation for the arc (left) and the s-curve (right). The figures in the second row show the curvature difference (left) and the shape differences (right) between our approach and nearest neighbor (■) / cubic (●) interpolation for arc (solid) and the s-curve (dashed) shape. Every measurement shows the average of 100 simulations.

Table 1. Results of the real test study: Mean and standard deviation of the measured distance (in mm) are listed for both shape types.

Shape	Distance	Nearest neighbor interpolation	Cubic interpolation	Proposed
Arc	d_{avg}	1.71	1.53	1.53
	d_{tip}	3.37	2.84	2.66
S-curve	d_{avg}	0.95	0.86	0.47
	d_{tip}	2.18	2.04	1.10

sensor positions. To assess the shape reconstruction quality, we compute the distances between reconstructed points x_i and measured ground truth x_i^{gt} located every 10 mm along the shape for $i = 1, \ldots, 8$ and ending at the tip with $i = 8$. We calculated the average distance $d_{\text{avg}} := \frac{1}{8} \sum_{i=1}^{8} \|x_i - x_i^{\text{gt}}\|_2$ and the tip distance $d_{\text{tip}} := \|x_8 - x_8^{\text{gt}}\|_2$. Furthermore, in the simulation study we compare computed curvature values and shape positions at interpolated positions between our method and the two other reconstructions with nearest neighbor and state-of-the-art cubic curvature interpolation [2, 6]. To this end, we compute $n = 1000$ curvature values c_j and positions x_j with 0.1 mm spacing for $j = 1, \ldots, n$ with $j = n$ as the tip position and we calculate the average curvature difference $d_{\text{curv}} := \frac{1}{n} \sum_{j=1}^{n} |c_j^{\text{our}} - c_j^{\text{other}}|$ and the average shape difference $d_{\text{shape}} := \frac{1}{n} \sum_{j=1}^{n} \|x_j^{\text{our}} - x_j^{\text{other}}\|_2$

3   Results

The results of the simulation study are summarized in Fig. 2. We highlight that the differences increase with the height parameter of the shape and that the differences are generally bigger in case of the s-curve. Furthermore, we see a significant variation among the results of the different methods. The results of our real-world experiment are summarized in Tab. 1 and Fig. 3 shows the

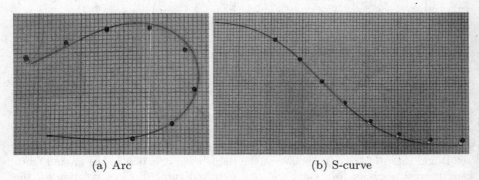

(a) Arc   (b) S-curve

Fig. 3. Image of the fiber (red line) with reconstructed shapes of different interpolation models: Nearest neighbor interpolation (blue dots), cubic spline (red dots), our proposed method (green dots).

reconstructed positions of the FBGs. Here the proposed method leads to lower errors than using nearest neighbor and cubic interpolation.

4   Discussion

We proposed a novel more realistic model for curvature interpolation, which is one error source for shape reconstruction. In our simulation study we analyzed the effects of our method for curvature estimation in comparison to nearest neighbor and common state-of-art cubic interpolation. Here, we showed that the proposed method has an influence on computed curvature values and reconstructed shapes, respectively. Furthermore, our new interpolation model systematically yields smaller reconstruction errors than the compared state-of-the art reference methods supporting the underlying motivation of the proposed model.

In future work we aim to carry over our averaging model to the computation of direction angles. Moreover, since the interpolation of the measured values is only one error source, future work will be the analysis of further errors, that can occur in the shape reconstruction pipeline.

Acknowledgement. This work was funded by the German Federal Ministry of Education and Research (BMBF, project Nav EVAR, funding code: 13GW0228C).

References

1. Park YL, Elayaperumal S, Daniel B, et al. Real-time estimation of 3-D needle shape and deflection for MRI-guided interventions. IEEE ASME Trans Mechatron. 2010;15(6):906–915.
2. Henken KR, Dankelman J, van den Dobbelsteen JJ, et al. Error analysis of FBG-based shape sensors for medical needle tracking. IEEE ASME Trans Mechatron. 2014;19(5):1523–1531.
3. Lee B. Review of the present status of optical fiber sensors. Opt Fiber Technol. 2003;9(2):57–79.
4. Henken K, Van Gerwen D, Dankelman J, et al. Accuracy of needle position measurements using fiber bragg gratings. Minim Invasive Ther Allied Technol. 2012;21(6):408–414.
5. Roesthuis RJ, Kemp M, van den Dobbelsteen JJ, et al. Three-dimensional needle shape reconstruction using an array of fiber bragg grating sensors. IEEE ASME Trans Mechatron. 2014;19(4):1115–1126.
6. Moore JP, Rogge MD. Shape sensing using multi-core fiber optic cable and parametric curve solutions. Opt Express. 2012;20(3):2967–2973.
7. Cui J, Zhao S, Yang C, et al. Parallel transport frame for fiber shape sensing. IEEE Photonics J. 2018;10(1):1–12.
8. Shi C, Luo X, Qi P, et al. Shape sensing techniques for continuum robots in minimally invasive surgery: a survey. IEEE Trans Biomed Eng. 2017;64(8):1665–1678.

On the Characteristics of Helical 3D X-Ray Dark-Field Imaging

Lina Felsner[1], Shiyang Hu[1], Veronika Ludwig[2], Gisela Anton[2],
Andreas Maier[1], Christian Riess[1]

[1]Pattern Recognition Lab, Computer Science, Univ. of Erlangen-Nürnberg
[2]Erlangen Centre for Astroparticle Physics, Univ. of Erlangen-Nürnberg
lina.felsner@fau.de

Abstract. The X-ray dark-field can be measured with a grating interferometer. For oriented structures like fibers, the signal magnitude depends on the relative orientation between fiber and gratings. This allows to analytically reconstruct the fiber orientations at a micrometer scale. However, there currently exists no implementation of a clinically feasible trajectory for recovering the full 3D orientation of a fiber. In principle, a helical trajectory can be suitable for this task. However, as a first step towards dark-field imaging in a helix, a careful analysis of the signal formation is required. Towards this goal, we study in this paper the impact of the grating orientation. We use a recently proposed 3D-projection model and show that the projected dark-field scattering at a single volume point depends on the grating sensitivity direction and the helix geometry. More specifically, the dark-field signal on a 3D trajectory always consists of a linear combination of a constant and an angular-dependent component.

1 Introduction

X-ray phase-contrast is an interferometric imaging technique that is compatible with clinical requirements. It can be implemented with a Talbot-Lau interferometer via a set of gratings between a medical X-ray source and detector (Fig. 1). This interferometer creates an attenuation image, a differential phase image and a dark-field image. The dark-field image measures small-angle scattering of fibrous structures. The strength of the anisotropic dark-field signal depends on the relative orientation of a fiber to the gratings [1, 2].

In recent years, several medical applications of the dark-field signal were investigated, for example for tumor detection, e.g., in the lung [3, 4], or the anisotropic reconstruction of the brain fiber connectivity [5].

Several algorithms were proposed for anisotropic dark-field reconstruction in 2D and 3D [6, 7, 8, 9, 10, 11]. 2D methods [2, 6] reconstruct the projection of the fiber-orientation in one plane. 3D reconstructions are based on various models. One approach is to compute the 3D tensor indirectly from two 2D vectors [7], others are X-ray tensor tomography [8], to fit a scattering ellipsoid [9], or to estimate spherical harmonics [10]. All these methods rely on iterative reconstruction.

Recently, Schaff *et al.* proposed a non-iterative approach [11]. They aligned the grating bars perpendicular to the rotation axis, such that the sensitivity direction is parallel to the rotation axis. This way, the projection of the fiber onto the sensitivity direction is constant for the scan, and a standard filtered back-projection (FBP) can be used for a 2D reconstruction. 3D fiber orientations are then estimated by combining reconstructions from multiple trajectories. However, all these models rely on specialized, quite complex trajectories, which prohibits their use for medical applications.

In this paper, we make first steps towards a novel approach for 3D dark-field imaging. The idea is to use a 3D helix trajectory. While, in principle, a helix allows recovery of 3D information, it is necessary to closely examine the associated dark-field signal model, which is subject of this work. The dark-field model and projection models in 2D and 3D are presented in Sec. 2. We investigate the helical trajectory in more detail. In Sec. 3, we evaluate the dark-field signal for different helical trajectories, followed by a discussion in Sec. 4.

2 Materials and methods

The dark-field model is described below. Its characteristics in a 2D and 3D scanning trajectory are presented in Sec. 2.1 and Sec. 2.2, respectively.

Our examinations are based on the 3D dark-field model proposed in [12]. However, in this work we will limit ourself to only one fiber. Moreover, we will not consider the full model, but consider only the projections of the associated Gaussian scatter function. The dark-field signal then consists of an isotropic part that is constant in all directions, and an anisotropic part that depends on the viewing and grating sensitivity direction.

The observed dark-field signal d from a single Gaussian scattering function is defined as

$$d = d_{\mathrm{iso}} + d_{\mathrm{aniso}}(\boldsymbol{s}^\top \boldsymbol{v})^2 \tag{1}$$

where d_{aniso} describes anisotropic the scattering strength of the object, and d_{iso} the isotropic part. The anisotropic signal is modeled as the inner product of a

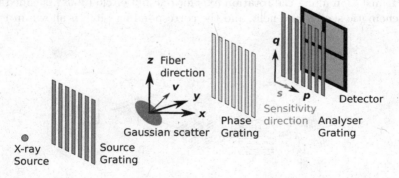

Fig. 1. Sketch of setup and coordinate systems. The global coordinate system is denoted as $\{\boldsymbol{x}, \boldsymbol{y}, \boldsymbol{z}\} \in \mathbb{R}^3$ and the detector coordinate system is given as $\{\boldsymbol{p}, \boldsymbol{q}\} \in \mathbb{R}^2$.

scattering fiber vector v and sensitivity direction s. In this work, we assume that s and v are normalized to 1. Both vectors are shown in Fig. 1.

2.1 Dark-field with 2D trajectories

Existing dark-field projections were only described for 2D trajectories [6, 11]. There, the grating alignment is either parallel to the rotation axis [6] (Fig. 2), left) or perpendicular to it [11] (Fig. 2, middle). For the following specific descriptions we use the coordinate system(s) defined in Fig. 1.

If the gratings are aligned parallel to the rotation axis, the sensitivity direction is parallel to the trajectory and given as $s = (1,0)^\top$. The measured dark-field signal is then the projection of v in the x-y-plane. This results in a sinusoidal function that depends on the rotation angle. Since the sensitivity direction is given by the vector p (Fig. 1) we denote this special case as s_p.

If the gratings are aligned parallel to the trajectory, the sensitivity direction is parallel to the rotation axis $s = (0,1)^\top$. In this case, the projection of the fiber on the z-axis is measured, which leads to a dark-field signal that is constant during tomography. This case is denoted as s_q.

In principle, the gratings could also be oriented diagonally (Fig. 2, right). In this case, the observed dark-field signal is a linear combination of s_p and s_q. The sensitivity direction s is then given by

$$s = A \cdot s_p + B \cdot s_q \tag{2}$$

2.2 Dark-field with a 3D helical trajectory

Unlike 2D trajectories, the reconstruction plane of a 3D trajectory is not necessarily perpendicular to the rotation axis. Then, the observed dark-field signal is a non-trivial linear combination of s_p and s_q. We now apply this reasoning to the medically relevant special case of a helix trajectory. Here, the X-ray system is rotating around the object, with an offset along the rotation axis. The amount of the translation along the rotation axis for one full circle (360°) is called pitch h. A schematic sketch of a helix and the corresponding pitch is shown in Fig. 2.

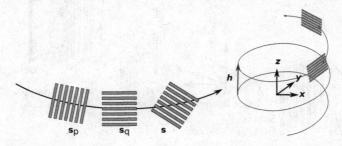

Fig. 2. Grating directions are described with respect to the trajectory (left) and Helix (right).

The helix describes a continuous path, and hence for the case that the sensitivity direction is aligned with the trajectory, the sensitivity is given by

$$s = A \cdot (1, 0)^\top + B \cdot (0, 1)^\top = (A, B)^\top \tag{3}$$

Here, the helix-specific parameters A and B, are

$$A = -\alpha \cdot \sqrt{1 - B^2} B \qquad\qquad = \beta \cdot \frac{2}{\pi} \tag{4}$$

where α is the signed rotation angle between two consecutive projections and β is the signed rising angle of the helix. Thus, the behavior of the dark-field projection in a helix is defined by the sensitivity direction and the helix pitch.

3   Experiments and results

We show the behavior of the 3D dark-field on helix pitch and grating orientation for simulated data. The fiber in our experiments is defined by the parameters $d_{\mathrm{iso}} = 1$, $d_{\mathrm{aniso}} = 1.73 = \sqrt{3}$ and $v = (1, 1, 1)$ and it is centered at the rotation axis. We will consider six different trajectory settings, which differ in the trajectory or the sensitivity direction. We simulate a cone-beam geometry and define the sensitivity vector s to always be perpendicular on the ray direction r. This corresponds to a curved detector, which slightly simplifies the interpretation of the results. The setup geometry always has a source-isocenter distance of 600 mm and source-detector distance of 1200 mm. The 2D circle trajectories (Fig. 3(a,b)) consist of 360° with angular increment of 1.5°. The helical trajectories (Fig. 3(c-f)) also with angular increment of 1.5°, with pitch h_1 or h_2.

3.1   Experiment 1

We investigate two cases of a circular trajectory. First, the gratings are perpendicular to the trajectory (Fig. 3(a)), i.e., with sensitivity direction s_p. Second, the gratings are parallel to the trajectory (Fig. 3(b)), i.e., with sensitivity direction s_q. The resulting dark-field signal is shown in Fig. 4 for sensitivity direction s_p in red and sensitivity direction s_q in blue. While the dark-field signal with direction s_p varies across the tomographic angles, the dark-field signal with direction s_q is constant.

3.2   Experiment 2

In this experiment, the dark-field signal for helical trajectories with different pitches are compared. We set the pitches h_1 to the detector height $h_2 = 0.5 \cdot h_1$ and $h_3 = 2 \cdot h_1$. For gratings parallel to the trajectory, this variation of detector pitch visualized in Fig. 3(c) and Fig. 3(d). The resulting intensity variations are shown in (Fig. 5, left). Here, black, red, and blue show the intensity profiles for pitches h_1, h_2, h_3, respectively. The variations in the curves show that the amplitude, and hence the anisotropic part of the signal, increases with the pitch. However, this dependency scales not linearly. Note also that the fiber is observed over a smaller angular range with increasing pitch.

Fig. 3. Experiments. (a,b) circle trajectory (c–f) helical trajectory. For each scanning mode the grating orientation and rotation axis is shown.

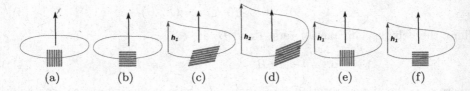

(a)   (b)   (c)   (d)   (e)   (f)

3.3 Experiment 3

For pitch h_1, we evaluate the sensitivity directions shown in Fig. 3(c), 3(e) and 3(f). The resulting intensity profiles are shown in (Fig. 5, right), where the black, red, and blue curves correspond to the directions in Fig. 3(c), 3(e) and 3(f), respectively. Unlike the case of gratings parallel to the trajectory in Exp. 1, none of these grating orientations leads to a constant signal: the 3D helix trajectory always leads to a (non-trivial) linear combination of s_p and s_q.

4 Discussion

We showed that the dark-field signal behaves differently for 2D and 3D trajectories. On 3D trajectories, we necessarily observe a linear combination of the two 2D base cases. This leads to a mixture of a constant and a varying signal component. For the particular case of a helical trajectory, we validated these findings with simulation experiments. We believe that understanding the dark-field signal in a helix opens the perspective to implement orientation-sensitive tomographic systems that are much more practical for scanning patients. As a next step the complete 3D projection model described in [12] shall be evaluated with a helical trajectory. For future work we will investigate an algorithm that incorporates trajectory-dependent information to simultaneously reconstruct the scatter directions and isotropic signal components.

Acknowledgement. The authors acknowledge funding from the German Research Foundation (DFG).

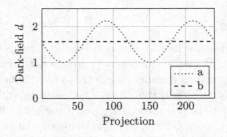

Fig. 4. Line plot of dark-field with a circular trajectory. Intensity profiles in red and blue correspond to grating orientations in Fig. 3(a) and 3(b), respectively.

Fig. 5. Line plot of dark-field for different helical trajectories. The corresponding grating orientations are shown in Fig. 3(c-f).

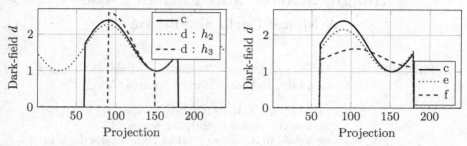

(a) Helical trajectory with different pitch. $h_2 = 0.5 \cdot h_1$ and $h_3 = 2 \cdot h_1$.

(b) Helical trajectory with different sensitivity directions.

References

1. Jensen TH, Bech M, Bunk O, et al. Directional X-ray dark-field imaging. Phys Med Biol. 2010;55(12):3317.
2. Revol V, Kottler C, Kaufmann R, et al. Orientation-selective X-ray dark field imaging of ordered systems. J Appl Phys. 2012;112(11):114903.
3. Scherer K, Yaroshenko A, Bölükbas DA, et al. X-ray dark-field radiography-in-vivo diagnosis of lung cancer in mice. Sci Rep. 2017;7(1):402.
4. Hellbach K, Baehr A, Marco F, et al. Depiction of pneumothoraces in a large animal model using X-ray dark-field radiography. Sci Rep. 2018;8(1):2602.
5. Wieczorek M, Schaff F, Jud C, et al. Brain connectivity exposed by anisotropic X-ray dark-field tomography. Sci Rep. 2018;8.
6. Bayer FL, Hu S, Maier A, et al. Reconstruction of scalar and vectorial components in X-ray dark-field tomography. Procs Nat Acad Sci. 2014;111(35):12699–12704.
7. Hu S, Riess C, Hornegger J, et al. 3D tensor reconstruction in X-ray dark-field tomography. Proc BVM. 2015; p. 492–497.
8. Malecki A, Potdevin G, Biernath T, et al. X-ray tensor tomography. Europhys Lett. 2014;105(3):38002.
9. Vogel J, Schaff F, Fehringer A, et al. Constrained X-ray tensor tomography reconstruction. Optics Express. 2015;23(12):15134–15151.
10. Wieczorek M, Schaff F, Pfeiffer F, et al. Anisotropic X-ray dark-field tomography: a continuous model and its discretization. Phys Rev Lett. 2016;117(15):158101.
11. Schaff F, Prade F, Sharma Y, et al. Non-iterative directional dark-field tomography. Sci Rep. 2017;7(1):3307.
12. Hu S, Felsner L, Maier A, et al. A 3-D projection model for X-ray dark-field imaging. arXiv:181104457. 2018;.

Effects of Tissue Material Properties on X-Ray Image, Scatter and Patient Dose
A Monte Carlo Simulation

Philipp Roser[1,3], Annette Birkhold[2], Xia Zhong[1], Elizaveta Stepina[2], Markus Kowarschik[2], Rebecca Fahrig[2], Andreas Maier[1,3]

[1]Pattern Recognition Lab, FAU Erlangen-Nürnberg
[2]Siemens Healthcare GmbH, Forchheim
[3]Erlangen Graduate School in Advanced Optical Technologies (SAOT)
philipp.roser@fau.de

Abstract. With increasing patient and staff X-ray radiation awareness, many efforts have been made to develop accurate patient dose estimation methods. To date, Monte Carlo (MC) simulations are considered golden standard to simulate the interaction of X-ray radiation with matter. However, sensitivity of MC simulation results to variations in the experimental or clinical setup of image guided interventional procedures are only limited studied. In particular, the impact of patient material compositions is poorly investigated. This is mainly due to the fact, that these methods are commonly validated in phantom studies utilizing a single anthropomorphic phantom. In this study, we therefore investigate the impact of patient material parameters mapping on the outcome of MC X-ray dose simulations. A computation phantom geometry is constructed and three different commonly used material composition mappings are applied. We used the MC toolkit Geant4 to simulate X-ray radiation in an interventional setup and compared the differences in dose deposition, scatter distributions and resulting X-ray images. The evaluation shows a discrepancy between different material composition mapping up to 20% concerning directly irradiated organs. These results highlight the need for standardization of material composition mapping for MC simulations in a clinical setup.

1 Introduction

Over the last years, the amount of X-ray guided diagnostic and interventional procedures has increased steadily, raising the awareness of dose-induced deterministic and stochastic risks for the patient as well as the treating medical staff. Therefore, efforts are made to determine and visualize the distribution of absorbed dose and scattered radiation in the context of the interventional suite and hybrid operating room using Monte Carlo (MC) methods [1]. Recently, MC simulation of photon transport gained additional boost with deep convolutional neural networks being established to be state of the art in most X-ray imaging classification and regression tasks, such as landmark detection or segmentation.

With novel architectures emerging on a daily basis, the demand for diverse training and testing data intensifies. Since medical data is treated sensitively, there is a constant lack of sufficient data. Although efforts are made to build open source databases, there exist prominent problems, such as scatter reduction [2], hindering the collection of accurate ground truth data without imitating existing solutions, such as anti-scatter grids. Therefore, realistic simulation of these problems has become a fundamental step to build learning solutions to real-world problems. However, to push deep learning from research to clinical application, the training data must be valid to a certain measure. There is, however, a multitude of parameters affecting the outcome of MC simulations in an unintuitive way, such as modeling the energy spectrum or biasing the particle source. To obtain valid and realistic results, it is mandatory to be aware of all sources of uncertainty concerning modeling the clinical setup. In this study, the impact of variations in the tissue material properties on resulting X-ray image, scattered radiation and patient dose are determined using Monte Carlo simulation.

2   Materials and methods

2.1   Phantom model geometry and material parameters

To study the effect on material composition mapping, we use the geometry of the voxel phantom Golem provided by the Institute for Radiation Protection [1]. The Golem phantom consists of 220 slices with 256×256 voxels each, ranging from the vertex down to the toes of a normally shaped, 176 cm adult male. It is segmented into 122 organ and tissue labels. Three different, voxel-wise material composition mappings are used to assign material properties to the associated labels for MC simulation. A material is defined by its volumetric mass density and the fraction of mass of elementary components. Two material composition mappings reference the commonly used anthropomorphic dosimetry phantoms RANDO (Alderson [2]) and CIRS (ATOM [3]), respectively. The Alderson mapping (AM1) includes real bone (cortical) and an approximation of the lungs besides a mixture to represent soft tissue as the main component of the human body. The Atom mapping (AM2) includes bone, soft and lung (inhale) equivalent tissues. The third material mapping serves as reference mapping (RM) and is modeled to resemble a living adult male, following the material specifications proposed by the International Commission on Radiological Protection (ICRP) [4] standard. It comprises adipose, soft, skin, brain, bone (cortical), muscle and lung (inhale) tissue.

---

[1] www.helmholtz-muenchen.de/iss/index.html
[2] www.rsdphantoms.com/rt_art.htm
[3] www.cirsinc.com/products/all/33/atom-dosimetry-verification-phantoms/
[4] www.icrp.org

2.2   Detector model

The simulated $320 \times 237.5 \, \text{mm}^2$ flat panel detector has a resolution of 256×190 pixels. To reduce variance, it consists of Cesium-Iodide with a 20 mm thickness to absorb all incoming photons. We consider the detector as an ideal detector with a linear detector response curve, no electron noise or defect pixels. No processing is applied to the resulting image from the detector.

2.3   Simulation of experimental setup

The simulation is implemented in the general purpose MC toolkit Geant4 [3], which offers a high degree of customizability and flexibility allowing for arbitrary experiment configuration and quantity scoring. Furthermore, Geant4 provides an interface to materials as defined by the ICRP, alongside arbitrary material compositions.

The phantom is centered in the origin of the world coordinate system, the particle source is placed in 800 mm distance ante-posterior to the phantom, such that the prostate lies approximately in the center of the emitted X-ray beam. The particle source is circularly shaped with a radius of 0.3 mm and collimated resulting in 7.6 ° for both aperture angles. Emitted photon vertices are sampled using cosine-weighting to obtain homogeneous fluence with respect to a sphere surface. The underlying energy spectrum of the photon shower is modeled considering a tungsten anode, 70 kV peak voltage and 2.7 mm Aluminum self-filtration using Boone's algorithm [4]. The flat panel detector is placed in 1300 mm distance to the photon source perpendicular to the central X-ray direction. Particle interactions that may occur at the given energy spectrum are considered, including the photo electric effect, Rayleigh scattering and Compton scattering for photons and ionization and Bremsstrahlung for electrons. All processes are modeled adhering to the Livermore model for low energy physics [5]. Primary photons and secondary particles are tracked until their associated kinetic energy in consumed completely to satisfy energy preservation and assure accurate results.

To obtain stable dose and scatter distributions 9×10^8 primary photons are emitted, for X-ray image generation 51×10^8, respectively. Dose distributions are scored with respect to the dose D absorbed by each voxel measured in Gy. To quantify scatter distributions and X-ray images, the incident radiant energy R in J is tracked. The simulation is carried out in batches of 10^8 primaries in order to bring variance to the initial random seed and to split the computation to several nodes of the high performance computing (HPC) cluster. Each batch computation lasts on average 3.5 h, however multiple batches are processed in parallel. The resulting dose distributions have the same resolution as the associated phantom volumes. To score the scatter distributions, a $8 \, \text{m}^3$ volume comprising $100 \times 100 \times 100$ isotropic voxels is placed surrounding the phantom and material parameters of air defined by ICRP are applied. No interventional table is considered. We performed simulations using aforementioned configurations for each mapping. The simulation result employing RM are considered as base line, results of AM1 and AM2 are compared to this reference.

3   Results

3.1   Scatter and dose distributions

Fig. 1a-c show the distributions of scattered radiation in the patient environment ($\log_{10}$; coronal slices) using the three material mappings. The deviation maps of the percentage difference to RM for AM1 and AM2 are depicted in Fig. 1e. Distribution of scattered radiation in both AM simulations shows high overall agreement with the RM results; however, concerning specific regions deviations of 20% to 50% were determined. Fig. 2 shows an axial slice of the phantom dose distribution simulation results for RM (a), AM1 (b) and AM2 (c). Deviation maps of the dose distribution for AM1 and AM2 are depicted in Fig. 2e and show similar deviations from the reference as the scattered radiation. For a set of directly irradiated organs (bladder, colon, prostate, skin, testes) the total dose was determined. Fig. 3 shows the dose ratio between AMs and RM for these dose sensitive organs. Correlating the AMs to the RM, introduces a deviation of up to 20% for the prostate at a reference dose of 72% of the peak dose measured. For organs within 19% to 30% of the peak dose, a deviation of 3% to 29% can be observed.

3.2   X-ray images

Fig. 4 shows the detector image results of the simulation and associated deviation maps. Although the images are similar in general, the deviation maps disclose

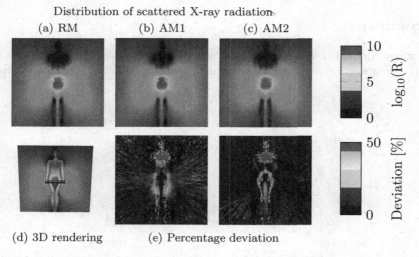

Distribution of scattered X-ray radiation
(a) RM   (b) AM1   (c) AM2

$\log_{10}(R)$

Deviation [%]

(d) 3D rendering   (e) Percentage deviation

Fig. 1. Coronal view of the scatter distributions associated with each material composition mapping. (e) Corresponding percentage deviation maps with respect to RM. (d) Spatial relationship between scatter maps and phantom. Scatter distributions are shown in logarithmic domain. The identifier R refers to the radiant energy entering a voxel in J.

Fig. 2. (a)-(c) Axial view of the deposited X-ray dose distribution associated with each set of material properties. (e) Corresponding percentage deviation maps with respect to RM. (d) Spatial relation between dose maps and phantom. The dose distributions are shown in the logarithmic domain. The identifier D refers to the dose absorbed by a voxel in Gy.

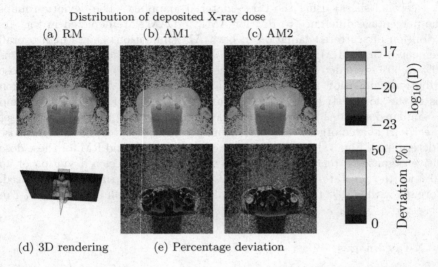

Distribution of deposited X-ray dose

(a) RM   (b) AM1   (c) AM2

(d) 3D rendering   (e) Percentage deviation

major differences concerning all tissue types. Future studies may evaluate if these differences are in a diagnostic relevant range.

4   Summary

This study highlights variances in MC simulation results when using different material composition mapping for the same phantom geometry. We showed, that

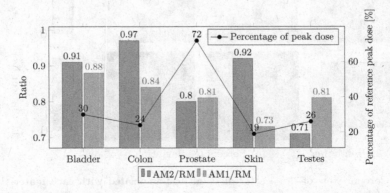

Fig. 3. Ratios of total organ dose between different material composition mappings (AM1, AM2) and the reference (RM) for five directly irradiated organs. The absolute organ doses in Gy for the RM are given by the black plot.

Fig. 4. Primary photon contribution to X-ray images generated with respect to 51×10^8 primary particles. No processing is applied, the raw radiant energy incident at the detector is tracked.

Dose distribution

(a) RM   (b) AM1   (c) AM2

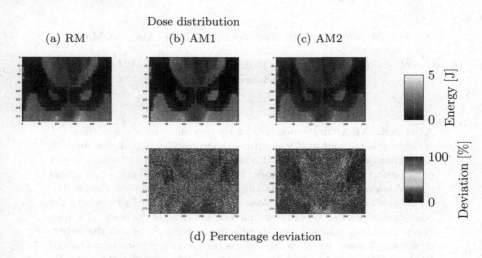

(d) Percentage deviation

the material composition mapping affects X-ray dose, scatter as well as created image to a certain extent. Therefore, for quantitative analysis and comparison between experimental and simulation studies these variances have to be considered. A more detailed standardization of material parameters might be needed. This need for standardization is further emphasized as MC simulations are potentially used to generate training data for deep learning methods.

Acknowledgement. The concepts and information presented in this paper are based on research and are not commercially available.

References

1. Loy Rodas N, Padoy N. Seeing is believing: increasing intraoperative awareness to scattered radiation in interventional procedures by combining augmented reality, Monte Carlo simulations and wireless dosimeters. Int J Comput Assist Radiol Surg. 2015;10(8):1181–1191.
2. Maier J, Berker Y, Sawall S, et al. Deep scatter estimation (DSE): feasibility of using a deep convolutional neural network for real-time x-ray scatter prediction in cone-beam CT. Procs SPIE. 2018;10573:1–6.
3. Agostinelli S, Allison J, et al KA. Geant4: a simulation toolkit. Nucl Instr Meth Phys Res A. 2003;506(3):250–303.
4. Boone JM, Seibert JA. An accurate method for computer-generating tungsten anode x-ray spectra from 30 to 140 kV. Med Phys. 1997;24(11):1661–1670.
5. Cullen DE, Hubbell JH, Kissel L. EPDL97: the evaluated photon data library, 97 Version; 1997.

Isocenter Determination from Projection Matrices of a C-Arm CBCT

Ahmed Amri, Bastian Bier, Jennifer Maier, Andreas Maier

Department of Computer Science 5, Pattern Recognition, FAU Erlangen-Nürnberg
ahmed.amri@fau.de

Abstract. An accurate position of the isocenter of a cone-beam CT trajectory is mandatory for accurate image reconstruction. For analytical backprojection algorithms, it is assumed that the X-ray source moves on a perfectly circular trajectory, which is not true for most practical clinical trajectories due to mechanical instabilities. Besides, the flexibility of novel robotic C-arm systems enables new trajectories where the computation of the isocenter might not be straight forward. An inaccurate isocenter position directly affects the computation of the redundancy weights and consequently affects the reconstructions immediately. In this work, we compare different methods for computing the isocenter of a non-ideal circular scan trajectory and evaluate their robustness in the presence of noise. The best results were achieved using a method based on a least-square-based fit. Furthermore, we show that an inaccurate isocenter computation can lead to artifacts in the reconstruction result. Therefore, this work highlights the importance of an accurate isocenter computation with the background of novel upcoming clinical trajectories.

1 Introduction

C-arm cone-beam computed tomography is an established modality in medical imaging for various applications in diagnostic and interventional imaging. Novel robotic systems offer a great flexibility of trajectories for image acquisition, allowing to scan objects in horizontal or vertical configuration [1]. In these, the X-ray source and the detector rotate around the object and 2D projection images from different directions are acquired, allowing for 3D object reconstruction. In theory, these trajectories correspond to a perfect circle, in reality, mechanical instabilities introduce non-idealities, also referred to as a system "wobble". In order to perform image reconstruction, these trajectories are calibrated using an offline calibration scan with a calibration phantom [2] that yields a set of projection matrices.

A common reconstruction algorithm is the filtered backprojection-based FDK-algorithm [3]. For a short scan, Parker redundancy weights [4] have to be applied on the projection images. These weights account for redundant rays that are measured twice. They are defined dependent on the angle of the current projection matrix that is part of a perfect circular trajectory. To this end, in a first step, the isocenter, e.g. the rotation center of the C-arm, is calculated, which acts as reference for the computation of the angles. If the isocenter is corrupted, this results in wrong angles and consequently in errors in the computation of the redundancy weights. This potentially introduces artifacts in the reconstruction, which decrease the value of these images for diagnosis or further processing [5]. One solution to find the isocenter is to fit a circle to the trajectory [6]. In this approach, the axes of rotations between consecutive frames are determined. From this set of axes, a mean axis of rotation is computed. Afterwards, a cylinder is fitted parallel to the mean axis of rotation to all X-ray source positions. Additionally, a plane is fitted orthogonal to the axis of rotation to all X-ray source positions. The intersection of the plane with the cylinder is defined as the effective isocenter. However, this approach showed to be error-prone in the presence of non-idealities in the trajectory. The aim of this paper is to investigate the robustness of different isocenter computations. We further show also how this might affect the image quality.

2 Materials and methods

2.1 Background: the projection matrix

An X-ray system can be modeled as a basic pinhole camera [7]: a world point is mapped onto a 2D image, which can be represented by a 3×4 homogeneous projection matrix $\mathbf{P}$. A homogeneous 3D point $\widetilde{\mathbf{q}} \in \mathbb{P}^4$ can be mapped from world space to a homogeneous 2D point $\widetilde{\mathbf{p}} \in \mathbb{P}^3$ in camera space by $\widetilde{\mathbf{p}} = \mathbf{P} \cdot \widetilde{\mathbf{q}}$. $\mathbf{P}$ can be decomposed into intrinsic and extrinsic parameters. The extrinsic parameters define the orientation of the camera (X-ray source) and are given by the rotation $\mathbf{R} \in \mathbb{R}^{3 \times 3}$ and the translation $\mathbf{t} \in \mathbb{R}^3$. The intrinsic parameters depend only on internal parameters of the system. These parameters can be expressed as a 3×3 matrix $\mathbf{K}$, where $\mathbf{f_x}$ and $\mathbf{f_y}$ are the focal lengths and $\mathbf{p_u}$ and $\mathbf{p_v}$ are the coordinates of the principal point. α is the skew parameter. $\mathbf{P}$ is then represented as

$$\mathbf{P} = \underbrace{\begin{pmatrix} \mathbf{f_x} & \alpha & \pm\mathbf{p_u} \\ 0 & \mathbf{f_y} & \pm\mathbf{p_v} \\ 0 & 0 & \pm 1 \end{pmatrix}}_{\mathbf{K}} \cdot \left(\mathbf{R} \mid \mathbf{t} \right) \tag{1}$$

The projection matrix has some important properties: The *camera center* $\mathbf{C}$, or source position, is the 3D position of the X-ray sources. $\mathbf{C}$ can be directly computed from $\mathbf{R}$ and $\mathbf{t}$: $\mathbf{C} = -\mathbf{R}^\top \cdot \mathbf{t}$ The *principal axis* is the line passing through the camera center and perpendicular to the image plane [7]. The *principal point* $\left(\mathbf{p_u}, \mathbf{p_v} \right)^\top$ is the intersection of the principal ray with the image plane. It can be read out from the last column of $\mathbf{K}$.

2.2   Isocenter computation methods

Method 1 The first method is based on a heuristic: It uses the fact that the isocenter should be the intersection of all principal rays. Therefore, we randomly select two projection matrices, calculate their principle rays, and compute their intersection point. This step is repeated 150 times and the final isocenter is the average over all calculated intersection points.

Method 2 In this method, a sphere is fitted through all X-ray source positions using the following objective function

$$\mathbf{X} = \arg\min_{\mathbf{X}} \left(\sum_{j=1}^{N} (\mathbf{C_j} - \mathbf{X})^{\top} (\mathbf{C_j} - \mathbf{X}) - \mathbf{d^2} \right)^2 \tag{2}$$

Where $\mathbf{X}$ is the isocenter, $\mathbf{N}$ is the number of projection matrices, $\mathbf{d}$ is the source to isocenter distance, which is a system configuration. X is initialized with the result from Method 1. The optimization is then solved with a gradient descent algorithm.

Method 3 This method computes the isocenter by solving a least-square problem. The isocenter is the smallest squared distance to all principle rays [8]

$$\begin{pmatrix} u_j \\ v_j \\ 1 \end{pmatrix} \cdot \xi_{\mathbf{j}} = \mathbf{P_j} \cdot \begin{pmatrix} \tilde{x} \\ \tilde{y} \\ \tilde{z} \\ 1 \end{pmatrix} = \begin{bmatrix} \tilde{p}_{j,1}^{\top} \; p_{j,14} \\ \tilde{p}_{j,2}^{\top} \; p_{j,24} \\ \tilde{p}_{j,3}^{\top} \; p_{j,34} \end{bmatrix} \begin{pmatrix} \tilde{x} \\ \tilde{y} \\ \tilde{z} \\ 1 \end{pmatrix} \tag{3}$$

where ξ_j is a homogeneous term, $\tilde{\mathbf{p}}_{\mathbf{j,m}}^{\top} = (\mathbf{P_{j,m1}}, \mathbf{P_{j,m2}}, \mathbf{P_{j,m3}})$ is the j-th projection and $\mathbf{m}$ is a matrix row number. Eliminating ξ_j produces

$$\begin{bmatrix} u_j \cdot \tilde{p}_{j,3}^{\top} - \tilde{p}_{j,1}^{\top} \\ v_j \cdot \tilde{p}_{j,3}^{\top} - \tilde{p}_{j,2}^{\top} \end{bmatrix} \cdot \begin{pmatrix} \tilde{x} \\ \tilde{y} \\ \tilde{z} \end{pmatrix} = \begin{pmatrix} -u_j \cdot p_{j,34} + p_{j,14} \\ -v_j \cdot p_{j,34} + p_{j,24} \end{pmatrix} \tag{4}$$

The remaining unknowns are $(\tilde{x}, \tilde{y}, \tilde{z})$, and with $\mathbf{j} = \mathbf{N}$ projections we therefore have sufficient information to solve the equation using SVD

$$\begin{pmatrix} \tilde{x} \\ \tilde{y} \\ \tilde{z} \end{pmatrix} = \begin{bmatrix} u_1 \cdot \tilde{p}_{1,3}^{\top} - \tilde{p}_{1,1}^{\top} \\ v_1 \cdot \tilde{p}_{1,3}^{\top} - \tilde{p}_{1,2}^{\top} \\ u_2 \cdot \tilde{p}_{2,3}^{\top} - \tilde{p}_{2,1}^{\top} \\ v_2 \cdot \tilde{p}_{2,3}^{\top} - \tilde{p}_{2,2}^{\top} \\ ... \\ u_N \cdot \tilde{p}_{N,3}^{\top} - \tilde{p}_{N,1}^{\top} \\ v_N \cdot \tilde{p}_{N,3}^{\top} - \tilde{p}_{N,2}^{\top} \end{bmatrix}^{-1} \cdot \begin{pmatrix} -u_1 \cdot p_{1,34} + p_{1,14} \\ -v_1 \cdot p_{1,34} + p_{1,24} \\ -u_2 \cdot p_{2,34} + p_{2,14} \\ -v_2 \cdot p_{2,34} + p_{2,24} \\ ... \\ -u_N \cdot p_{N,34} + p_{N,14} \\ -v_N \cdot p_{N,34} + p_{N,24} \end{pmatrix} \tag{5}$$

Method 4 This method uses SVD to find the isocenter. We define an equation that holds for all points $\mathbf{X}$ on the principal ray [9]

$$(\mathbf{I} - \mathbf{v} \cdot \mathbf{v}^\top) \cdot \mathbf{X} =^! (\mathbf{I} - \mathbf{v} \cdot \mathbf{v}^\top) \cdot \mathbf{C} \tag{6}$$

$\mathbf{I}$ is the identity matrix and $\mathbf{v}$ is the view direction. The left side is the projection of a point $\mathbf{X}$ onto the plane with the normal vector $\mathbf{v}$ and the right side is the projection of the X-ray source position $\mathbf{C}$ onto the same plane. The equation is only satisfied if $\mathbf{X}$ lies on the principal ray. There are an infinite number of points on this ray. However, if we set this equation for all projection matrices and solve it with the SVD, we will end up with a unique solution that corresponds to the isocenter

$$\begin{pmatrix} \mathbf{A_1} \\ \mathbf{A_2} \\ ... \\ \mathbf{A_N} \end{pmatrix} \cdot \mathbf{X} = \begin{pmatrix} \mathbf{b_1} \\ \mathbf{b_2} \\ ... \\ \mathbf{b_N} \end{pmatrix} \tag{7}$$

Where $\mathbf{A_j}$ is a 3×3 matrix and $\mathbf{b_j}$ is a 3×1 vector $\mathbf{A_j} = \mathbf{I} - \mathbf{v_j} \cdot \mathbf{v_j}^\top$ $\mathbf{b_j} = (\mathbf{I} - \mathbf{v_j} \cdot \mathbf{v_j}^\top) \cdot \mathbf{C_j}$

2.3   Experiments

We aim to evaluate the effect of noise on the isocenter computation. Therefore, we added a different amount of Gaussian noise onto a perfect circular trajectory and computed their deviation to the true center position. This is done using the following three steps: (1) Add the noise to $\mathbf{C}$ to get a new noisy camera center $\mathbf{C_{new}}$. (2) Compute a new translation vector $\mathbf{t}$: $\mathbf{t_{new}} = -\mathbf{R} \cdot \mathbf{C_{new}}$. (3) compute the new projection matrix $\mathbf{P_{new}} = \mathbf{K}[\mathbf{R}|\mathbf{t_{new}}]$. As accuracy measure, we calculated the distance of the computed isocenter to the reference isocenter position $(0, 0, 0)$. Fig. 1 shows a perfect circular trajectory, a trajectories with noise, and a real clinical calibrated trajectory.

3   Results

The results of the noise experiment are summarized in Tab. 1. If no noise is added (first row), all methods perform equally well with a distance to the true isocenter

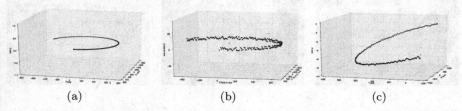

(a)   (b)   (c)

Fig. 1. Ideal trajectory without (a) and with $\pm 5\,\text{mm}$ (b) noise addition vs. real calibrated clinical trajectory (c).

Table 1. Distance of computed to reference isocenter in mm using ideal projections.

Noise [mm]	Method 1	Method 2	Method 3	Method 4
0	1.410^{-10}	4.810^{-13}	2.310^{-15}	3.810^{-14}
0.5	0.051	0.051	0.029	0.030
1	0.109	0.104	0.057	0.060
3	0.343	0.330	0.162	0.167
5	0.538	0.490	0.275	0.294

which lies in the range of rounding errors. Augmenting the noise intervals from 0.5 mm to ±5 mm, the distance to a reference isocenter increases for all tested methods. For the highest amount of noise, the best method deviates only by 0.257 mm, which corresponds to Method 3. Method 1 and Method 2 perform worse with an error of 0.538 mm and 0.490 mm, respectively.

In a second step, we show how these different methods impact the image reconstruction of a real clinical supine acquisition of a knee. As an example, we show the reconstruction results using the worst (sphere fitting) and the best isocenter computation method (least-square approach) in Fig. 2(a) and 2(b), respectively. Closely focusing on the bone edge at the patella, indicated with the red arrow in both images, shows the effect on the reconstructions: While using the more accurate isocenter computation leads to a clearly visible bone outline, the edge vanished and gets blurred in the other case. This subtle difference can also be seen in their difference image shown in Fig. 2(c). Note, that the artifact origins mostly from one distinct direction (horizontally). This direction corresponds to the last acquired projection images, that are, in consequence of an inaccurate isocenter computation, weighted with suboptimal Parker weights. This leads to a loss of information in that direction.

4   Discussion and conclusion

Isocenter computation can have an effect on the image quality of reconstructions of C-arm cone-beam CT scans. An inaccurate isocenter leads to non ideal

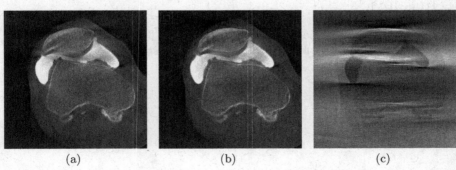

| (a) | (b) | (c) |

Fig. 2. Reconstruction using two different Isocenter computation methods: (a) with and (b) without artifact; (c) difference.

Parker-weights, that consequently might result in a loss of information. This is because the measured projection images are weighted with suboptimal weights, or in the extreme case even with zero. Thus, a robust isocenter computation is indispensable. Therefore, we investigated the robustness of four different methods in the presence of noise. We found that methods based on a least-square fit outperform methods based on fitting of lines and spheres. The results indicate that these methods are able to cope with the C-arm "wobble". Further, these methods might also be a candidate to compute the isocenter for other planar trajectories, such as ellipses. We showed that an isocenter determination is critical on the reconstruction result. Subtle differences in the reconstruction might already significantly reduce the diagnostic values of such. Further, possible postprocessing steps, e.g. segmentation of bones in order to compute cartilage thickness [5], are prone to such directional errors in the images. Therefore, our comparison can help to improve the reconstruction quality, also for other trajectories and novel trajectories in the future.

References

1. Maier A, Choi JH, Keil A, et al.; International Society for Optics; Photonics. Analysis of vertical and horizontal circular C-arm trajectories. Phys Med Imaging. 2011;7961:796123.
2. Jia F, Li Y, Xu H, et al.; IEEE. A simple method to calibrate projection matrix of c-arm cone-beam ct. Proc Biomed Eng Biotech. 2012; p. 682–685.
3. Feldkamp LA, Davis L, Kress JW. Practical cone-beam algorithm. Josa A. 1984;1(6):612–619.
4. Parker DL. Optimal short scan convolution reconstruction for fan beam CT. Med Phys. 1982;9(2):254–257.
5. Maier J, Black M, Bonaretti S, et al. Comparison of different approaches for measuring tibial cartilage thickness. J Integ Bioinf. 2017;14(2).
6. Navab N, Bani-Hashemi A, Nadar MS, et al.; Springer. 3D reconstruction from projection matrices in a C-arm based 3D-angiography system. Int Conf Med Image Comput Comput-Assist Interv. 1998; p. 119–129.
7. Hartley R, Zisserman A. Multiple View Geometry in Computer Vision. Cambridge University Press; 2003.
8. Choi JH, Maier A, Keil A, et al. Fiducial marker-based correction for involuntary motion in weight-bearing C-arm CT scanning of knees. II. experiment. Med Phys. 2014;41.
9. Fieselmann A, Ritschl L. Isocenter determination for arbitrary planar cone-beam CT scan trajectories. Proc Intl Mtg Image Form. 2016; p. 241–4.

Improving Surgical Training Phantoms by Hyperrealism

Deep Unpaired Image-to-Image Translation from Real Surgeries

Sandy Engelhardt[1,3], Raffaele De Simone[2], Peter M. Full[2], Matthias Karck[2], Ivo Wolf[3]

[1]Faculty of Computer Science, Mannheim University of Applied Sciences, Germany
[2]Department of Cardiac Surgery, Heidelberg University Hospital, Germany
[3]Dep. of and Graphics, Magdeburg University, Germany
s.engelhardt@hs-mannheim.de

Current 'dry lab' surgical phantom simulators are a valuable tool for surgeons which allows them to improve their dexterity and skill with surgical instruments. These phantoms mimic the haptic and shape of organs of interest, but lack a realistic visual appearance. In this work, we present an innovative application in which representations learned from real intraoperative endoscopic sequences are transferred to a surgical phantom scenario. The term *hyperrealism* is introduced in this field, which we regard as a novel subform of surgical augmented reality for approaches that involve real-time object transfigurations. For related tasks in the computer vision community, unpaired cycle-consistent Generative Adversarial Networks (GANs) have shown excellent results on still RGB images. Though, application of this approach to continuous video frames can result in flickering, which turned out to be especially prominent for this application. Therefore, we propose an extension of cycle-consistent GANs, named *tempCycleGAN*, to improve temporal consistency. The novel method is evaluated on captures of a silicone phantom for training endoscopic reconstructive mitral valve procedures. Synthesized videos show highly realistic results with regard to 1) replacement of the silicone appearance of the phantom valve by intraoperative tissue texture, while 2) explicitly keeping crucial features in the scene, such as instruments, sutures and prostheses. Compared to the original CycleGAN approach, temp-CycleGAN efficiently removes flickering between frames. The overall approach is expected to change the future design of surgical training simulators since the generated sequences clearly demonstrate the feasibility to enable a considerably more realistic training experience for minimally-invasive procedures. The work was presented at MICCAI 2018 [1]. A supplemental video is available here[1].

References

1. Engelhardt S, De Simone R, Full PM, et al. Improving surgical training phantoms by hyperrealism: deep unpaired image-to-image translation from real surgeries. Proc MICCAI. 2018; p. 747–755.

---

[1] https://youtu.be/qugAYpK-Z4M

Evaluation of Spatial Perception in Virtual Reality within a Medical Context

Jan N. Hombeck, Nils Lichtenberg, Kai Lawonn

Institute for Computational Visualistics, University of Koblenz-Landau
jhombeck@uni-koblenz.de

Abstract. This paper compares three different visualization techniques to improve spatial perception in virtual reality applications. In most virtual reality applications, spatial relations cannot be sufficiently estimated to make precise statements about the locations and positions of objects. Especially in the field of medical applications, it is crucial to correctly perceive the depth and structure of a given object. Thus, visualization techniques need to be developed to support the spatial perception. To address this, we carried out a user study to evaluate different visualization techniques and deal with the question of how glyphs influence spatial perception in a virtual reality application. Therefore, our evaluation compares arrow glyphs, heatmaps with isolines and pseudo-chromadepth in terms of improving the spatial perception within virtual reality. Based on the study results it can be concluded that spatial perception can be improved with the help of glyphs, which should motivate further research in this area.

1 Introduction

Virtual reality (VR) describes the idea to transfer a user into an almost real world. This VR experience covers everything from playing virtual games through educational purposes up to military applications and beyond. As technology advances, more and more applications are being developed to improve medical education and surgical planning in VR [1, 2]. These new applications also bring new challenges with them. Although stereoscopic VR improves spatial perception compared to conventional computer monitors, the spatial perception is still not as accurate as in the real world and therefore leads the user to inaccurate spatial estimations. These inaccuracies are unfavorable for medical training or preparation purposes. Especially for medical applications it is important that the spatial relations are recognized as accurately as possible to minimize errors during the interaction in the virtual environment. In order to train new surgeons or to support operation planning the spatial perception needs to improve. Most existing techniques to improve spatial perception are designed for common computer monitors and are therefore not suitable or not yet evaluated for VR applications. To support VR environments, which are based on surgery planning and training, this paper evaluates different approaches to improve the spatial perception within a virtual reality training application for liver ablation. There-fore a new glyph design will be compared to a spatial encoding by heatmaps and depth encoding by pseudo-chromadepth (PCD) [3]. Note that depth is a strong contributor to spatial perception. In summary, this work contributes to an improvement of spatial perception in VR and evaluates existing, monoscopic methods within a virtual reality application for liver ablation.

2   Materials and methods

This paper attempts to illustrate ways to improve spatial perception in VR. Through this improvement we want to reduce the error that occurs when nav-igating precisely in critical areas, i.e., areas close to a tumor or close to the vasculature. To achieve these goals we use the HTC Vive and an application that can simulate a simplified liver ablation in virtual reality. The liver mesh used in this application is obtained from medical volume data. For better vis-ibility and ease of use, we scaled the vessel model by a factor of ten w.r.t. its real-world size, resulting in a mesh size of approximately 1.5 m in virtual space. We always refer to this scaled scene if not stated otherwise. Our method is di-vided into three different types of visualization, as shown in Fig. 1. First arrow gylphs, second heatmap with isolines and third PCD.

2.1   Glyph design

According to Ward [4], the most important geometrical properties of glyphs are shape, size, orientation and position where the most important appearance at-tributes are color, texture and transparency. With this in mind we aim to achieve an optimal distance encoding based on these attributes. Therefore we combine the concept of color glyphs [5] and arrow glyphs [6] and adjust them to our needs. To ensure a clear orientation, all arrowheads point from a certain point, e.g., a tumor or needlepoint towards the vascular structure. As shown in Fig. 2, the shape of the glyph can be divided into two levels, it changes according to the current glyph length and its quantity. For more distant regions, the shape was designed in such a way that absolute distances of 2 cm are displayed using small orbs. In addition, the glyph has a fixed width of 1 cm. The length corresponds to the current distance value. If the quantity of glyphs increases or the distance to the vessel decreases, a different arrow glyph without additional absolute dis-tance encoding is used. Otherwise, due to the limited resolution of the HMD,

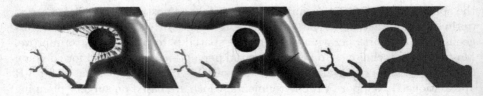

Fig. 1. Vessel with arrow glyphs, heatmap with isolines and PCD (left to right).

these areas may no longer be optimally represented by the glyphs. This resulting shape is stored in a texture and is then projected onto a view aligned quad. The color of the glyphs is an encoding of distance, e.g, the distance between the tip of a needle or a tumor position and the surface of the vessel. Here, the color is initialized with RGB values $(0.2, 0, 1)$ as blue for the maximum distance and with $(1,0,0.2)$ as red for a minimum distance [3]. The color values C are calculated as follows

$$C(d) = \begin{cases} red & \text{if } d < d_{\min} \\ (\frac{d}{d_{\max}} \cdot red) + (1 - \frac{d}{d_{\max}} \cdot blue) & \text{if } d_{\min} < d < d_{\max} \\ blue & \text{if } d > d_{\max} \end{cases} \qquad (1)$$

where d is the current length of the arrow glyph, $d_{\min}$ the shortest and $d_{\max}$ the longest possible glyph length. To prevent glyphs from simply appearing or disappearing, a gentle fading of the glyphs is achieved through transparency. Thus two different considerations were taken into account. First, the length of the glyph and second, the angle between the surface of the vessel and the glyph itself. Based on these two attributes a transparency value can be calculated. Thereby the sharper the angle or the greater the distance to the vessel surface, the more transparent the glyph is displayed. Depending on the mesh quality, the spatial vertex density is far too high to consider each vertex as a possible glyph location. While using the vertices of the mesh as anchor points for the arrow glyphs, the number of vertices has to be considerably reduced and at the same time a homogeneous distribution of the vertices must be ensured, as otherwise glyphs of different densities may occur in some areas, resulting in an inconsistent appearance of the glyphs. To obtain a consistent distribution of sample points across the mesh an implementation of the algorithm by Lichtenberg et al. [7] is used. Due to the periodic nature of the result, it is possible to extract near-uniformly distributed sample points.

2.2 Heatmap design

The arrow glyphs are designed to fill the empty space between the vessel and a point in three dimensional space. To evaluate a different approach of distance encoding, we have chosen heatmaps as an additional visualization technique. Heatmaps do not use the empty space between two points to encode its distance,

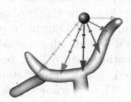 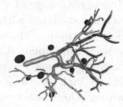

Fig. 2. Arrow glyphs with different shape, size and transparency.

Fig. 3. All eight distinct positions used for the evaluation.

but rather encode the distance directly on the mesh surface. Therefore the color of the mesh is changed according to the distance between a certain point and the vessel surface. To avoid visual overload, the heatmap is only displayed in critical areas. Therefore, a maximum distance was empirically set to $a/10$, where a is the mesh bounding sphere diameter. Anything beyond this distance is displayed in the original color and is not affected by the heatmap. The color value for the minimum distance has been set to a value of $(1, 0, 0.2)$, equal to the arrow glyphs. The maximum distance value is based on the primary mesh color. This ensures a smooth blend between the heatmap and the basic mesh color. The color interpolation between these values is similar to Equation 1. For consistency reasons these values are also modified with a Phong shading. Since it is difficult to encode quantitative values as distance with color alone, we add five isolines in the same region to get a better spatial impression of the critical areas.

2.3   Pseudo-chromadepth design

The heatmap and arrow glyphs are able to determine the relative distances between the vessel structure and a specific point in 3D space. In addition to these relative distance encodings, we aim to improve spatial perception through depth perception and encode the mesh depth directly with the PCD presented by Ropinski et al. [3]. The PCD encodes the depth information by means of color within a hue spectrum from red through magenta to purple and blue. The color of the mesh does not change according to the distance from a specific point to the surface, but rather encodes the depth of the mesh itself. In our work, the color of the vessel surface, tumor and needle tip changes depending on the position in the bounding box of the vessel and the view direction. The depth of different objects can therefore be aligned by matching colors. The color of the mesh is determined as described in Equation 1. In this case, the outermost point of the volume, which is nearest to the viewer, is red, while the point furthest away receives the color blue. For the purpose of this study we combine the depth-enhancing method of PCD with stereoscopic rendering.

2.4   Experiment

To confirm the hypothesis that spatial perception can be further improved in virtual reality, we conducted a quantitative comparative study with 17 volunteers with an age average of 24 years. The majority of participants were male computer science students without special medical skills. For this evaluation arrow glyphs, a heatmap with additional isolines and the PCD from Ropinski et al. [3] have been implemented and compared with a default Phong shading. As test environment, we used a virtual reality application with a liver vessel and added eight distinct positions represented by a red sphere. These spheres are scattered around the vessel tree, as shown in Fig. 3. The experiment was divided into two phases. During the first phase, called the preparation phase, the subject was displayed one of these spheres using a randomly selected method of visualization. After a detailed examination and once the subject was certain about

Table 1. Average results of all measurements for each visualization technique with standard deviation.

	Phong	Heatmap	Glyph	PCD	∅
Deviation (cm)	1.81 ± 0.13	1.97 ± 0.12	**1.52 ± 0.10**	1.75 ± 0.12	1.76 ± 0.12
Preparation (s)	**4.24 ± 3.89**	5.00 ± 4.74	5.06 ± 4.75	5.22 ± 4.50	4.85 ± 4.65
Execution (s)	**3.89 ± 1.94**	5.54 ± 3.48	5.56 ± 5.13	4.01 ± 2.71	4.75 ± 3.40

the proper position of the sphere, the sphere was removed. During the second stage, the execution phase, the subject was asked to place a new sphere at the previously examined position. In the process the time needed to orientate and estimate the position of the sphere, the time necessary to place the new sphere and the deviation from the original sphere position were determined.

3   Results

Each participant evaluated a total of 32 different combinations of sphere and visualization technique. The average results of all measured values for each visualization can be seen in Tab. 1. From all 544 measurements, the arrow glyph has the lowest deviation (1.52 cm) to be followed by the PCD (1.76 cm), Phong shading (1.81 cm) and heatmap combined with isolines (1.97 cm). The time required for preparation reveals that the participants were given a spatial impression of the sphere most quickly without visual stimuli (4.24 s). The same applies to the execution time, where Phong shading performed best with 3.89 s. We further performed an ANOVA test to determine a significant difference between the visualization techniques. The null hypothesis states that the arithmetic mean of the levels of the independent variable (i.e., the visualization techniques) are equal. Considering all measurements individually, we obtain $F(3, 540) = 3.055$ and $p = 0.0281$. Therefore we can reject the null hypothesis and state that the difference between the visualization techniques is statistically significant. In an additional two-way ANOVA, we investigated the impact of individual subject performance by considering the subjects as an additional independent variable. The interaction of both variables yield $F(48, 476) = 1.89$ and $p < 0.0001$. The significance of the visualization techniques was obtained as $F(3, 476) = 4, 17$ and $p = 0, 006$ and for the subjects as $F(16, 476) = 10.63$ and $p < 0.0001$. While we look at difference within groups, only glyph ↔ Phong ($p < 0.033$), glyph ↔ heatmap ($p < 0.00028$) and glyph ↔ PCD ($p < 0.049$) are significantly different by the Holm-Bonferroni post hoc analysis.

4   Discussion

In conclusion, considering Tab. 1, we can state that arrow glyphs can improve spatial perception in VR. The slightly increased orientation and execution time may be explained by an additional need to visually decode the distance information of the arrow glyphs in combination with the Phong shading. As the scenario is not designed to achieve results as quickly as possible but as accurately as possible, it is more important to minimize the error than to optimize the time required. The ANOVA test can be interpreted as a hint that subjects performed quite differently, but were nonetheless distinctly influenced by the visualization technique. A follow-up study should therefore investigate further factors that influence the subjects' precision.

Comparing the arrow glyphs with the default Phong shading, it can be observed that glyphs minimize the error by an average of 16 %. With the use of PCD, the error was also lowered by 3.3 %. It is surprising that a lot of time was needed for the initial orientation, whereas the placement of the sphere was very quick. This can be justified by the unique style of this visualization. As soon as the visualization is fully grasped, the placement is carried out in an intuitive way. The heatmap has achieved the lowest results in this study. Both the time required and the occurring error were higher than in other visualizations. During the experiment, we found that the subjects mainly used the contour of the isolines to navigate within the liver vessel, while no attention was paid to which exact isoline was used. The participants often matched wrong isolines. This may explain the increased error values of the heatmap with isolines. Depending on the surgical requirements, the visualizations can be useful for specific tasks. Arrow glyphs could improve navigation through a vascular structure as they have direct connections to the surface, while heatmaps or PCD could improve interaction with external structures such as tumors, since no additional geometry is generated. Since we have concluded that an improvement of spatial perception in VR can be achieved, we intend to conduct additional studies to determine which task can be best improved by which visualization technique.

Acknowledgement. The work was supported by the German Research Foundation (DFG) project LA 3855/1-1.

References

1. Huber T, Paschold M, Hansen C, et al. New dimensions in surgical training: immersive virtual reality laparoscopic simulation exhilarates surgical staff. Surg Endosc. 2017;31(11):4472–4477.
2. Mastmeyer A, Fortmeier D, Handels H. Evaluation of direct haptic 4d volume rendering of partially segmented data for liver puncture simulation. Sci Report. 2017;7(1):671.
3. Ropinski T, Steinicke F, Hinrichs K. Visually supporting depth perception in angiography imaging. Smart Graph Symp. 2006; p. 93–104.
4. Ward MO. A taxonomy of glyph placement strategies for multidimensional data visualization. Inf Vis. 2002;1(3-4):194–210.
5. Levkowitz H. Color icons-merging color and texture perception for integrated visualization of multiple parameters. IEEE Conf Vis. 1991; p. 164–170.
6. Wittenbrink CM, Pang AT, Lodha SK. Glyphs for visualizing uncertainty in vector fields. IEEE Trans Vis Comput Graph. 1996;2(3):266–279.
7. Lichtenberg N, Smit N, Hansen C, et al. Real-time field aligned stripe patterns. Comput Graph. 2018;74:137–149.

Simulation von Radiofrequenzablationen für die Leberpunktion in 4D-VR-Simulationen

Niclas Kath, Heinz Handels, Andre Mastmeyer

Institut für Medizinische Informatik, Universität zu Lübeck
mastmeyer@imi.uni-luebeck.de

Kurzfassung. Radio-Frequenz-Ablationen spielen eine wichtige Rolle in der Therapie von malignen Leberherden. Die Navigation einer Nadel zur Läsion stellt eine Herausforderung für den auszubildenden und auch für den intervenierenden Arzt dar. Daher ist es wünschenswert, Trainings- und Planungssysteme basierend auf medizinischen Bilddaten und Methoden der visuo-haptischen Virtual-Reality-Simulation anzubieten. In diesem Papier wird eine Methode zur Simulation von Ablationen an der Nadelspitze für einen bestehenden VR-Simulator nach erfolgreicher Nadelnavigation zum Läsionsherd vorgestellt. Ein verbessertes Modell wurde echtzeitfähig (CUDA) umgesetzt, evaluiert und erreicht hochperformant robustere und sicherere Planungsergebnisse als die Literatur.

1 Einleitung

Die Leber ist die größte Drüse des Menschen und erledigt die Schadstoffreinigung des Blutes. Sie ist sehr stark durchblutet (20% des Herzzeitvolumens). Dies führt zu einem erhöhten Streurisiko von Lebermetastasen neben den primären Tumoren, welche als hepatozelluläre Karzinome bekannt sind und aus bösartigen Mutationen der Leberzellen entstehen. Daneben treten in der Leber die selteneren Colangiokarzinome an den Gallengängen auf.

Bei der maximal-invasiven Leberteilresektion wird der tumorös betroffene Teil der Leber großzügig entfernt. Dies gelingt in der Nähe der Leberarterien nur erschwert. Bei solchen Tumoren ist die risikoärmere Radiofrequenzablation (RFA) möglich. Hierbei wird die Leberläsion punktiert und das Gewebe an der Nadelspitze erhitzt. Ab einer Temperatur von $42.5°C$ kommt es zur Denaturierung der Proteine innerhalb einer Zelle, was zum Absterben der erwärmten Zellregion führt.

Minimal-invasive Eingriffe wie die Leberpunktion können durch die jüngste Leistungssteigerung von Computern und Grafikkarten mit Methoden der Virtual-Reality (VR) simuliert werden. Dies verbessert potenziell die ärztliche Ausbildung sowie die Vorbereitung und Planung chirurgischer Eingriffe. Im Rahmen dieser Arbeit soll für einen existierenden visuo-haptischen VR-Simulator [1, 2, 3, 4, 5, 6] die RFA mit einem effizient parallel berechenbaren und im Vergleich zur Literatur [7] wie hier gezeigt besseren Temperaturmodell auf Grundlage der Pennes-Bioheat-Gleichung simuliert werden. Neu ist die effiziente Cuda- und Finite-Differenzen-basierte Berechnung, eine Verbesserung des Modells bez. eines Goldstandards [7] und ein konservativeres, sichereres Planungsergebnis.

2   Material und Methoden

Die virtuellen Körpermodelle wurden als Segmentierungsbilder mit existierenden Methoden modelliert [8, 9, 10]. Den Segmentierungsregionen wird ein struktur-spezifischer Temperaturwert zugewiesen, welcher bspw. für die temperaturab-führenden Blutgefäße eine Temperatur von zeitkonstant 37 °C aufweist. Dieses Temperaturregionenbild bildet die Zeititerationsgrundlage für die Simulation der RFA nach Positionierung der Nadelspitze in einer Läsion.

Das Modell für die Temperaturausbreitung ist die Pennes-Bioheat-Gleichung [7], diese lautet in dieser Arbeit

$$\rho c_p \frac{\partial T}{\partial t} = \nabla(K \nabla T) + w_b c_b (T_a - T) + Q_m \tag{1}$$

Im Unterschied zu [7] wird der Wärmewiderstand und der Gewebezustands-koeffizient nicht, dafür jedoch die metabolische Wärmequelle berücksichtigt. Hierbei stehen ρ für die spezifische Dichte der Leber ($1079 \frac{kg}{m^3}$), c_p für die Wär-mekapazität der Leber ($3540 \frac{J}{kg °C}$), t für die Zeit in Sekunden (s), K für die thermische Leitfähigkeit der Leber ($0.52 \frac{W}{m °C}$), T für die Temperatur (°C), w_b für die Durchblutungsrate der Leber ($16.687 \frac{ml}{min \, kg}$), c_b für die Wärmekapazität des Blutes ($3617 \frac{J}{kg °C}$), T_a für die Temperatur des Blutes ($37°C$) und Q_m für die metabolische Wärmegenerierung des Gewebes ($10714 \frac{W}{m^3}$) [11].

Für den 3D-Bildbereich lässt sich die partielle Differentialgleichung schreiben als

$$\rho c_p \frac{\partial T}{\partial t} = K \cdot \left(\frac{\partial^2 T}{\partial x^2} + \frac{\partial^2 T}{\partial y^2} + \frac{\partial^2 T}{\partial z^2} \right) + w_b c_b (T_a - T) + Q_m \tag{2}$$

Das in dieser Arbeit vorgestellte Modell rechnet auf diskreten 3D-Bilddaten. Daher wird die Gl. 2 mit der Finite-Differenzen-Methode (FDM) näherungsweise diskretisiert

$$\frac{\partial^2 (T_i)}{\partial x^2} = \frac{T(x_{i+1}) - 2T(x_i) + T(x_{i-1})}{(\Delta x)^2} \tag{3}$$

Δx steht für den Voxelabstand mit dem Index i an den benachbarten x-Stützstel-len $i-1$, i und $i+1$ in Millimetern. Mit den xyz-Richtungsindizes i, j und k lässt sich Gl. 2 in den 3D-Raum überführen

$$\rho c_p \frac{T_{i,j,k}^{n+1} - T_{i,j,k}^n}{\Delta t} = K \cdot (\frac{T_{i-1,j,k}^n - 2T_{i,j,k}^n + T_{i+1,j,k}^n}{(\Delta x)^2} + \frac{T_{i,j-1,k}^n - 2T_{i,j,k}^n + T_{i,j+1,k}}{(\Delta y)^2}$$

$$+ \frac{T_{i,j,k-1}^n - 2T_{i,j,k}^n + T_{i,j,k+1}^n}{(\Delta z)^2}) + (w_{b_{i,j,k}} c_{b_{i,j,k}} (T_a^n - T_{i,j,k}^n) + Q_{m_{i,j,k}})$$

$$\tag{4}$$

Hierbei gibt $T_{i,j,k}^n$ (Temperaturbild) die Temperatur des Voxels an der Stelle i, j, k im Bildkoordinatensystem zum Zeititerationsindex n an. Dieser kann mit equidistanten Zeitabständen in Sekunden umgerechnet werden.

Der Zeitschritttemperaturunterschied aus Gl. 4 wurde in CUDA umgesetzt, um die Berechnungen in Echtzeit auf der GPU durchführen zu können und wird iterativ auf das ursprüngliche Temperaturbild ($n = 0$) addiert.

2.1 Randbedingungen

Die Randbedingungen für die Voxel-Positionen an den Leberrändern werden im Rahmen dieser Arbeit idealisiert als komplett isolierend angenommen. Es findet keine Wärmediffusion an den Rändern der Leber statt. Für die Leberblutgefäße wird vereinfachend angenommen, dass sich diese nicht erwärmen (konst. $37°C$), da die Wärme stets vom Blutfluss abtransportiert wird. Dies wird in Form von entsprechenden, richtungsabhängigen Neumann-Randbedingungen (Temperaturkonstanzforderung über der Zeit) an den Lebergrenzen eingebracht.

2.2 Berücksichtigung der Atembewegung

Bei der Simulation einer Leberpunktion wird auch die Bewegung des Thoraxes während des Atmens berücksichtigt [1, 2]. Die verwendeten Temperaturbilder werden im Referenzraum X mit einem diffeomorphen Bewegungsvektorfeld $\hat{u}$ in den Atmungswölbungsraum x deformiert (Abb. 1) $I\left(\mathbf{x}_t\right) = I_{\text{ref}}\left(\mathbf{x}_t + \hat{u}^{-1}(\mathbf{x}_t, t)\right)$

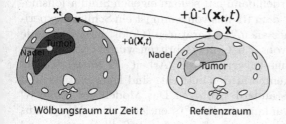

Wölbungsraum zur Zeit t Referenzraum

Abb. 1. Mit zeitvarianten diffeomorphen Bewegungsfeldern $\hat{u}$ besteht eine bijektive Beziehung zwischen Referenz- und Wölbungsraum. Die Simulation der Punktion [3] und der Ablationszonenausbreitung kann somit effizient im invarianten Referenzraum erfolgen und Atembewegung durch Projektion in den Wölbungsraum dargestellt werden [1, 2].

2.3 Evaluationsmethode

Zur Modelloptimierung und zur Überprüfung der Ergebnisse wurde die hier vorgeschlagene Temperaturausbreitungssimulation mit der Simulation und *in vitro* Messungen an echtem Gewebe von Linte et al. [7] verglichen. Zum Vergleich der Modelle wurde das Modell dieser Arbeit auf einem Temperaturbild mit der Leberregion in $380 \times 420 \times 271$ Voxeln und $0.5\,\text{mm}^3$ Voxelgröße berechnet. Die $2.5\,\text{mm}$ Geometrie der Nadelspitze wurde analog zu [7] als Voxel-Halbkugel modelliert durch fünf Voxel in xy-Richtung und drei Voxel in z-Richtung. Die Leistung der Methode wird mit der Anzahl der Bilder pro Sekunde, Frames per Second (FPS) vermessen. Die Grafikkarte für die Zeitmessungen war eine Nvidia GTX 1080 GPU. Verschiedene $x \times y \times z$-Thread pro Block-Konfigurationen wurden bewertet.

Tabelle 1. Vergleich vorhergesagter Temperaturen mit dem Goldstandard in 5 mm Abstand von der Nadelspitze mit $90°C$ (Δ-Fehler absolut; m-Mittelwert; σ-Standardabweichung).

Zeit	Modell		In vitro	Δ	
	hier	[7]	[7]	hier	[7]
0s	$37,00°C$	$37,0°C$	$37,0°C$	N/A	N/A
11,2s	**$37,28°C$**	**$37,3°C$**	$37,1°C$	**$0,18°C$**	**$0,2°C$**
19,6s	$38,06°C$	$37,4°C$	$38,8°C$	$0,74°C$	$1,4°C$
30,8s	$39,08°C$	$38,8°C$	$39,7°C$	$0,62°C$	$0,9°C$
39,2s	$39,71°C$	$40,3°C$	$40,4°C$	$0,69°C$	$0,1°C$
50,4s	$40,39°C$	**$41,6°C$**	$40,8°C$	$0,41°C$	**$0,8°C$**
58,8s	$40,81°C$	**$44,2°C$**	$41,4°C$	$0,59°C$	**$2,8°C$**
m	$39,22°C$	**$39,9°C$**	$39,7°C$	$0,54°C$	$1,0°C$
σ	$1,36°C$	$2,67°C$	$1,56°C$	$0,21°C$	$1,0°C$

3   Ergebnisse

3.1   Simulation der Temperaturausbreitung

Linte [7] hat in einem klinisch relevanteren in vitro Experiment die Temperaturverteilung bei einer Ablation mit $90°C$ im Abstand von 5 mm von der Nadelspitze in Präparaten gemessen. Diese wurden dann mit seinem eigenen Simulationsmodell vorhergesagt. Der Versuch mit dem Radius von 5 mm ist ein Schlüsselexperiment, da hier bei den in vitro gemessenen Temperaturen (Goldstandard) gerade nicht die Denaturierungsschwelle von $42.5°C$ überschritten wurde (Abb. 2).

Damit liegen die Temperaturmodellwerte dieser Arbeit im Mittel $0.54°C$ von den in vitro [7] bestimmten Temperaturen entfernt, sind konservativer und schwanken weniger um den Goldstandard (Abb. 2). Das Modell von Linte [7] liegt im Mittel bei größerer Schwankungsbreite $1°C$ entfernt. Das Modell aus dieser Arbeit modelliert die Temperaturgrenze für sterbende Zellen genauer und robuster als das Vergleichsmodell [7]. Bei kleineren Fehlern liegt das vorgestellte Modell als auch die in vitro bestimmten Temperaturen unterhalb der Schwelle von $42.5°C$ und weist einen systematisch ähnlicheren Temperaturkurvenverlauf zum Goldstandard auf. Die Ablation an einer temperaturabführenden Leberarterie wird in Abb. 3 gezeigt. Es wird rechts im Bild die Asymmetrie der gelben Hitzezone an der Leberarterie durch den Wärmeabtransport deutlich.

Abb. 2. Zeitlicher Verlauf der Temperaturen: Tendenzielle Überschätzung der Zelltodzone in Linte et al. [7].

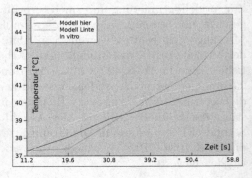

Konf.	t_{6000} [s]	t_1 [s]	FPS [Hz]
$64 \times 3 \times 3$	10,8	0,00180	556
$256 \times 3 \times 1$	12,3	0,00205	488
$1024 \times 1 \times 1$	12,23	0,00205	490

Tabelle 2. Kernel-Konfigurationen (Konf.) als $x \times y \times z$-Threads pro Block; Laufzeiten t_{6000} für 6000 Bilder, die daraus resultierende Zeit pro Bild t_1 sowie die Frames per Second (FPS).

3.2 Rendering-Performance

Die Performance der Simulation wurde durch mehrfachen Aufruf und Messung des Zeitverhaltens des CUDA-Kerns geprüft. Dabei wurden drei verschiedene Kernel-Aufrufkonfigurationen ($x \times y \times z$-Threads pro Block) getestet. Für den Vergleich der Laufzeiten wurden 6000 Iterationsbilder der Temperaturausbreitung berechnet.

Alle Kernel-Konfigurationen erreichen weit über 24 Bilder pro Sekunde (FPS) für eine flüssige Darstellung bewegter Bilder. Damit können alle Konfigurationen für die Echtzeitsimulation der Temperaturausbreitung verwendet werden. Die etwa 12% schnellere Laufzeit der Konfiguration mit $64 \times 3 \times 3$ Threads pro Block ist in der Ausnutzung des geteilten Speichers von CUDA für die Berechnung der finiten Differenzen begründet.

4 Diskussion

Das vorgestellte Modell simulierte Einzelbilder mit einer weit übererfüllenden Frequenz (FPS>24 Hz, ×23) für den VR-Simulator [12]. Den Goldstandard im Auge behaltend wurde im Unterschied zu [7] als Ergebnis der qualitativen Modelloptimierungen der Gewebezustandskoeffizient und der Wärmewiderstand nicht, jedoch die metabolische Wärmegenerierung der Leber berücksichtigt. Die Wärmezone lag näher an der Realität, d.h. der Radius der Wärmezone >42,5°C stimmt bei kleineren Fehlern mit den in vitro [7] bestimmten Vergleichswerten besser und im Zeitverlauf gleichförmiger überein. Die systematische Unterschätzung in Abb. 2 bedeutet eine konservativere Planung und ist rezidivsicherer als eine Überschätzung. Im Rahmen dieser Arbeit wurde eine hocheffiziente, präzise

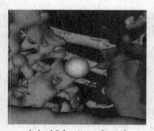 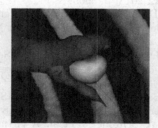 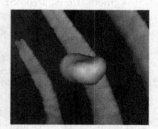

(a) Ablation distal   (b) Ablation proximal   (c) Abl. prox. ohne Gefäß

Abb. 3. Hitzezone (42.5°C, gelb) ohne Einfluss der temperaturabführenden Leberarterie. Hierbei entsteht eine kugelförmige Denaturierungszone (a). Ausbreitung der Temperatur direkt an der Leberarterie, wodurch sich die Form der Zone an die Leberarterie anpasst (b). Die Ausbreitungszone mit ausgeblendeter Leberarterie (c).

Methode zur Simulation der Bioheat-Gleichung vorgeschlagen. Diese modifiziert unter Plausibilitätsaspekten einige Terme innerhalb der Gleichung. Zur einer gefäßnahen Lage der Ablation (proximal) lagen uns leider keine in vitro Daten in [7] o. ä. vor. Trotz der Plausibilitätsannahmen wurde im Vergleich zum in vitro Experiment eine höhere Realitätsnähe und Robustheit erreicht. Interessant wäre zukünfig auch die Simulation der Brachytherapieintervention [13].

Danksagung. Drittmittel: DFG: HA 2355/11-2; Nvidia GPU Grant 2018 (A. Mastmeyer)

Literaturverzeichnis

1. Fortmeier D, Wilms M, Mastmeyer A, et al. Direct visuo-haptic 4D volume rendering using respiratory motion models. IEEE Trans Haptics. 2015;8(4):371–383.
2. Mastmeyer A, Fortmeier D, Handels H. Evaluation of direct haptic 4D volume rendering of partially segmented data for liver puncture simulation. Nat Sci Rep. 2017;7(1):1–15.
3. Mastmeyer A, Wilms M, Fortmeier D, et al. Real-time ultrasound simulation for training of US-guided needle insertion in breathing virtual patients. Stud Health Technol Inform: Med Meets Virtual Real 22 - MMVR. 2016;220:219–226.
4. Mastmeyer A, Fortmeier D, Handels H. Direct haptic volume rendering in lumbar puncture simulation. Stud Health Technol Inform: Med Meets Virtual Real 19 - MMVR. 2012;173:280–286.
5. Fortmeier D, Mastmeyer A, Handels H. GPU-based visualization of deformable volumetric soft-tissue for real-time simulation of haptic needle insertion. Procs BVM. 2012; p. 117–122.
6. Fortmeier D, Mastmeyer A, Handels H. An image-based multiproxy palpation algorithm for patient-specific VR-simulation. Stud Health Technol Inform. 2014; p. 107–113.
7. Linte C, Camp J, Holmes D, et al. Toward modeling of radio-frequency ablation lesions for image-guided left atrial fibrillation therapy: model formulation and preliminary evaluation. Stud Health Technol Inform. 2013;184(11):261–267.
8. Mastmeyer A, Fortmeier D, Maghsoudi E, et al.; International Society for Optics; Photonics. Patch-based label fusion using local confidence-measures and weak segmentations. Proc SPIE. 2013; p. 86691N–1–11.
9. Mastmeyer A, Fortmeier D, Handels H. Efficient patient modeling for visuo-haptic VR simulation using a generic patient atlas. Comput Methods Programs Biomed. 2016;132:161–175.
10. Mastmeyer A, Fortmeier D, Handels H; International Society for Optics; Photonics. Random forest classification of large volume structures for visuo-haptic rendering in CT images. Proc SPIE. 2016;9784:97842H–1–8.
11. Hasgall P, Gennaro F, Baumgartner C, et al.. IT'IS database for thermal and electromagnetic parameters of biological tissues. IT'IS Foundation; 2018.
12. Fortmeier D, Mastmeyer A, Schröder J, et al. A virtual reality system for PTCD simulation using direct visuo-haptic rendering of partially segmented image data. IEEE J Biomed Health Inform. 2016;20(1):355–366.
13. Mastmeyer A, Pernelle G, Ma R, et al. Accurate model-based segmentation of gynecologic brachytherapy catheter collections in MRI-images. Med Image Anal. 2017;42:173–188.

Abstract: An SVR-Based Data-Driven Leaflet Modeling Approach for Personalized Aortic Valve Prosthesis Development

Jannis Hagenah[1], Tizian Evers[1], Michael Scharfschwerdt[2], Achim Schweikard[1], Floris Ernst[1]

[1]Institute for Robotics and Cognitive Systems, University of Lübeck
[2]Department of Cardiac Surgery, University Hospital Schleswig-Holstein, Lübeck
hagenah@rob.uni-luebeck.de

While the aortic valve geometry is highly patient-specific and studies indicate its high influence on the circulation, state-of-the-art valve prostheses are not aiming at reproducing this individual geometry. One challenge in manufacturing personalized prostheses is the imaging of the thin leaflets in their curved 3D shape as well as the mapping from this shape to the planar 2D leaflet shape that is cut out of the fabrication material. Even in the gold standard imaging modality (transesophageal ultrasound), the leaflets are barely visible. Hence, we present a machine learning approach to estimate the individual leaflet shape from the image information on the shape of the surrounding tissue, i.e. the aortic root.

Thus, a database was set up to derive and evaluate valve leaflet shape models [1] . First, 3D ultrasound images of ex-vivo porcine valves were acquired under physiologically realistic pressure. In these images, geometric key features were identified manually to describe the individual geometry of the root. In a second step, the valves' leaflets were cut out, spread on an illuminated plate and photographed in this state. From these images, the leaflet shape was extracted using edge detection.

This database allows the derivation of a data-driven leaflet model utilizing non-linear support vector regression (SVR), aiming on a mapping from the geometric key features to the leaflet shape. Additionally, an existing, hand-crafted geometric leaflet shape model was evaluated on the dataset to evaluate its performance regarding personalization. The data-driven approach provided an acceptable leaflet shape estimation (0.61 mm ASCD) and clearly outperformed the existing model (2.21 mm ASCD). Hence, machine learning is capable of estimating the individual leaflet shape from sparse image data. This presents an important step towards personalized aortic valve prostheses.

References

1. Hagenah J, Evers T, Scharfschwerdt M, et al. An SVR-based data-driven leaflet modeling approach for personalized aortic valve prosthesis development. Comput Cardiol. 2018; p. accepted.

Mitral Valve Quantification at a Glance
Flattening Patient-Specific Valve Geometry

Pepe Eulzer[1], Nils Lichtenberg[1], Rawa Arif[2], Andreas Brcic[3], Matthias Karck[2], Kai Lawonn[1], Raffaele De Simone[2], Sandy Engelhardt[4]

[1]Institute for Computational Visualistics, University of Koblenz-Landau
[2]Department of Cardiac Surgery, Heidelberg University Hospital
[3]Department of Anaesthesiology, Heidelberg University Hospital
[4]Department of Computer Science, Mannheim University of Applied Sciences
eulzer@uni-koblenz.de

Abstract. Malfunctioning mitral valves can be restored through complex surgical interventions, which greatly benefit from intensive planning and pre-operative analysis from echocardiography. Visualization techniques provide a possibility to enhance such preparation processes and can also facilitate post-operative evaluation. In this work we extend current research in this field, building upon patient-specific mitral valve segmentations that are represented as triangulated 3D surface models. We propose a 2D-map construction of these models, which can provide physicians with a view of the whole surface at once. This allows assessment of the valve's area and shape without the need for different viewing angles and scene interaction. Clinically highly relevant pathology indicators, such as coaptation zone areas or prolapsed regions are color coded on these maps, making it easier to fully comprehend the underlying pathology. Quality and effectiveness of the proposed methods were evaluated through a user survey conducted with domain experts. We assessed pathology detection accuracy using 3D valve models in comparison to the developed method. Classification accuracy increased by 2.8 % across all tested valves and by 10.4 % for prolapsed valves.

1 Introduction

Treatment of mitral valve (MV) defects often requires complex therapies, including catheter-based interventions or repair surgeries on the valve. For diagnostic purposes and treatment decisions, transesophageal echocardiography (TEE) is the standard clinical modality and especially 3D probes are a valuable tool to recapitulate the surgeon's view on the valve. However, the volume visualizations that are part of most standard clinical care workstations are not capable of showing important clinical pathology indicators at a glance. Thus, more enhanced visualization techniques should be added to the cardiologist's and cardiac surgeon's toolbox for improved clinical assessment and surgical planning.

The mitral valve, consisting of four different parts, has a rather complicated three-dimensional configuration that is difficult to fully comprehend on volume rendered TEE images. At the same time, flat representations of anatomical structures are becoming increasingly popular in the domain of medical visualizations. Such 2D representations allow the assessment of a whole object in a single view. Practically all flattening techniques are projection-based and rely on mesh parameterization, i.e., the creation of bijective mappings between a parameter domain in $\mathbb{R}^2$ and a triangulated surface embedded in $\mathbb{R}^3$. A general overview of mesh parameterization techniques can be found in [1].

A recent state of the art report [2] reviews a variety of medical visualization techniques focused on planar representations. Flat depictions have been proposed for the circulatory system, the colon, the brain and the bones. A 2D representation of aortic valve prostheses has been introduced as well [3]. Properties like stent compression were assessed after implantation in order to analyze complication co-occurrences. In contrast, our approach targets facilitation of pre-operative MV analysis. Beyond that, we propose a planar view of patient specific MVs through global parameterization that preserves original structure in terms of tissue area and shape. Therefore, we use a boundary-free approach while fixing certain landmarks in the parameter space, enhancing overall comparability.

2   Materials and methods

As we target patient-specific maps, we rely on an already existing semi-automatic method to extract MV surface models from 4D ultrasound scans [4], consisting of annulus and leaflets. This segmentation algorithm provides separate triangulations for both MV leaflets and the annulus across the time-steps captured during a full cardiac cycle. Anatomical markers (Fig. 1) are already embedded in the representation and can be utilized during the flattening. Chordae tendineae and papillary muscles are not part of these models.

The quality of a flattening technique can be determined through metrics describing the amount of (inevitable) distortions. Usually, parameterization methods either focus on preserving angles (conformal) or area (equiareal) of an input mesh [5]. Fulfillment of both characteristics would result in an isometric or length-preserving parameterization. It is desirable that a 2D-view of the MV is close to isometric or at least equiareal. Retaining the proportions of the MV is

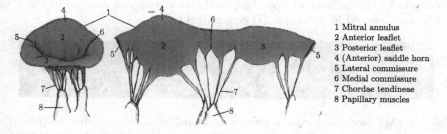

1 Mitral annulus
2 Anterior leaflet
3 Posterior leaflet
4 (Anterior) saddle horn
5 Lateral commissure
6 Medial commissure
7 Chordae tendineae
8 Papillary muscles

Fig. 1. MV similar to depictions in anatomy books with closed (left) and flattened valve (right), cut along the lateral commissure. Important anatomical features are marked.

a primary goal of our method, which should enable the possibility of area and length quantification on the flattened surface. Further, a physician using the 2D-view should develop an intuition for its orientation and scale. Hence, apart from minimizing distortions, the 2D-view should also target comparability across different data sets through a uniform appearance. Lastly, spatial context should be preserved, i.e., the relation between the 3D- and 2D-domain should be clear.

The general idea of the proposed flattening algorithm is to cut the MV along its lateral commissure and to unroll it along its diameter. This results in a perspective similar to the valve's depiction in textbooks [6] (Fig. 1, right side). In our algorithm we split the flattening process into three steps: annulus parameterization, leaflet initialization and relaxation. The shape of the annulus can give important hints during pathology analysis, therefore we first parameterize it as a curve, independent from the MV leaflets. Its configuration will remain unchanged during all further steps, preserving the annulus shape and arc length and increasing comparability across different data sets.

The annulus' height is plotted along the v- and its length along the u-axis of the 2D-view (Fig. 2). The correspondence of the u-axis in 3D is a reference plane through the annulus curve. An intuitive approach to compute it would be the least-squares method, resulting in a plane with minimal distances to points on the annulus. However, due to unfavorable distribution of annulus points in the model, this approach does not always lead to good results, i.e., the annulus' height is over- or underestimated (cf. dotted line in Fig. 2). Therefore, we employ a landmark-based approach, defining the annulus plane through three points: the two commissure points on the annulus, which form a natural axis through the MV and the barycenter of the posterior annulus, which usually approximates a planar layout. The resulting 2D view now allows to compare the annulus curve in relation to the u-axis, i.e. the location and height of the anterior saddle horn can be assessed in relation to the rest of the curve (Fig. 2, white line).

The leaflet geometry is placed below the annulus, ajar to the appearance of Fig. 1. First, a valid configuration is initialized, i.e., a leaflet layout without self-intersections or triangle-flips. We furthermore exploit the spline-like parallel lines which proceed vertically across the 3D surface representation. They are interpreted as iso-u curve approximations and points of each line are mapped to a shared u-coordinate while the distance between points is preserved in v-direction. The iso-u line corresponding to the saddle horn is marked in Fig. 2 on the 3D surface and in its initial 2D configuration.

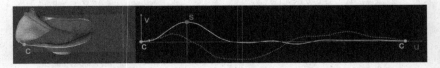

Fig. 2. 3D MV model and annulus plane constructed by a landmark-method (left). Parameterization of annulus (right) using a landmark- (white) and least-squares-method (yellow). Lateral commissure (c) and saddle horn (s) including its iso-u line are marked.

After all vertices are initialized they are iteratively optimized towards a more isometric parameterization. We target to minimize an energy term describing the distortion amount of the mesh's edge lengths. If the 3D mesh consists of vertices $\mathbf{p}_i$, corresponding to uv-coordinates $\mathbf{q}_i$ and the set N_i contains the indices of all neighbors of $\mathbf{p}_i$, a per-vertex length energy can be described as

$$E_l = \frac{1}{|N_i|} \sum_{j \in N_i} \frac{||\mathbf{q}_i - \mathbf{q}_j||}{||\mathbf{p}_i - \mathbf{p}_j||} + \frac{||\mathbf{p}_i - \mathbf{p}_j||}{||\mathbf{q}_i - \mathbf{q}_j||} \tag{1}$$

We use an iterative Euler method to minimize this energy, modelling the mesh edges in 2D as a network of springs. The vertices are displaced each iteration in the direction of a summed spring force calculated based on the model's edge lengths. A similar method was proposed to simulate mitral valve closure [7]. After the parameter space has been established, a variety of parameters can be color-mapped onto the 2D and 3D surface. We implemented two mappings: The first one shows an approximated coaptation zone, where we used a 2 mm distance threshold between anterior and posterior leaflet to determine the parts of the surface that collide. The other one is similar to a height-map. It marks areas of the MV which are above and below the annulus-plane. All mappings are applied to both, the 3D- and 2D-view, which are always rendered side-by-side.

3   Evaluation

To evaluate the employed optimization step, we performed measurements concerning area, angle and edge-length deformation using 50 MV models and compared the results before and after the spring relaxation method. Furthermore, we assessed the capabilities of the proposed visualization in a user study conducted with one visualization expert, two cardiac surgeons and one anesthetist. After an introductory video subjects were given a point-localization task, where they were asked to mark corresponding points in the 3D- and 2D-view. The main task was designed to simulate clinical decision making. Within an interactive prototype of our implementation participants were subsequently shown 40 MV models in two alternating formats: half of the models were only displayed in 3D (without color-coding) and half in a combined 3D/2D-view (with color-coding). In the latter, participants could access the coaptation and the height map (Fig. 3). Participants were asked to assign each valve to a category: normal, prolapsed or functional mitral regurgitation. The participants were not told that actually there were only 20 distinct MV models. Each model was shown twice in a randomized order, once in each view format, making direct comparison possible. Participants were further instructed to mark their confidence in their classification on a Likert-scale from one (not confident) to five (very confident).

4   Results

Evaluation of the relaxation step showed that we could optimize the average edge-length energy E_l from 0.78 before the relaxation to 0.07 afterwards (de-

Table 1. Averaged results of the pathology identification task per participant P regarding accuracy A_i, confidence C_i and time T_i comparing the 3D-only-view ($i = 0$) and the proposed 3D/2D combination ($i = 1$).

P	A_0	A_1	C_0	C_1	T_0	T_1
1	78.9 %	84.2 %	3.89	4.16	11.5 s	15.4 s
2	68.4 %	73.7 %	4.37	4.53	14.0 s	15.7 s
3	78.9 %	89.5 %	4.58	4.84	15.9 s	12.6 s
4	84.2 %	73.7 %	3.00	3.00	13.9 s	13.2 s
Total	77.6 %	80.3 %	3.96	4.13	13.8 s	14.2 s

viation from its possible minimum). Similar improvements were found for area distortion, however, measured angle energy remained relatively constant.

Two examples of the resulting visualization can be seen in Fig. 3. The upper row shows a healthy MV with a closed coaptation zone and no prolapsing parts. The lower row shows a pathological MV, and visual analysis of the 2D maps provide a much more detailed understanding of the pathology: in the 3D-view it is not clearly visible whether the valve fully closes or not. In contrast to that, the 2D-coaptation view indicates a part where the leaflets do not touch. Beyond that, the height map illustrates the extent of prolapsing areas very well, i.e. tissue which surpasses the annulus plane in systole is marked in red.

Within the first task of the user survey, all points were correctly assigned to each other in both views. Furthermore, the user survey showed an increase in the pathology detection rate of 3 out of 4 participants when they had access to the flattened MV, including the coaptation and prolapse color maps (Tab. 1). A total average of 2.6 % increased accuracy was measured. Most noticeably, global detection accuracy for prolapsed valves rose from 83.3 to 93.8 %. The time required for one classification averaged at about 14 s, regardless of the view mode. Participants were slightly more confident in their decisions when using the combined view. Average confidence (discrete scale from 1 to 5) rose from 3.96 to 4.13. When making incorrect classifications, participants reported an average confidence of 3.53 in both view-modes. For correct classifications, average confidence increased from 4.08 (3D-only) to 4.28 (3D/2D).

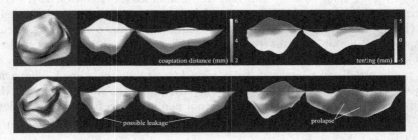

Fig. 3. Combined 3D/2D view with color-mapping. Healthy valve (top), prolapsed valve (bottom). Left to right: 3D coaptation, 2D coaptation, 2D height mapping.

5   Discussion

We presented an approach for flattening patient-specific MV models, resulting in a consistent depiction across data sets. The visualization targets facilitation of clinical MV analysis, a process that appears to benefit from the proposed 2D-view with color-maps. This is underlined by the increased pathology detection rate measured in our survey, which holds especially true for prolapsed valves. The coaptation zone can be assessed at a glance, as well as the prolapsed valve area. A landmark-based parameterization of the annulus makes comparison of height deviations possible. Low area and edge-length distortions of the leaflet geometry allow size quantification of the flattened MV. The evaluation shows that spatial context is preserved as the domain experts had no difficulties understanding 3D/2D-correspondence. Participants claimed pathologies were easier to identify and MV analysis was facilitated when the 2D-view was provided. A possible drawback of our method is low generalizability. The approach is specific towards the MV and our implementation relies on a specific model representation [4].

In the future we plan to extend the planar MV view by inclusion of functional information. Samples over the whole cardiac cycle could be visualized in 2D at once, simplifying assessment of annulus shape variation.

Acknowledgement. The work was supported by the German Research Foundation (DFG) project 398787259, EN1197/2-1, DE 2131/2-1.

References

1. Hormann K, Polthier K, Sheffer A. Mesh parameterization: theory and practice. Course presented at ACM SIGGRAPH; 2008.
2. Kreiser J, Meuschke M, Mistelbauer G, et al. A survey of flattening-based medical visualization techniques. Comput Graph Forum. 2018;37(3):597–624.
3. Born S, Sündermann SH, Russ C, et al. Stent maps: comparative visualization for the prediction of adverse events of transcatheter aortic valve implantations. IEEE Trans Vis Comp Graph. 2014;20(12):2704–2713.
4. Engelhardt S, Lichtenberg N, Al-Maisary S, et al. Towards automatic assessment of the mitral valve coaptation zone from 4D ultrasound. Funct Imaging Mod Heart. 2015;9126:137–145.
5. Grossmann N, Köppel T, Gröller E, et al. VisualFlatter: visual analysis of distortions in the projection of biomedical structures. Eurographics Workshop Vis Comput Biomed. 2018; p. 167–177.
6. Carpentier A, Adams DH, Filsoufi F. Carpentier's Reconstructive Valve Surgery. Maryland Heights, Missouri: Saunders/Elsevier; 2010.
7. Hammer PE, Perrin DP, Pedro J, et al. Image-based mass-spring model of mitral valve closure for surgical planning. Proc SPIE. 2008;6918:69180Q.

Fully-Deformable 3D Image Registration in Two Seconds

Daniel Budelmann[1], Lars König[1], Nils Papenberg[1], Jan Lellmann[2]

[1]Fraunhofer Institute for Medical Image Computing (MEVIS), Lübeck
[2]Institute of Mathematics and Image Computing, Universität zu Lübeck
daniel.budelmann@mevis.fraunhofer.de

Abstract. We present a highly parallel method for accurate and efficient variational deformable 3D image registration on a consumer-grade
graphics processing unit (GPU). We build on recent matrix-free variational approaches and specialize the concepts to the massively-parallel
manycore architecture provided by the GPU. Compared to a parallel
and optimized CPU implementation, this allows us to achieve an average speedup of 32.53 on 986 real-world CT thorax-abdomen follow-up
scans. At a resolution of approximately 256^3 voxels, the average runtime
is 1.99 seconds for the full registration. On the publicly available DIR-lab
benchmark, our method ranks third with respect to average landmark
error at an average runtime of 0.32 seconds.

1 Introduction

Image registration – i.e., finding a dense correspondence map between images or
volumes taken at different points in time or under different conditions – is still
a crucial component of many clinical and research pipelines: compensating for
patient movement and breathing in radiological follow-up and radiation therapy,
monitoring progression of degenerative diseases, 3D reconstruction from slices
in histopathology, and many others. It is made particularly challenging by the
typically large, three-dimensional nature of the data, highly non-convex energies,
and runtime requirements of clinical practice.

Towards reducing runtime, the authors of [1, 2] propose a highly accurate
non-rigid registration model with applications in follow-up imaging in radiology
and liver ultrasound tracking, and introduce a parallel algorithm for the CPU.
They also include a preliminary GPU implementation for the 2D case provided
by [3]. To achieve sub-second runtimes, we extend these ideas to a fast, matrix-
free, parallel algorithm that solves the variational, regularized problem for full
3D image registration on the GPU.

2 Materials and methods

2.1 Model

Regarding the model, we follow [2]: We seek a three-dimensional deformation
vector field $y \in \mathbb{R}^{3\overline{m}^y}$, $\overline{m}^y := m_x^y m_y^y m_z^y$, discretized on a deformation grid with

dimensions $m_x^y \times m_y^y \times m_z^y$, which deforms a template image $\mathcal{T} \in \mathbb{R}^{\overline{m}}$ to be similar to a reference image $\mathcal{R} \in \mathbb{R}^{\overline{m}}$, $\overline{m} := m_x m_y m_z$, both discretized on an image grid with dimensions $m_x \times m_y \times m_z$.

To find y, we numerically minimize an objective function $\mathcal{J}(y) : \mathbb{R}^{3\overline{m}^y} \to \mathbb{R}$, consisting of distance measure $\mathcal{D}$ and smoothing term $\mathcal{S}$, weighted by $\alpha > 0$

$$y^* := \arg \min_{y \in \mathbb{R}^{3\overline{m}^y}} \mathcal{J}(y) \quad \mathcal{J}(y) := \mathcal{D}(\mathcal{R}, \mathcal{T}(P(y))) + \alpha \mathcal{S}(y) \tag{1}$$

Here $P : \mathbb{R}^{3\overline{m}^y} \to \mathbb{R}^{3\overline{m}}$ denotes the grid conversion $Py =: \hat{y}$, which converts the deformation y from the deformation grid to the image grid, before it is used to interpolate the deformed template image $\mathcal{T}(P(y))$ on the image grid.

For the distance measure, we use the well-known normalized gradient field (NGF), which is particularly suitable for multi-modal images [4]. It focuses on intensity changes and compares the angles of the image gradients. To encourage smooth deformations, we employ the curvature-based regularization term $\mathcal{S}(y)$ introduced by [5], which penalizes the Laplacian of the deformation field components y_i via $(\Delta y_i)^2$.

For solving (1) numerically and robustly without accurate initialization, we use the Limited-Memory Broyden-Fletcher-Goldfarb-Shanno algorithm described in [6], embedded in a multi-level (coarse-to-fine) approach.

2.2 Parallelization

We chose to implement our method on the GPU using the CUDA toolkit, which allows working close to the hardware and fine-tuning.

Performance on the GPU is tightly coupled to a high occupancy, defined as the number of running threads divided by the number of potentially running threads that the device can handle. Using a large number of registers per thread decreases occupancy [7], therefore, we keep the number of variables per thread low and split large functions (kernels) into smaller ones.

We generally used single-precision (32 bit) floating variables due to the faster computations and only half the number of required registers compared to double precision (64 bit) [7].

For the multi-level approach, reference and template images need to be downsampled to various resolutions. The CUDA framework provides CUDA streams, which enable concurrency between GPU computations and memory transfers between host and GPU [7]. This allows to run the pyramid generation and data transfer for reference and template image in parallel.

Evaluating the distance term
$\mathcal{D}(y) : \mathbb{R}^{3\overline{m}^y} \to \mathbb{R}$ and its gradient requires two grid conversions and a gradient computation

1. convert the deformation y to the image grid, denoted by P: $\hat{y} := P(y)$
2. compute the distance measure $\mathcal{D}$ and its gradient $\nabla \mathcal{D}(\hat{y})$, and
3. convert $\hat{y}$ and $\nabla \mathcal{D}(\hat{y})$ to the deformation grid by applying $P^\top$

In the following sections, we discuss the details of each step and its implications for the implementation with CUDA.

We denote by $\nabla \mathcal{R}_i$ and $\nabla \mathcal{T}_i(P(y))$ the gradients of the reference and deformed template image at the i-th image grid point and discretize the NGF distance measure as a sum over grid points

$$\mathcal{D}_{\mathrm{NGF}}(y) = \frac{\overline{h}}{2} \sum_{i=1}^{\overline{m}} \left(1 - \left(\frac{\langle \nabla \mathcal{T}_i(P(y)) \nabla \mathcal{R}_i \rangle + \tau \varrho}{||\nabla \mathcal{T}_i(P(y))||_\tau ||\nabla \mathcal{R}_i||_\varrho} \right)^2 \right) \tag{2}$$

with voxel volume $\overline{h} = h_x h_y h_z$ as product of the image grid spacings, the smoothed norm function $|| \cdot ||_\varepsilon = \sqrt{\langle \cdot, \cdot \rangle + \varepsilon^2}$, and the modality-dependent parameters $\tau, \varrho > 0$ to filter the gradient image for noise. Following [1], we can parallelize the computation of the distance measure function value directly over the terms in the sum.

Applying derivative-based numerical optimization methods such as L-BFGS requires frequent evaluation of the gradient $\nabla \mathcal{D}$. The chain rule yields $\nabla \mathcal{D}_{\mathrm{NGF}}(y) = \frac{\partial \psi}{\partial \mathcal{T}} \frac{\partial \mathcal{T}}{\partial P} \frac{\partial P}{\partial y}$ with the reduction function $\psi : \mathbb{R}^{\overline{m}} \to \mathbb{R}$.

Evaluating the gradient using the chain rule by computing the gradient parts and multiplying step-by-step is expensive in terms of (intermediate) memory required. We avoid this by relying on the matrix-free methods introduced by [2].

Following the approach proposed by [1], we separate the deformation grid resolution $\overline{m}^y$ and the image resolution $\overline{m}$. This allows to save memory and speed up the registration by discretizing the deformation on a coarser grid while preserving all information in the input images.

For optimal performance, a (surprisingly) crucial step in computing the distance measure and its gradient is conversion between the two grids, i.e., computing matrix-vector products with P and $P^\top$. Applying P is directly parallelizable when using trilinear interpolation [1]. However, applying $P^\top$ with a coarser deformation grid produces possible write conflicts introduced when summing up values from multiple points on the higher-resolution image grid in order to obtain a value for a single point on the lower-resolution deformation grid.

To account for this issue, the authors of [1] introduced a red-black scheme, where all odd slices are computed in parallel, followed by all even slices. However, the author of [3] observed a poor utilization of GPU cores with this method. Therefore they computed every slice, row, and column in parallel, and used atomic operations to avoid write conflicts.

We introduce a different method, which is not based on the red-black-scheme and free of write conflicts: Each thread computes a deformation grid point independently by summing the corresponding image domain points

$$y = \sum_{i \in \Omega_1} \sum_{j \in \Omega_2} \sum_{k \in \Omega_3} \omega \cdot \hat{y}_{i,j,k} \tag{3}$$

Here, ω is the local weight and Ω_i are the corresponding indices of $\hat{y}$ for each dimension, which are determined beforehand, separately for each dimension. While there is a certain overhead in computing the weights ω this way, in our case it was found that the overall runtime is still faster due to the higher parallelism.

Table 1. Mean runtimes and standard deviations, averaged over 986 thorax-abdomen registrations. Finest image resolutions were approximately 256^3, 128^3, 64^3 and 32^3. Compared to the CPU-based OMP implementation, we achieve an average speedup of 32.53 with average runtimes of less than 2 seconds, which opens up new application scenarios for clinical use and interactive registration.

	256^3	128^3	64^3	32^3
Ours (s)	**1.99 ± 0.87**	0.56 ± 0.14	0.39 ± 0.08	0.36 ± 0.08
OMP (s)	66.94 ± 39.36	8.11 ± 3.21	2.24 ± 0.69	1.62 ± 0.43
Speedup	**32.53 ± 10.04**	14.06 ± 2.56	5.64 ± 0.68	4.51 ± 0.40

3   Results

We investigated the accuracy and speed of our method in comparison to state-of-the-art alternatives from the DIR-Lab 4DCT benchmark [8, 9]. We also compared to an Open Multi-Processing–(OMP–)based implementation of the same model on the CPU proposed in [2], which is already one to two orders of magnitude faster than a matrix-based implementation using the MATLAB FAIR toolbox [4].

All experiments were performed using an NVIDIA GeForce GTX 1080Ti GPU and an Intel Core i7-6700K CPU.

3.1   Radboud follow-up CT dataset

In order to investigate the performance of our method on high-resolution 3D data, we measured the average runtime over 986 registrations on a dataset of follow-up thorax abdomen CT scans provided by the Radboud University Medical Center, Nijmegen, Netherlands. The images have resolutions in the range of $512^2 \times \{72, \ldots, 1577\}$. As full image resolution was slightly out of reach due to memory restrictions of the GPU, we evaluated our approach on half, quarter, eighth and sixteenth resolution per dimension.

For the highest resolution, average runtime was 1.99 seconds, with an average speedup of 32.53 compared to the CPU-based parallel OMP implementation (Tab. 1). On the lower resolutions, our method achieves sub-second runtimes at a speedup of about one order of magnitude. A majority of the runtime on the lower resolutions is spent on the multi-level creation, due to the large memory transfer and downsampling.

It is prudent to ask whether moving from double precision to single precision on the GPU introduces differences due to rounding. In fact, we observed that this can have an effect (Fig. 1, Tab. 2). However, it typically only occurs when there are no clear correspondences, such as in regions of the colon with different content, or when the examination table is visible in one of the two scans. In these areas, there is no strong objective function gradient in either direction during optimization, so that numerical differences have a larger impact. However, we argue that if such areas were to be registered accurately, a more elaborate model that accounts for the possible removal of structures would have to be employed in any case.

3.2   DIR-Lab 4DCT benchmark

For a comparison to the state of the art, we evaluated our method on the DIR-Lab 4DCT dataset [8, 9], consisting of ten CT scan pairs of the lung in fully-inhaled and fully-exhaled state. Resolutions are in the range of $256^2 \times \{94, \ldots, 112\}$ for the first five images and $512^2 \times \{120, \ldots, 136\}$ for the last five images. We set the deformation grid to one quarter of the image resolution.

Accuracy of the final registration was measured by the average landmark error (LME) over 300 expert-annotated landmarks for each dataset (Fig. 2). Our OMP implementation scores only slightly behind the best-performing pTVreg method at an average LME of 0.92 mm vs. 0.93 mm and places second-best overall in terms of accuracy.

Our GPU implementation follows closely due to the single precision computations and achieves third place overall in terms of accuracy at an LME of 0.94 mm. Moreover, it is about one order of magnitude faster than all other methods in the benchmark for which runtimes could be obtained. Compared to the only method with better accuracy (pTVreg), it is approximately 400 times faster, at an average of 0.32 seconds per full 3D registration.

4   Discussion

We introduced a new method for non-linear registration using the GPU, which is highly efficient while maintaining state-of-the-art accuracy. We compared it to an optimized CPU implementation and achieved speedups up to a factor of 32.53 ± 10.04 at runtimes under 2 seconds, while placing third with respect to accuracy in the DIR-Lab 4DCT benchmark. We believe that such low overall runtimes will open up new application scenarios for clinical use, such as interactive registration and real-time organ tracking, and will further clinical adoption of fully-deformable, non-rigid registration methods.

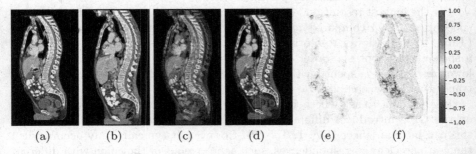

(a)   (b)   (c)   (d)   (e)   (f)

Fig. 1. (a,b) Sagittal slices of reference and template image; (c) overlay image before registration; (d) after deformable registration, the overlay image clearly highlights morphological differences; (e) the difference image between GPU- and OMP-based registration results shows slight variations in regions with few unambiguous correspondences, such as the colon; (f) final registration result with differences highlighted in color. Image courtesy of Radboud University Medical Center, Nijmegen, Netherlands.

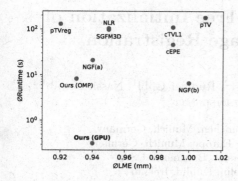

Fig. 2. Comparison of average landmark error (LME) in mm and runtime based on the DIR-Lab dataset. Shown are the algorithms with smallest average LME.

	∅ LME [mm]	∅ Runtime
Ours (GPU)	**0.94±1.10**	0.32 s
NGF(b)	1.00±1.07	6.56 s
Ours (OMP)	**0.93±1.07**	8.24 s
NGF(a)	0.94±1.07	20.90 s
cEPE	0.99±1.13	46 s
SGFM3D	0.95±1.07	98 s
NLR	0.95±1.07	104.19 s
cTVL1	0.99±1.09	110 s
pTVreg	**0.92±1.06**	130 s
pTV	1.01±1.12	180 s
LMP	0.95±1.07	N/A
isoPTV	0.95±1.15	N/A

Table 2. Comparison of average landmark error (LME) in mm and runtime based on the DIR-Lab dataset. While achieving state-of-the-art accuracy, our method is faster by orders of magnitude and provides fully deformable 3D registrations in 0.32 seconds on average.

References

1. König L, Rühaak J. A fast and accurate parallel algorithm for non-linear image registration using normalized gradient fields. Proc ISBI. 2014; p. 580–583.
2. König L, et al. A matrix-free approach to parallel and memory-efficient deformable image registration. SIAM J Sci Comput. 2018;40(3):B858–B888.
3. Meike M. GPU-basierte nichtlineare Bildregistrierung [mathesis]. 2016;.
4. Modersitzki J. FAIR: Flexible Algorithms for Image Registration. Proc SIAM; 2009.
5. Fischer B, Modersitzki J. A unified approach to fast image registration and a new curvature based registration technique. Linear Algebr Appl. 2004;380:107–124.
6. Nocedal J. Updating quasi-newton matrices with limited storage. Math Comput. 1980;35(151):773–782.
7. Wilt N. The CUDA Handbook: A Comprehensive Guide to GPU Programming. Addison-Wesley; 2013.
8. Castillo R, et al. A framework for evaluation of deformable image registration spatial accuracy using large landmark point sets. Phys Med Biol. 2009;54(7):1849–1870.
9. Castillo E, et al. Four-dimensional deformable image registration using trajectory modeling. Phys Med Biol. 2009;55(1):305–327.

Abstract: Landmark-Free Initialization of Multi-Modal Image Registration

Julia Rackerseder[1], Maximilian Baust[2], Rüdiger Göbl[1], Nassir Navab[1,3],
Christoph Hennersperger[1,4]

[1]Technische Universität München, Munich, Germany
[2]Konica Minolta Laboratory Europe, Munich, Germany
[3]Johns Hopkins University, Baltimore, USA
[4]Trinity College Dublin, Dublin, Ireland
julia.rackerseder@tum.de

To achieve convergence, nonlinear deformable image registration tasks of partial-view 3D ultrasound and MRI, as often seen in US guided interventions or retrospective studies thereof, need to be initialized. In clinical practice corresponding 3D landmarks are selected in both images. Performing this depends on the geometrical understanding of the targeted anatomy and the modality-specific appearance and is thus prone to error. Therefore, in [1] we propose a novel landmark-free initialization procedure that is robust in terms of target area overlap (pixels where target area and US volume are superimposed before initialization) as well as image overlap (pixels where MRI and US are superimposed). The method only requires N low-resolution coarse segmentations as input, which in most cases can be obtained automatically or with minimal user interaction, such as few pre-labeled pixels. A euclidean distance transform is applied to these N label maps, creating a multi-class distance map for both images. This leads to a minimization problem, where these maps are registered by optimizing our proposed similarity measure via a modified gradient descent scheme, which prevents unstable behaviour. The proposed method was evaluated, showing a success rate of 100% for registration tasks with initial target area overlap over 10%. It also converges for all cases with image overlap of 30% or more.

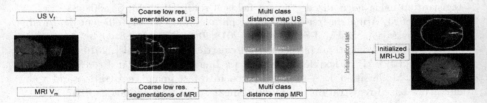

Fig. 1. Graphical overview of the method.

References

1. Rackerseder J, Baust M, Göbl R, et al. Initialize globally before acting locally: enabling landmark-free 3D US to MRI registration. Proc MICCAI. 2018; p. 827–835.

Enhancing Label-Driven Deep Deformable Image Registration with Local Distance Metrics for State-of-the-Art Cardiac Motion Tracking

Alessa Hering[1,2], Sven Kuckertz[1,3], Stefan Heldmann[1], Mattias P. Heinrich[3]

[1]Fraunhofer MEVIS, Lübeck
[2]Diagnostic Image Analysis Group, Radboud UMC, Nijmegen, Netherlands
[3]Institute of Medical Informatics, University of Lübeck
alessa.hering@mevis.fraunhofer.de

Abstract. While deep learning has achieved significant advances in accuracy for medical image segmentation, its benefits for deformable image registration have so far remained limited to reduced computation times. Previous work has either focused on replacing the iterative optimization of distance and smoothness terms with CNN-layers or using supervised approaches driven by labels. Our method is the first to combine the complementary strengths of global semantic information (represented by segmentation labels) and local distance metrics that help align surrounding structures. We demonstrate significant higher Dice scores (of 86.5 %) for deformable cardiac image registration compared to classic registration (79.0 %) as well as label-driven deep learning frameworks (83.4 %).

1 Introduction

Image registration aims to align two or more images to achieve point-wise spatial correspondence. This is a fundamental step for many medical image analysis tasks and has been a very active field of research for decades. In deformable image registration approaches, non-rigid, non-linear deformation fields are established between a pair of images, such as cardiac cine-MR images. Typically, image registration is phrased as an unsupervised optimization problem w.r.t. a spatial mapping that minimizes a suitable cost function by applying iterative optimization schemes. Due to substantially increased computational power and availability of image data over the last years, learning-based image registration methods have emerged as an alternative to energy-optimization approaches.

1.1 Prior work on CNN-Based deformable registration

Compared to other fields relatively little research has yet been undertaken in deep-learning-based image registration. Only recently have the first deep-learning based image registration methods been proposed [1, 2, 3], which mostly aim to learn a function in form of a CNN that predicts a spatial deformation warping a moving image to a fixed image. We categorize these approaches into *supervised*

[1], *unsupervised* [2, 4] and *weakly-supervised* [3] techniques based on how they train the network.

The supervised methods use ground-truth deformation fields for training. These deformation fields can either be randomly generated or produced by classic image registration methods. The main limitation of these approaches is that their performance is limited by the performance of existing algorithms or simulations. In contrast, the unsupervised method do not require any ground-truth data. The learning process is driven by image similarity measures or more general by evaluating the cost function of classic variational image registration methods. An important milestone for the development of these methods was the introduction of the spatial transformer networks [5] to differentiably warp the moving image during training. Weakly-supervised methods also do not rely on ground-truth deformation fields but training is still supervised with prior information. The labels of the moving image are transformed by the deformation field and compared within the loss function with the fixed labels. All anatomical labels are only required during training.

1.2 Contributions

We propose a new deep-learning-based image registration method that learns a registration function in form of a CNN to predict a spatial deformation that warps a moving image to a fixed image. In contrast to previous work, we propose the first weakly-supervised approach, which successfully combines the strengths of prior information (segmentation labels) with an energy-based distance metric within a comprehensive multi-level deep-learning based registration approach.

2   Materials and methods

Let $\mathcal{F}, \mathcal{M} : \mathbb{R}^2 \to \mathbb{R}$ denote the fixed image and moving image, respectively, and let $\Omega \subset \mathbb{R}^2$ be a domain modeling the field of view of $\mathcal{F}$. We aim to compute a deformation $y : \Omega \to \mathbb{R}^2$ that aligns the fixed image $\mathcal{F}$ and the moving image $\mathcal{M}$ on the field of view Ω such that $\mathcal{F}(x)$ and $\mathcal{M}(y(x))$ are similar for $x \in \Omega$.

Fig. 1. Illustration of the training process. For convenience, there is only one output deformation field shown instead of three. While application after the training only flows represented by red-dotted lines and red parts are required.

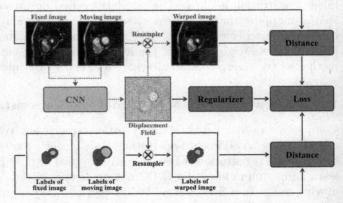

Inspired by recent unsupervised image registration methods (e.g. [2, 1]), we do not employ iterative optimization like in classic registration, but rather use a CNN that takes images $\mathcal{F}$ and $\mathcal{M}$ as input and yields the deformation y as output (Fig. 1). Thus, in the context of CNNs, we can consider y as a function of input images $\mathcal{F}, \mathcal{M}$ and trainable CNN model parameters θ to be learned, i.e. $y(x) \equiv y(\theta; \mathcal{F}, \mathcal{M}, x)$. During the training, the CNN parameters θ are learned so that the deformation field y minimizes the loss function

$$\mathcal{L}(\mathcal{F}, \mathcal{M}, b_{\mathcal{F}}, b_{\mathcal{M}}, y) = \delta \cdot \mathcal{D}(\mathcal{F}, \mathcal{M}(y)) + \alpha \cdot \mathcal{R}(y) + \beta \cdot \mathcal{B}(b_{\mathcal{F}}, b_{\mathcal{M}}(y)) \quad (1)$$

with so-called distance measure $\mathcal{D}$ that quantifies the similarity of fixed image $\mathcal{F}$ and deformed moving image $\mathcal{M}(y)$, regularizer $\mathcal{R}$ that forces smoothness of the deformation and a second distance measure $\mathcal{B}$ that quantifies the similarity of fixed segmentation $b_{\mathcal{F}}$ and warped moving segmentation $b_{\mathcal{M}}(y)$. The parameters $\delta, \alpha, \beta \geq 0$ are weighting factors. For convenience, we set $\delta = 1$. Note that the segmentations are only used to evaluate the loss function and not used as network input and are therefore only required during training. We use the edge-based normalized gradient fields distance measure [6]

$$\mathcal{D}(\mathcal{F}, \mathcal{M}(y)) = \frac{1}{2} \int_{\Omega} 1 - \frac{\langle \nabla \mathcal{M}(y(x)), \nabla \mathcal{F}(x) \rangle_{\epsilon}^2}{\|\nabla \mathcal{M}(y(x))\|_{\epsilon}^2 \|\nabla \mathcal{F}(x)\|_{\epsilon}^2} \, dx$$

with $\langle f, g \rangle_{\epsilon} := \sum_{j=1}^{2} f_j g_j + \epsilon^2 \, \|f\|_{\epsilon} := \sqrt{\langle f, f \rangle_{\epsilon}}$ so-called edge parameter $\epsilon > 0$ and curvature regularizer $\mathcal{R}(y) = \frac{1}{2} \int_{\Omega} \sum_{j=1}^{2} \|\Delta y_j\|^2 \, dx$ [6]. The similarity of the segmentation masks is measured using a sum of squared differences of the one-hot-representation of the segmentations $\mathcal{B}(y) = \frac{1}{2} \int_{\Omega} \|b_{\mathcal{M}}(y(x)) - b_{\mathcal{F}}(x))\|^2 dx$

2.1 Architecture and training

Our architecture is illustrated in Fig. 2. Our network architecture basically follows the structure of a UNet [7], taking a pair of fixed and moving images as

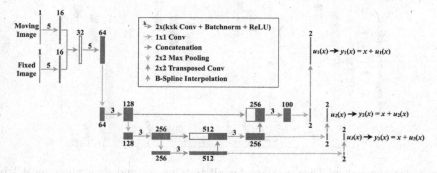

Fig. 2. Proposed UNet based architecture of our CNN. Each blue box represents a multi-channel feature map whose width corresponds corresponds to the number channels which is denoted above or below the box.

input. However, we start with two separate, yet shared processing streams for the moving and fixed image. The CNN generates a grid of control points for a B-spline transformer, which output is a full displacement field to warp a moving image to a fixed image. During training, the outputs of the network are three deformation fields of different resolutions. We compute the overall loss as a weighted sum of the network outputs on this different resolution levels. This design decision is inspired by the multi-level strategy of classic image registration. During inference, only the deformation field on the highest resolution is used.

2.2 Experiments

We perform our experiments on the ACDC dataset [8]. It contains cardiac multi-slice 2D cine-MR images of 100 patients captured at end-diastole (ED) and end-systole (ES) time point, amounting to 951 2D images per cardiac phase. The dataset includes annotations for left and right ventricle cavity and my-ocardium of a clinical expert. We only use slices that contain all labels, i.e. 680 2D images pairs. All images are cropped to the region of interest with a size of 112×112 pixels. Image intensities are normalized to a range of $[0, 1]$ For data augmentation we slightly deform the images and segmentations to increase the number of image pairs by a factor of 8.

Training is performed as a k-fold cross-validation with $k = 10$, which divides our dataset patient-wise. The network is trained for 40 epochs on a GTX 1080 in Pytorch in ≈ 0.5 hours using an ADAM optimizer with a learning rate of 10^{-3} and a batch size of 30. We empirically choose the regularization parameter $\alpha = 10^3$, the boundary-loss weight $\beta = 5 \cdot 10^4$ and edge parameter $\epsilon = 0.1$ in the loss function. To evaluate our registration we use the computed deformation field to propagate the segmentation of the moving image and measure the volume overlap using the Dice coefficient. We compare our method with a classic multi-level image registration model similar to [6] which iteratively minimizes the loss function without the use of segmentation data.

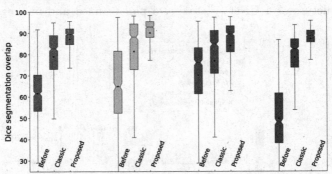

Fig. 3. Comparison of Dice overlaps for all test images and each anatomical label (brown: average of all labels, yellow: left ventricle cavity (vc), red: right vc, and green: myocardium). For each one the distributions of Dice coefficients before, after classic and after our proposed registration are shown.

Table 1. The quantitative effect of variations of the weighting within the loss function $\mathcal{L} = \delta \cdot \mathcal{D} + \alpha \cdot \mathcal{R} + \beta \cdot \mathcal{B}$ is shown when varying one parameter and fixing the others to their empirically determined optimal values. Besides the resulting Dice coefficient the percentage of pixels in which foldings $(\det(\nabla y) \leq 0)$ occur is depicted.

opt. →	$\delta = 1$		$\alpha = 10^3$		$\beta = 5 \cdot 10^4$		Colormap
	Dice	Folding	Dice	Folding	Dice	Folding	87%
$\times 10^2$	0.1%	78.2%	75.4%	0.0%	86.0%	0.6%	86%
$\times 10^1$	83.1%	0.7%	83.5%	0.2%	87.2%	0.1%	85%
							84%
	86.5%	0.0%	86.5%	0.0%	86.5%	0.0%	83%
$\times 10^{-1}$	85.9%	0.0%	87.0%	0.2%	85.3%	0.1%	82%
$\times 10^{-2}$	85.5%	0.1%	87.2%	0.4%	81.6%	0.4%	81%
$\times 0$	83.4%	0.1%	0.0%	40.6%	81.9%	0.4%	<80%

3 Results

As shown in Fig. 3, our proposed method outperforms the classic multi-level image registration approach compared by the average Dice coefficient. Our method achieves an average improvement from 79.0 % (classic) and 83.4 % (label-driven [3]) to 86.5 % across all three labels in terms of Dice accuracy while reducing the computation time drastically from 3.583 s (classic) to 0.006 s per image pair. Not only the average Dice score of our approach is higher for every anatomical label, but also the variation is reduced (Fig. 3). Fig 4 shows two example image pairs and the registration results, demonstrating the ability of our method to compensate large local deformations.

In comparison to the method of Krebs [4] which uses the same dataset and

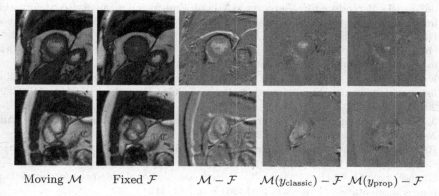

Moving $\mathcal{M}$ Fixed $\mathcal{F}$ $\mathcal{M} - \mathcal{F}$ $\mathcal{M}(y_{\text{classic}}) - \mathcal{F}$ $\mathcal{M}(y_{\text{prop}}) - \mathcal{F}$

Fig. 4. Example input images $\mathcal{M}$ and $\mathcal{F}$, difference image of the input images (third column), of fixed image and the warped image after classic registration (fourth column) and of fixed image and warped image after our proposed registration (fifth column). White and black indicate a great difference, while grey means similar images.

present comparable Dice coefficients of unregistered images, our method yields an improvement from 78.3 % to 81.9 % (when considering unsupervised approaches $\beta = 0$). As illustrated in Tab. 1, our choice of weighting parameters within the loss function (1) leads to a compromise between maximizing the Dice score and keeping the percentage of foldings low.

4   Discussion

We have presented a new weakly-supervised deep-learning-based method for image registration that replaces iterative optimization steps with deep CNN-layers. Our approach advances the state-of-the-art in CNN-based deformable registration by combining the complementary strengths of global semantic information (supervised learning with segmentation labels) and local distance metrics borrowed from classical medical image registration that supports the alignment of surrounding structures. We have evaluated our technique on dozens of cardiac multi-slice 2D cine-MR images and demonstrate substantial improvements compared to classic image registration methods both in terms of Dice coefficient and execution time. We also demonstrated the importance of integrating both unsupervised (distance measure $\mathcal{D}$) supervised (boundary term $\mathcal{B}$) learning objectives into a unified framework and achieve state-of-the-art Dice scores of 86.5 %.

Acknowledgement. M.P.H. acknowledges partial funding of this work through DFG grant HE 7364/1-2

References

1. Rohé MM, Datar M, Heimann T, et al.; Springer. SVF-Net: learning deformable image registration using shape matching. Proc MICCAI. 2017; p. 266–274.
2. de Vos BD, Berendsen FF, Viergever MA, et al. End-to-end unsupervised deformable image registration with a convolutional neural network. Proc MICCAI Workshop DLMIA, ML-CDS. 2017; p. 204–212.
3. Hu Y, Modat M, Gibson E, et al. Weakly-supervised convolutional neural networks for multimodal image registration. Med Image Anal. 2018;49:1–13.
4. Krebs J, Mansi T, Mailhé B, et al. Unsupervised probabilistic deformation modeling for robust diffeomorphic registration. Proc MICCAI Workshop DLMIA, ML-CDS. 2018; p. 101–109.
5. Jaderberg M, Simonyan K, Zisserman A, et al. Spatial transformer networks. Adv Neural Inf Process Sys. 2015; p. 2017–2025.
6. Rühaak J, Heldmann S, Kipshagen T, et al. Highly accurate fast lung CT registration. Proc SPIE. 2013;8669:86690Y.
7. Ronneberger O, Fischer P, Brox T. U-Net: convolutional networks for biomedical image segmentation. Proc MICCAI. 2015; p. 234–241.
8. Jodoin PM, Lalande A, Bernard O. Automated cardiac diagnosis challenge (ACDC); 2017. Accessed: 2018-09-24. Available from: https://www.creatis.insa-lyon.fr/Challenge/acdc/databases.html.

Respiratory Deformation Estimation in X-Ray-Guided IMRT Using a Bilinear Model

Tobias Geimer[1,2,3], Stefan B. Ploner[1], Paul Keall[4], Christoph Bert[2,3],
Andreas Maier[1,2]

[1]Pattern Recognition Lab, Friedrich-Alexander-Universität Erlangen-Nürnberg
[2]Erlangen Graduate School of Advanced Optical Technologies, FAU ER-N
[3]Department of Radiation Oncology, Universitätklinikum Erlangen, FAU ER-N
[4]ACRF Image X Institute, The University of Sydney, Australia
tobias.geimer@fau.de

Abstract. Driving a respiratory motion model in X-ray guided radiotherapy can be challenging in treatments with continuous rotation such
as VMAT, as data-driven respiratory signal extraction suffers from angular effects overlapping with respiratory changes in the projection images.
Compared to a linear model trained on static acquisition angles, the bilinear model gains flexibility in terms of handling multiple viewpoints at
the cost of accuracy. In this paper, we evaluate both models in the context of serving as the surrogate input to a motion model. Evaluation is
performed on the 20 patient 4D CTs in a leave-one-phase-out approach
yielding a median accuracy drop of only 0.14 mm in the 3D error of
estimated vector fields of the bilinear model compared to the linear one.

1 Introduction

In intensity modulated radiotherapy (IMRT) the radiation beams are shaped to
closely envelope the tumor region. With the linear accelerator (LINAC) rotating
around the patient, a therapeutic dose is accumulated within the malignent
cells while healthy tissue is spared. Treatment is either performed from predefined angles (Step&Shoot) or in a continuous rotation (VMAT). Requiring a
complex dose optimization planned on pre-treatment (4D) CT, intra-fractional
respiratory motion can hinder accurate dose delivery. To compensate, a gimbaled
beam following the tumor motion [1] coupled with respiratory motion models [2]
have found success in image-guided radiotherapy (IGRT).

A motion model comprises a motion representation trained from 4D CT,
e.g. via principal component analysis (PCA). Correspondence is established
to a highly-correlated surrogate available in the treatment room, from which
the internal motion is inferred. Among surrogate sources, many LINACs come
equipped with an on-board imager to provide kV fluoroscopy. In this context, X-
ray guided RT shares similarities with cone-beam CT reconstruction where respiratory signal extraction from X-ray projections is prominent. Most data-driven
approaches [3] provide only a 1D signal insufficient for a low reconstruction error of the PCA-based motion representation [2]. While unsupervised learning on

X-ray fluoroscopy [4] yields multiple respiratory features, they are restricted to static acquisition and only applicable to Step&Shoot but not to continuously rotating VMAT. Recently, Geimer et al. [5] presented a bilinear decoupling of angular and respiratory variation in rotational X-ray scans. Based on digitally reconstructed radiographs (DRRs), a rotational and respiratory feature representation is learned. While it was shown that the decoupled respiratory features can drive a respiratory motion model, no quantitative evaluation was performed against comparable PCA-based models. With the bilinear model being an extension to the static case, this paper aims to provide insight into how much accuracy is potentially sacrificed to gain independence from the trajectory angle.

2 Material and methods

2.1 Respiratory motion models

McClelland et al. [2] identify four components, (1) the representation of the motion to be described, (2) the choice of surrogate signal and processing thereof, (3) a correlation model linking surrogate to motion, and (4) a fitting method to determine model parameters from training data. In the following, we will give a possible choice of these components for X-ray guided RT and demonstrate how the bilinear fluoroscopic model can slot in as the surrogate component.

Motion representation Given F binned volumes $v_j \in \mathbb{R}^{N^3}$, $j \in \{1, \ldots, F\}$ in a 4D CT, B-spline based deformable image registration (DIR) over the entire lung w.r.t. the end-exhale phase (0_{In}) yields displacement vector fields (VF) $d_j \in \mathbb{R}^{3N^3}$ (1), where N is the arbitrary dimension of the volume. In order to suppress noise and prevent overfitting, PCA is often applied resulting in a low-dimensional representation $\{\tilde{\Theta}, \bar{d}\}$, where $\tilde{\Theta} = \left(\tilde{\theta}_1, \ldots, \tilde{\theta}_f\right) \in \mathbb{R}^{3N^3 \times f}$, $f \ll F$, are the first f eigenvectors and $\bar{d}$ is the mean VF. As a result, every d_j can be expressed as a linear combination by the respiratory PC scores $\tilde{a}_j \in \mathbb{R}^f$ up to a residual error $\epsilon \in \mathbb{R}^{N^3}$

$$d_j = \tilde{\Theta}\, \tilde{a}_j + \bar{d} + \epsilon \tag{1}$$

Static X-ray surrogate An X-ray projection $p_{i,j} \in \mathbb{R}^{N^2}$ of volume v_j under the acquisition angle ϕ_i is given by the X-ray transform $R_i \in \mathbb{R}^{N^2 \times N^3}$, such that $p_{i,j} = R_i v_j$, where N again denotes arbitrary dimension of projection images and/or volume. An analogous decomposition to (1) for the volume v_j yields

$$p_{i,j} = R_i \left(\Theta a_j + \bar{v}\right) = \Theta_i^R a_j + \bar{p}_i \tag{2}$$

Here, $\Theta_i^R \in \mathbb{R}^{N^2 \times f}$ describes respiration-induced variation observable in the 2D projections under the specific angle ϕ_i. Consequently, such a PCA decomposition can be trained on the 4D CT forward projected under said acquisition angle.

Correlation model A popular model in literature for the correlation between internal and surrogate scores $\tilde{A}, A \in \mathbb{R}^{F \times f}$ is multi-linear regression (MLR) [6]

$$W = \underset{\hat{W}}{\mathrm{argmin}} \left(\frac{1}{2}||\hat{W}A - \tilde{A}||_2^2 + \alpha \frac{1}{2}||\hat{W}||_2^2 \right) \tag{3}$$

with the Moore-Penrose pseudoinverse as the closed-form solution.

2.2 Bilinear model for rotational X-ray

A static angle model as described in (2.1) is unable to explain variation caused by rotation. As an extension to the linear case, a bilinear model can decouple angular and respiratory variation into distinct feature spaces [5], such that a projection $p_{i,j}$ at angle ϕ_i and respiratory phase t_j can be written as

$$p_{i,j} = \mathcal{M} \times_1 a_j \times_2 b_i \tag{4}$$

where $a_j \in \mathbb{R}^f$, $b_i \in \mathbb{R}^g$ are respiratory and rotational feature weights, and $\mathcal{M} \in \mathbb{R}^{N^2 \times f \times g}$ is a model tensor trained from DRRs of a prior 4D CT. $\times_k$ denotes the kth mode product [7]. Bilinear training and application will be outlined in the following. For a detailed derivation we refer the reader to [5].

Model training Simulating a circular scan that mimics the VMAT arc the F volumes v_j are projected at G angles ϕ_i, $i \in \{1, \ldots, G\}$. Higher-order SVD [7] is applied to the data tensor $\mathcal{P} \in \mathbb{R}^{N^2 \times F \times G}$ such that $\mathcal{P} = \mathcal{M} \times_1 A \times_2 B$, where $A \in \mathbb{R}^{F \times f}$ and $B \in \mathbb{R}^{G \times g}$ contain the model weights of the training set.

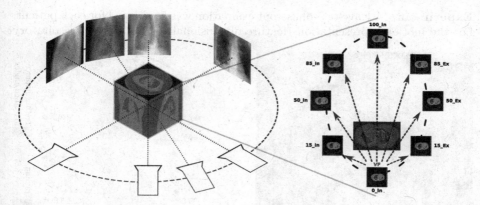

Fig. 1. Illustration of the bilinear decoupling idea. Respiratory changes are inherently 3-dimensional, but can only be observed in 2D when projected according to the X-ray transform, where they overlap with angular changes due to rotation.

Weight estimation Both rotational and respiratory bilinear weights need to be determined for a new projection image $p(t, \phi)$ at unknown respiratory state t. While the acquisition angle is known, the corresponding rotational weights $\boldsymbol{b}(\phi)$ are not. However, given similarity between neighboring views, we adopt the B-spline interpolation of [5] interpolate $\boldsymbol{b}(\phi)$ from the training weights $\boldsymbol{B}$. Mode-multiplying $\boldsymbol{b}(\phi)$ into $\mathcal{M}$ removes the angular variation and yields

$$\mathcal{M}_\phi^R = \mathcal{M} \times_2 \boldsymbol{b}(\phi) \in \mathbb{R}^{N^2 \times f \times 1} \quad \rightarrow \quad \boldsymbol{M}_\phi^R \in \mathbb{R}^{N^2 \times f} \qquad (5)$$

an angle-dependent model matrix such that $p(\phi, t) = \boldsymbol{M}_\phi^R \boldsymbol{a}_t$ as in (2).

2.3   Performance comparison

Data We evaluate the performance of the linear and bilinear surrogate model on the 4D CTs of 20 patients being treated for lung carcinoma or metastasis at the University Hospital Erlangen. Each 4D CT consists of $F = 8$ volumes reconstructed at respiratory states 0 %, 15 %, 50 %, 85 %, 100 % inhale, and 85 %, 50 %, 15 % exhale. DIR of these volumes provided the VF for training the patient-specific PCA-based internal motion representation as described in (2.1). For training the bilinear surrogate model, each phase was forward projected along a circular trajectory according to the Vero SBRT (Brainlab AG, Munich, Germany) geometry at $G = 60$ angles in steps of 6° from 0° to 354°. For testing, additional DRRs were created at ten angles ϕ_k every 38.7° starting at 3°. The interval was chosen to ensure varying distances to neighboring training angles. (2) illustrates the choice of training and testing angles, including °-distances.

Experiments A leave-one-phase-out evaluation was performed for each patient. For the motion representation (feature dimensionality $f = 4$) each respiratory

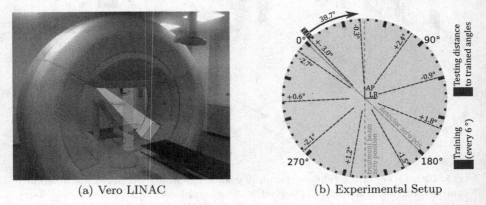

(a) Vero LINAC   (b) Experimental Setup

Fig. 2. (a) Vero with kV imager mounted on the same ring gantry, offset by 45° to the MV treatment beam. (b) Bilinear training at every 6° (blue) with test angles (red) every 38.7° starting at 3°, resulting in varying distances to neighboring training angles.

phase was subsequently removed prior to PCA. The linear surrogate model with $f = 4$ was trained from the DRRs of each test angle directly minus the left-out phase. In contrast, the bilinear model was trained on the $G = 60$ training angles without the left-out phase and $g = 40$ as rotational dimensionality ensuring flexibility towards rotation. Here, $f = 5$ as the 1st bilinear component is near constant and represents the shift towards the mean due to missing mean normalization [5]. Finally, the regression matrices were computed between internal scores and the two different surrogate features of the training set.

The projection $p_{k,j}$ for left-out phase t_j and test angle ϕ_k is then fed to both surrogate models, with the bilinear model also requiring the angle ϕ_k. The extracted weights are regressed to an internal representation a_j and the VF is reconstructed according to (1). Estimation accuracy is reported based on the voxelwise euclidean error to the ground truth VF from DIR.

3   Results

Average accuracy over all 20 patients, 10 angles, and 8 phases was 1.13 ± 0.58 mm (median: 0.78 mm) for the static model and 1.27 ± 0.67 mm (median: 0.89 mm) for the bilinear surrogate. Given 1600 observation per model, a Levene test was performed on the mean errors indicating significance at a p-value of $1.2e^{-6}$. (3) shows the average error over all patients displayed for individual angles and phases. Neither surrogate model is sensitive to the viewing angle. Estimation error outliers increased with the inhale state, which seems reasonable given that the 100_{In} state corresponds to largest VF magnitude. As seen in (4) displaying the mean error for individual patients average over all phases and angles, the estimation error mostly relies on the actual patient and the quality of the prior 4D CT. Overall, the bilinear surrogate model was only 0.14 mm worse on average than the linear model specifically trained for that particular test angle.

4   Discussion

The bilinear surrogate model performed only slightly worse than the one trained on static acquisition angles. This is unsurprising, as the static model has seen

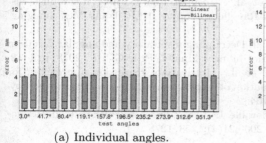

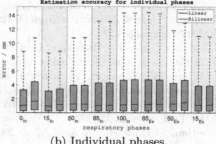

(a) Individual angles.   (b) Individual phases.

Fig. 3. Estimation error of the linear and bilinear model averaged for angles and phases.

Fig. 4. Average estimation error of the linear and bilinear model for individual patients.

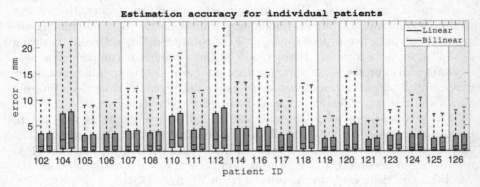

the test angle except for the test phase while the bilinear one is flexible over the entire trajectory. As such, the major gain in flexibility comes at the cost of only a small drop in accuracy. Similar to [5], the leave-one-out evaluation suffers from two shortcomings in assuming a perfect baseline registration between diagnostic 4D CT and the in-room patient, and no inter-fractional changes. However, the linear model also benefits from this simplification and, thus, the comparison is still valid. Relying on two distinct 4D CT per patient for training and testing can help model these conditions.

In conclusion, we showed in a retrospective patient study that a bilinear model operating on a circular X-ray sequence can be used to drive a respiratory motion model during continuously rotating VMAT treatments.

References

1. Akimoto M, Nakamura M, Miyabe Y, et al. Long-term stability assessment of a 4D tumor tracking system integrated into a gimbaled linear accelerator. J Appl Clin Med Phys. 2015;16(5):373–380.
2. McClelland JR, Hawkes DJ, Schaeffter T, et al. Respiratory motion models: a review. Med Image Anal. 2013;17(1):19–42.
3. Yan H, Wang X, Yin W, et al. Extracting respiratory signals from thoracic cone beam CT projections. Phys Med Biol. 2013;58(5):1447–64.
4. Fischer P, Pohl T, Faranesh A, et al. Unsupervised learning for robust respiratory signal estimation from X-Ray fluoroscopy. IEEE Trans Med Imaging. 2017;36(4):865–877.
5. Geimer T, Keall P, Breininger L, et al. Decoupling respiratory and angular variation in rotational X-ray scans using a prior bilinear Mmdel. Proc GCPR. 2018; p. 1–12.
6. Wilms M, Werner R, Ehrhardt J, et al. Multivariate regression approaches for surrogate-based diffeomorphic estimation of respiratory motion in radiation therapy. Phys Med Biol. 2014;59(5):1147–1164.
7. De Lathauwer L, De Moor B, Vandewalle J. A multilinear singular value decomposition. SIAM J Matrix Anal Appl. 2000;21(4):1253–1278.

Augmented Mitotic Cell Count Using Field of Interest Proposal

Marc Aubreville[1], Christof A. Bertram[2], Robert Klopfleisch[2], Andreas Maier[1]

[1]Pattern Recognition Lab, Computer Sciences, Friedrich-Alexander-Universität
Erlangen-Nürnberg, Germany
[2]Institute of Veterinary Pathology, Freie Universität Berlin, Germany
marc.aubreville@fau.de

Abstract. Histopathological prognostication of neoplasia including most
tumor grading systems are based upon a number of criteria. Probably
the most important is the number of mitotic figures which are most
commonly determined as the mitotic count (MC), i.e. number of mitotic
figures within 10 consecutive high power fields. Often the area with the
highest mitotic activity is to be selected for the MC. However, since mitotic activity is not known in advance, an arbitrary choice of this region
is considered one important cause for high variability in the prognostication and grading. In this work, we present an algorithmic approach that
first calculates a mitotic cell map based upon a deep convolutional network. This map is in a second step used to construct a mitotic activity
estimate. Lastly, we select the image segment representing the size of ten
high power fields with the overall highest mitotic activity as a region proposal for an expert MC determination. We evaluate the approach using
a dataset of 32 completely annotated whole slide images, where 22 were
used for training of the network and 10 for test. We find a correlation of
r=0.936 in mitotic count estimate.

1 Introduction

One important aspect of tumor prognostication in human and veterinary pathology is the proliferative rate of the tumor cells, which is assumed to be correlated
with the density of cells undergoing divison (mitotic figures) in a histology slide
and is applied as a criterion in almost all current tumor grading systems [1].
However, mitotic activity is known to have large inter-observer variances [2],
which consequentially strongly affects the histological grade assigned. One reason might be that the classification between mitotic and non-mitocic cells is not
clearly defined and varies across labs, schools and even individuals [1, 3]. Another important reason for this is, that the distribution of mitotic cells in the
slide is usually sparse with local changes in density across the specimen. In clinical practice, this sampling problem is dealt with by counting mitotic figures in
ten fields of view at a magnification of 400× (high power fields, HPF), resulting
in the mitotic count (MC). However, as shown previously [4], especially for low to
borderline mitotic counts, semi-random selection of those ten high power fields

is not sufficient for a reproducible MC determination. While examining larger areas would improve on this, it is not the method of choice given limited time budgets in pathology labs. As of this writing, completely algorithmic approaches for mitotic activity estimation lack the sensitivity and specificity that would be required to achieve clinical applicability. Further, purely algorithmic outcomes may be subject to hesitation from the pathology side, since automatic solutions that are not easily comprehensible for the medical expert, such as deep learning networks, may not be robust.

In this paper, we present an algorithmic approach that proposes a region of the area of 10 high power fields that is assumed to have the highest mitotic count within the slide. This has two positive aspects: While we still rely on the expertise of a pathologist to assess the actual mitotic activity, we limit the focus area to a defined field of interest in the image. Further, as this algorithmic answer will always be equal for the same image, it will allow us to differentiate the true inter-observer variance in an optimal setting when the area on the slide is already fixed. This region proposal will serve as an augmentation to the pathology expert.

A significant number of algorithmic approaches for mitosis detection have emerged very recently, most based on deep convolutional networks [5, 6], making use of transfer learning [7] and hard-negative example mining [5]. Typically, these algorithms use a two-stage approach, where in the first stage multiple regions of interest are detected and in a second stage classification is done according to being a mitotic figure or not. However, as also stated in the TUPAC challenge, automated identification of mitoses is only an intermediate step in tumor grading. F1-scores of up to 0.652 [6] have been achieved on the TUPAC challenge test data set. Current results are unlikely to reach clinical standards. Additionally, fully automated grading algorithms could run into acceptance problems, because robustness in a clinical workflow has yet to be proven.

2 Material

For this work, we annotated 32 histology slides of canine cutaneous mast cell tumors dyed with standard hematoxylin and eosin stain. The slides were digitized using a linear scanner (Aperio ScanScope CS2, Leica Biosystems, Germany) at a magnification of $400\times$ (resolution: $0.25 \frac{\mu m}{px}$). Contrary to popular other publicly available mitosis data sets, we did not pre-crop the whole slide images (WSI) but include all parts of the slide, including borders, which we consider important for a general applicability of the framework. All slides have been annotated by two pathologists using the open source annotation software SlideRunner [8]. Out of all cells annotated as mitotic figure, we only use those where both observers agreed upon being a mitotic figure. We arbitrarily chose 10 slides to be the test set, and 22 to be used for the training process. The data set includes slides of low, medium and high mitotic activity in both training and test set. In total, 45,811 mitotic cells have been annotated on all slides. To the best of our knowledge, this data set is unprecedented in size for any mitotic cell task and may serve as basis for many algorithmic improvements to the field.

3   Methods

We regard mitosis detection as an intermediate step needed to propose a region of interest that could either be representing the statistics of the complete slide, or, as typically intended, represents the region of highest mitotic activity. For this approach, however, it is valid to not consider the object detection task of mitotic figures, but rather to derive maps where mitotic cells are located.

3.1   Mitosis as segmentation task

For the purpose of field of interest proposal, we consider mitotic figure detection a segmentation task, with mitotic figures being represented by filled circles. This enables the use of concepts like the dice coefficient (intersection/union) for both, evaluation as well as for optimization.

3.2   High power field area proposal

We employ an approach based on prediction of mitotic activity (Fig. 1, upper path) and an estimation of a valid mask (Fig. 1, lower path), which will select image areas that are covered to a very large extent by tissue. A single HPF at field number 22 (i.e. the diameter of the eyepiece lens is 22 mm) is assumed to have an area of $A = 0.237$ mm^2 [1]. In order to find an area with the size of 10 HPF, we thus look for an moving average estimator with the following width w and height h in pixels (aspect ratio of 4/3 is assumed)

$$w = \frac{\sqrt{\frac{10 \cdot 4}{3} A}}{r} \cdot 1000 \frac{\mu m}{mm} \tag{1}$$

$$h = \frac{\sqrt{\frac{10 \cdot 3}{4} A}}{r} \cdot 1000 \frac{\mu m}{mm} \tag{2}$$

with r being the resolution of the scanner (in $\mu m/px$).

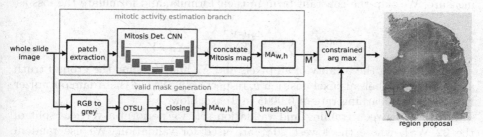

Fig. 1. Overview of the proposed approach for mitotic count region proposal. The upper path will derive singular mitotic annotations, followed by a moving average (MA) filter. The lower path derives an activity map of the image to exclude border regions of the image. Region proposal (red rectangle) shows result on slide taken from the test set with ground truth MC depicted as as green overlay.

Mitotic activity estimation For estimation of mitotic activity, the image is divided into overlapping (margin: $64\,px$) patches of size 512×512. The prediction of the network is being concatenated to yield a map of mitotic figure activity M.

Valid mask stimation In order to exclude regions of the image that are partly uncovered by specimen, we construct a binary mask of tissue presence from the WSI: The downsampled image is converted to grey-scale, then a binary threshold is performed using Otsu's adaptive method. A closing operator is applied to reduce thin interruptions of the tissue map, and a moving average filter of size $w \times h$ is being applied. Next, a thresholding with 0.95 is applied to retain only areas that are covered to at least 95 % with tissue, resulting in the valid mask M. Lastly, both masks are used to find the position of the maximum mitotic activity, constrained to image areas where the valid mask is nonzero.

3.3 Convolutional neural network (CNN) structure

We follow the popular U-Net architecture of Ronneberger *et al.* [9], which was successful in segmentation tasks in microscopy images, and use a network consisting of five stages, each containing two 2D convolutional layers with batch-normalization followed by a max pooling layer in the downsampling branch. The network then uses an upsampling branch and feeds information of the layers of matching resolution to the upsamling convolutions. Finally, a convolution layer with sigmoid activation function is being used.

The ground truth image map is being generated as filled circles around the actual annotation coordinates of each mitotic figure in the current image patch. This approach follows the original works by Cireşan *et al.* [5], where the CNN-based detector would receive a positive mitosis indication as ground truth if the closest annotation distance is less than a given radius.

Following Rahman & Wang [10], we directly use the intersection over union (IOU) for binary classification as optimization loss for our task. In heavily imbalanced problems such as our mitosis segmentation task, IOU will yield a balanced measure. We skip the constant term in their formula, and formulate the loss as

$$L_{IoU} = -\frac{\sum_{v \in V} (X_v + Y_v)}{\sum_{v \in V} (X_v + Y_v - X_v * Y_v)} \tag{3}$$

with V being the totality of all pixels and X_v and Y_v being the ground truth and predicted labels at pixel position v, respectively. We use the Adam optimizer with an initial learning rate of 0.0005 in TensorFlow.

To split between training and validation set, we perform a vertical split of the 22 WSI, where the lowest 20 % are used for validation. We use random rotation as augmentation. For training, we feed tuples of images to the network, representing three groups of images with different intentions. The first group consists of arbitrary image patches containing at least one mitotic figure. This group is responsible to not have a complete underrepresentation of the positive class in our data set. The second group represents hard negative examples. It consists of images that contain at least one mitosis candidate where both experts disagreed on the cell class or where cells have been classified by both experts as unable to classify. The third group is completely random picks of images on the slide. This group ensures also picking images that do not contain tissue with mitotic figures for images that do not contain a large number of mitoses as well as border or non-tissue regions on the slide.

4 Results

On the test set, we achieve a correlation coefficient in mitotic count estimate of $r = 0.936$, with partial over-estimation on a small part of the data set Fig. 2(a). The overall F1-score of the intermediate mitotic figure prediction task of the network is 0.662, the mean IOU is 0.495. Our test dataset shows a significant spread of the mitotic count within the specimen of the respective test slides, as indicated by the box-whisker-plot in Fig. 2(b). Some of the slides (1 to 3) have low mitotic count, reflecting a low low grade tumor, while others show clearly high-grade tumors (7-10). The slides with intermediate mitotic counts (4-6) are of special interest, since the ground truth MC ranges closely around the commonly used cut-off value of MC$\geq$7 and thus we would expect a higher variability of the assigned tumor grade if the same slide is assessed by multiple independent experts. The approach presented in this work chose for all relevant slides a position in the forth quartile of the ground truth MC (Fig. 2(b), red dashed line, for an example see image on the right of Fig. 1.

5 Discussion

The mitotic figure prediction network scored in the same order as other algorithms on other data sets that also do mitosis detection. However, while the

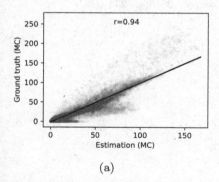

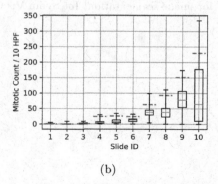

(a)   (b)

Fig. 2. a) Relation between ground truth mitotic count (MC) prediction and estimated MC prediction on test set (r=0.936) b) MC distribution on test slides (ground truth). Red dashed line marks ground truth MC for proposed position.

general problem of automatically identifying mitotic figures in WSI with sufficient accuracy for clinical application remains a challenge, the outcomes of these approaches might indeed serve as a surrogate for field of interest proposal and thus as a augmentation to the pathology expert. In future studies, it will have to be proven that clinical application of such augmentation methods will be able to reduce variability in MC determination.

References

1. Meuten DJ, Moore FM, George JW. Mitotic count and the field of view area. Vet Pathol. 2016;53(1):7–9.
2. Boiesen P, Bendahl PO, Anagnostaki L, et al. Histologic grading in breast cancer: reproducibility between seven pathologic departments. Acta Oncol. 2000;39(1):41–45.
3. Bertram CA, Gurtner C, Dettwiler M, et al. Validation of digital microscopy compared with light microscopy for the diagnosis of canine cutaneous tumors. Vet Pathol. 2018;55(4):490–500.
4. Bonert M, Tate AJ. Mitotic counts in breast cancer should be standardized with a uniform sample area. Biomed Eng Online. 2017;16(1):28.
5. Cireşan DC, Giusti A, Gambardella LM, et al. Mitosis detection in breast cancer histology images with deep neural networks. Proc MICCAI. 2013;16:411–418.
6. Paeng K, Hwang S, Park S, et al. A unified framework for tumor proliferation score prediction in breast histopathology. Deep Learn Med Image Anal Multimod Learn Clin Decis Support. 2017; p. 231–239.
7. Li C, Wang X, Liu W, et al. DeepMitosis: mitosis detection via deep detection, verification and segmentation networks. Med Image Anal. 2018;45:121–133.
8. Aubreville M, Bertram CA, Klopfleisch R, et al. SlideRunner - a tool for massive cell annotations in whole slide images. Proc BVM. 2018; p. 309–314.
9. Ronneberger O, Fischer P, Brox T. U-net - convolutional networks for biomedical image segmentation. Proc MICCAI. 2015;9351(Chapter 28):234–241.
10. Rahman MA, Wang Y. Optimizing intersection-over-union in deep neural networks for image segmentation. Int Symp Vis Comput. 2016; p. 234–244.

Feasibility of Colon Cancer Detection in Confocal Laser Microscopy Images Using Convolution Neural Networks

Nils Gessert[1], Lukas Wittig[2], Daniel Drömann[2], Tobias Keck[3], Alexander Schlaefer[1], David B. Ellebrecht[3]

[1]Institute of Medical Technology, Hamburg University of Technology
[2]Department of Pulmology, University Medical Centre Schleswig-Holstein
[3]Department of Surgery, University Medical Centre Schleswig-Holstein
nils.gessert@tuhh.de

Abstract. Histological evaluation of tissue samples is a typical approach to identify colorectal cancer metastases in the peritoneum. For immediate assessment, reliable and real-time in-vivo imaging would be required. For example, intraoperative confocal laser microscopy has been shown to be suitable for distinguishing organs and also malignant and benign tissue. So far, the analysis is done by human experts. We investigate the feasibility of automatic colon cancer classification from confocal laser microscopy images using deep learning models. We overcome very small dataset sizes through transfer learning with state-of-the-art architectures. We achieve an accuracy of 89.1% for cancer detection in the peritoneum which indicates viability as an intraoperative decision support system.

1 Introduction

Colorectal cancer is one of the most common types of cancer [1]. Due to metastatic spread, peritoneal carcinomatosis can occur in later stages which often leads to substantially shorter survival times [2]. Therefore, reliable detection of metastases is important. Typical imaging modalities such as magnetic resonance imaging and computed tomography currently lack the required resolution and intraoperative availability. Therefore, an intraoperative device using confocal laser microscopy (CLM) has been proposed [3] which offers submicrometer resolution.

In the above-mentioned study, colon carcinoma cells were implanted into the colon and peritoneum of ten rats. After seven days of tumor growth, laparotomy was carried out for subsequent in-vivo CLM. For each subject, healthy colon tissue, malignant colon tissue, healthy peritoneum and malignant peritoneum were scanned. The study showed that different organs, as well as malignant and non-malignant regions could be distinguished by experts.

To further improve the intraoperative assessment by CLM, image processing methods can be used for automatic and fast tissue characterization. Recently, deep learning methods have shown remarkable success for a variety of medical segmentation and classification tasks [4] where human-level performance was achieved [5].

We investigate the feasibility of deep learning-based colon cancer detection from CLM images. We consider several classification problems with the four classes "colon normal", "colon malignant", "peritoneum normal"and "peritoneum malignant". In particular, we investigate both the differentiability of organs and also of malignant and non-malignant tissue both for the colon and peritoneum. As we are dealing with a very small dataset we employ transfer learning which has been shown to improve performance for a variety of medical learning problems [6, 7]. We use the state-of-the-art models Densenet121 [8] and SE-Resnext50 [9] which are pretrained on the ImageNet dataset.

2 Methods

2.1 Dataset

The dataset we use was kindly provided to us by the authors of a previous study on CLM [3]. The dataset was acquired at the University Hospital Schleswig-Holstein in Lübeck using a custom intraoperative CLM device. The CLM device (Karl Storz GmbH & Co KG, Tuttlingen, Germany) covers a field of view of $300\mu m \times 300\mu m$ with a resolution of 384×384 pixels. The images were obtained from ten rats where colon adenocarcinoma cells had been implanted into the colon and peritoneum seven days before scanning. For each subject, images of healthy colon tissue (HC), malignant colon tissue (MC), healthy peritoneum tissue (HP) and malignant peritoneum tissue (MP) were obtained. In total, there are 533 images of class HC, 309 images of class MC, 343 images of class HP and 392 images of class MP which results in a total dataset size of 1577 images. Note, that for one subject there are no images of class HC and for one subject there are no images of class MP. Example cases for each class are shown in Fig. 1. The assignment of classes for each image was performed based on subsequent histological evaluation of resected tissue from the scanning area.

We split the dataset in a leave-one-subject-out cross-validation scheme, i.e., we consider ten different dataset splits where images from one subject are left out for evaluation. If a required class is missing, the subject's validation split is omitted. We consider three classification problems in total. First, we address the binary classification task HC versus HP which provides information on whether

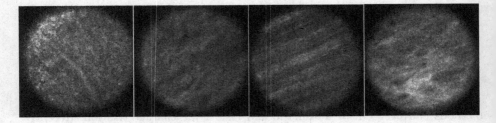

Fig. 1. Examples of the four different classes. From left to right, healthy colon tissue, malignant colon tissue, healthy peritoneum tissue and malignant peritoneum tissue.

the organs can be differentiated in principle. Next, we consider the learning problems HC versus MC and HP versus MP which investigates the feasibility of detecting malignant tissue from CLM images.

2.2 Models and training

We employ convolutional neural networks (CNNs) for the classification tasks at hand. The images are directly fed into a CNN which learns to extract relevant features and also perform classification at its output. We employ the two state-of-the-art architectures Densenet121 [8] and SE-Resnext50 [9]. Densenet121 follows the principle of densely connected layers, i.e., features computed within a convolutional layers are also reused in subsequent layers. In this way, the architecture is very efficient in terms of the number of learnable parameters as features are reused heavily. Considering the small dataset size at hand, this can be very beneficial. The SE-Resnext50 architecture is based on the Resnext principle [10] where feature extraction is performed by multiple, parallel paths. In addition, squeeze and excitation (SE) modules are incorporated into the model which perform a feature recalibration step. In standard convolutions the aggregation of features is learned implicitly through a summation. Instead, the SE modules explicitly model dependencies between learned features which increases the models' representational power. The building blocks of the two concepts are shown in Fig. 2.

To overcome the general lack of data, we use transfer learning, i.e. the models are pretrained on the ImageNet dataset. During training we fine tune all weights. For comparison, we also consider training from scratch. The pretrained models' input layer contains three channels. We put the gray-scale CLM images into one channel and set the other channels to zero. We cut off the last layer and add fully-connected layer with two outputs for binary classification.

During training, we use online data augmentation with unscaled random crops of size 224×224 from the original images of size 384×384. Also, we use random flipping along both dimensions and random changes in brightness and contrast. For stochastic gradient descent we employ Adam with a batch size of

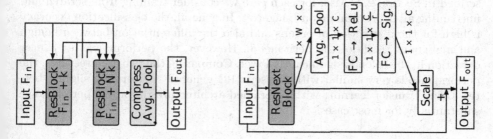

Fig. 2. The key concepts of the architecture we employ. The shown modules replace sets of standard convolutional layers in the architecture. Left, a Densenet [8] block is shown. Right, an SE block is shown for the Resnext architecture [9].

Table 1. The results of all our deep learning experiments. The mean values for leave-one-subject-out cross-validation are shown. Dense refers to the Densenet121 model, SE-RX refers to the SE-Resnext50 model. TL refers to transfer learning and SRC refers to training from scratch. For each training scenario, the best performing value is marked bold. All values are given in percent. The sensitivity is given with respect to the cancer class and for the case of organ differentiation it is given with respect to the peritoneum class.

		Accuracy	Sensitivity	Specificity	F1-Score
HC vs. HP	Dense TL	**90.8**	**80.2**	**93.9**	**91.7**
	Dense SRC	78.5	74.2	78.1	79.1
	SE-RX TL	89.3	78.6	90.3	90.5
	SE-RX SRC	70.8	77.9	67.3	72.6
HC vs. MC	Dense TL	**66.7**	74.1	64.8	**69.0**
	Dense SRC	60.0	**81.0**	50.7	63.6
	SE-RX TL	58.9	69.8	57.3	62.6
	SE-RX SRC	64.5	69.5	**67.1**	65.6
HP vs. MP	Dense TL	**89.1**	80.9	**87.2**	**90.0**
	Dense SRC	77.0	70.8	70.2	79.3
	SE-RX TL	83.2	72.5	86.9	84.9
	SE-RX SRC	77.3	**85.4**	64.7	77.6

40 and learning rate of 0.00001 and we train for 125 epochs. For evaluation, we use multi-crop evaluation with $N_c = 9$ crops. The predictions of all crops are averaged into a final prediction for each image. The models are implemented in PyTorch.

3 Results

All results are shown in Tab. 1. In terms of metrics, we report accuracy, sensitivity, specificity and the F1-score. For each of the three training scenarios, HC versus HP, HC versus MC and HP versus MP, we consider the architectures described in Section 2.2. Also, for each case we consider training from scratch and fine-tuning after pretraining on ImageNet. In general, the classification accuracy is high for the distinction of organs and also the differentiation between benign and malignant tissue of the peritoneum. However, the performance for cancer detection in the colon is significantly lower. Comparing the two architectures, the performance is very similar with Densenet121 generally performing slightly better. Using transfer learning with pretrained architectures improves performance substantially for most cases.

4 Discussion

In this study we investigate the feasibility of detecting colon cancer from confocal laser microscopy (CLM) images using deep learning models. This extends a previous study where the feasibility of cancer detection from CLM images by experts was shown [3]. Here, we use two state-of-the-art deep learning architectures to automatically detect cancer from CLM images. As a baseline, we consider the task of differentiating healthy tissue from the colon and the peritoneum. With an F1-score of 91.7, the best model, Densenet121, shows a high performance which indicates that different organs can be well distinguished in CLM images by deep learning models. It is notable that without pretraining performance drops substantially across all metrics. This highlights the effectiveness of transfer learning for a particularly small dataset [6]. Regarding the detection of malignant tissue in the peritoneum, the model performance is also very high with Densenet121 performing best. It is notable that Densenet121 generally performs better than SE-Resnext50 in our study while the latter clearly outperforms the former on the ImageNet dataset [9]. This is likely tied to Densenet121 having significantly fewer parameters which prevents overfitting with the small dataset. Also, the performance difference between training from scratch and transfer learning is larger for Densenet121. This indicates, that Densenet121 benefits more from the pretrained weights. Considering the detection of malignant tissue in the colon, the performance is significantly lower compared to the other tasks. It should be noted that the performance difference is most obvious in the specificity. Thus, most cases of cancer are detected but a lot of false positives occur as well. This might be tied to the heterogeneous appearance of the colon in different areas which makes the learning task very challenging due to the small dataset size. Also, carcinoma cells transform from healthy tissue via adenoma to carcinoma. Thus, healthy and malignant tissue can have a similar appearance which might complicate the learning problem.

Overall, we showed that automatic organ differentiation and cancer detection from CLM images is feasible using pretrained convolutional neural networks. For future work, more data could be acquired and the detection of malignant tissue in the colon area could be studied further.

References

1. Torre LA, Bray F, Siegel RL, et al. Global cancer statistics, 2012. CA: Cancer J Clin. 2015;65(2):87–108.
2. Franko J, Shi Q, Goldman CD, et al. Treatment of colorectal peritoneal carcinomatosis with systemic chemotherapy: a pooled analysis of north central cancer treatment group phase III trials N9741 and N9841. J Clin Oncol. 2012;30(3):263.
3. Ellebrecht DB, Kuempers C, Horn M, et al. Confocal laser microscopy as novel approach for real-time and in-vivo tissue examination during minimal-invasive surgery in colon cancer. Surg Endosc. 2018; p. 1–7.
4. Litjens G, Kooi T, Bejnordi BE, et al. A survey on deep learning in medical image analysis. Med Image Anal. 2017;42:60–88.
5. Esteva A, Kuprel B, Novoa RA, et al. Dermatologist-level classification of skin cancer with deep neural networks. Nature. 2017;542(7639):115.
6. Hoo-Chang S, Roth HR, Gao M, et al. Deep convolutional neural networks for computer-aided detection: CNN architectures, dataset characteristics and transfer learning. IEEE Trans Med Imaging. 2016;35(5):1285.

7. Gessert N, Lutz M, Heyder M, et al. Automatic plaque detection in IVOCT pullbacks using convolutional neural networks. IEEE Trans Med Imaging. 2018; p. 1–9.
8. Huang G, Liu Z, Weinberger KQ, et al. Densely connected convolutional networks. Proc CVPR. 2017;.
9. Hu J, Shen L, Sun G. Squeeze-and-excitation networks. Proc CVPR. 2018;.
10. Xie S, Girshick R, Dollár P, et al. Aggregated residual transformations for deep neural networks. Proc CVPR. 2017; p. 5987–5995.

Efficient Construction of Geometric Nerve Fiber Models for Simulation with 3D-PLI

Jan A. Reuter, Felix Matuschke, Nicole Schubert, Markus Axer

Institute of Neuroscience and Medicine (INM-1), Forschungszentrum Jülich
`j.reuter@fz-juelich.de`

Abstract. Three-dimensional (3D) polarized light imaging (PLI) is an unique technique used to reconstruct nerve fiber orientations of post-mortem brains at ultra-high resolution. To continuously improve the current physical model of 3D-PLI, simulations are powerful methods. Since the creation of simulated data can be time consuming, we developed a tool which enables fast and efficient creation of synthetic fiber data using parametric functions and interpolation methods. Performance tests showed that every component of the program scales linearly with the amount of fiber points while the reconstructed fiber cup phantom and optic chiasm-like crossing fiber models reproduce known effects known from 3D-PLI measurements.

1 Introduction

Three-dimensional (3D) polarized light imaging (PLI) is used to identify and reconstruct nerve fiber orientations in post-mortem brains with micrometer resolution. Unstained brain sections with a thickness of about 60 μm are illuminated by polarized light which allows the reconstruction of fiber orientations by measuring the birefringence of the myelin sheaths surrounding most of the axons in the brain [1].

The scattering of polarized light or complex intermingling nerve fiber constellations within individual voxels might cause misinterpretations of the local fiber orientations with the current physical model. Therefore, simulation methods were developed to further investigate the different scenarios while validating and improving the current analysis models [2, 3]. Since the creation of synthetic fiber data is very time-consuming, particularly for complex and large-scale fiber models, we developed a software tool that offers a simple and efficient way to create fiber bundles and at the same time gives the user a visual feedback of the created data sets.

2 Material and methods

3D-PLI reconstructs nerve fiber orientations based on measured signals emitted by myelin sheats surrounding the nerve fibers of histological brain sections. For the measurement, a polarimetric setup is used [1]. An unstained histological brain section with a thickness of $60\,\mu m$ is sandwiched between a combination of a linear polarizer and a quarter-wave retarder (below) and a linear polarizer (above) and illuminated by an LED light source. Each optical component is rotated by an angle of $\rho \in [0°, 10°, \ldots, 170°]$ with a camera recording the resulting light intensities. One scanned section series yields 18 gray-scale images where each pixel describes the locally measured light intensity. Analyzing the signal shows a sinusoidal curve with different amplitudes and phase shifts depending on the local fiber orientation per pixel. The Jones Matrix Calculus [4] provides a mathematical framework to describe the physical effects of optical components on traversing polarized light. It allows to derive physical pararmeters such as retardation and the in-plane and out-of-plane fiber directions. The latter paramters are used to reconstruct and visualize the fiber orientation at a given pixel by assigning each orientation to a specific color (using RGB or HSV color space). The result is a color coded fiber orientation map (FOM) for each histological brain section.

In order to better understand the underlying effects of the measurements and their influence on the reconstruction of the fiber orientations, a simulation method for 3D-PLI (SimPLI) was developed [2]. Based on user generated fiber models as a tubular structure, they enable the reconstruction of real tissue which is then used to create fiber orientation maps. The SimPLI algorithm can be described in three main steps [2]:

1. The created synthetic fiber model is converted to a vector field which describes the normalized tangential direction of the fiber at each voxel.
2. By using the Jones Matrix Calculus, the light intensity for every pixel is calculated. Each optical component is rotated nine times resulting in a gray-scale image series.
3. Image filters like blurring and noise are applied to simulate interferences caused by the camera and the measuring environment. The images are also scaled to match the measured resolution.

While simulations are possible with given synthetic fiber data, creation of this data is quite expensive without a proper tool. Changing a created data set by rotation, for example, requires the usage of scripts and does not grant a visual representation. The creation of a data set requires knowledge in programming languages itself, since large files cannot be created within an acceptable time frame. This can lead to errors within the synthetic tissue which are not visible until the simulation has finished. FiberFox [5], a fiber modeling tool specifically desgined for Magnetic Resonance (dMRI) simulations, allows to create synthetic fiber data sets with interpolation methods. However, the results are lacking the accuracy to adequately describe 3D-PLI data.

To enable fast and effective generation of synthetic fiber data, we developed a tool that allows the declaration of curves using parametric functions or interpolation methods. The generated fiber bundles are visualized in three-dimensional space so that the user can interact with them by rotating or moving the viewing angle. Once created, the data can be rotated, moved, duplicated and removed afterwards, providing fast creation of complex models. For editing larger amounts of fiber bundles, groups can be created to which the same operations can be applied to. Both groups and fiber bundles can be hidden from the view to enable more visibility when dealing with larger data sets. A fiber bundle created with parametric functions is represented by three functions for each axis as well as a minimum and maximum evaluation value defining the start and end point of a fiber bundle. Finally a radius has to be declared which can change over the defined course. Declaring fiber bundles by waypoints is done by describing four attributes for each point: the position in three-dimensional space as well as the current radius of the fiber bundle. methods can be used to smooth out finished curves and remove sharp edges between fiber points.

The software is implemented in C++ using Qt 5 and OpenGL 3.3 for rendering and interaction purposes. Fiber bundles are represented by filled cylinders with a given radius. Those are approximated by n-sided regular polygons where n is variable depending on the current frame rate for a fluent representation even if the performance of the given graphics card is limited or big data sets are shown. Just like in FOMs, fiber bundles are colored with their orientation vector. This allows comparisons between the original data and the results given by the simulation algorithms. For separation of distinct fiber bundles, a second color option is available where each fiber bundle is represented by a distingushable color chosen with pseudo-random values. Created models can be exported and imported in a file format where each data point is stored in combination with its radius. This format can be used for SimPLI without converting the data. The program GUI is shown in Fig. 2.

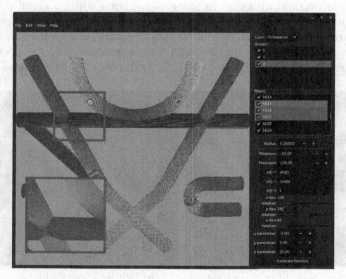

Fig. 1. Screenshot of the "FAConstructor"program. The reconstructed fiber cup phantom [6] is loaded and shown in the center which can be moved or rotated freely. On the right side created groups and fibers are gathered. More options can be accessed through context menus at the top bar.

3   Results

In order to show that data sets created with "FAConstructor" correspond to the results of previous simulations [2], two fiber models were created: a replica of both the fiber cup phantom and an optic chiasm. The fiber cup phantom is inspired by the the fiber configuration of a coronal human brain section [6]. Both crossing and splitting fibers in this data set are relevant for 3D-PLI as they represent common challenges of the measurement method. To reconstruct the model, seven fiber bundles were created by using functions as well as the manual input of waypoints. After filling the model by using equidistant seed points on a triangular grid, 10.149 fibers are determined. To reconstruct splitting fibers, multiple bundles within the same area were created. While all collisions which were caused by the overlapping of the fibers were removed before the simulation by treating all sections of the fibers as capsules and pressing colliding parts tangentially apart while maintaining their respective orientation, the number of fibers leads to an increased density compared to the crossing fiber bundle. The simulation result is shown in Fig. 3 (a). The previously mentioned area shows a deep green color with edges colored in many different colors. Other crossing regions show colors not represented by either of the crossing bundles. The remaining areas present an orientation matching with the color bubble in the lower right corner.

As crossing fibers are a common challenge, a synthetic dataset inspired by an optic chiasm of a hooded seal [2] was created as well. Here, most of the fibers maintain their original direction in the crossing area while a small part bends and stays on the same side after leaving the crossing. Therefore, the central area features many crossing fibers. Four fiber bundles were created for this synthetic data set, two crossing fiber bundles and two remain on their respective side. Filling the synthetic fiber bundles yields 1290 fibers. Fig. 3 (b) shows the sim-

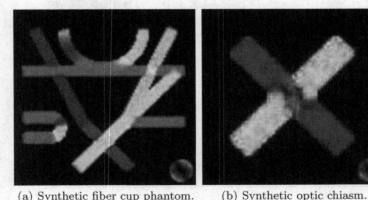

(a) Synthetic fiber cup phantom.   (b) Synthetic optic chiasm.

Fig. 2. Fiber orientation map of synthetic created fiber bundles after simulation with SimPLI. Both figures show the effects of extinction or misinterpretation due to the existence of multiple fibers at the same pixel.

ulation results. The crossing area shows darker and red spots while other areas are visualized in a single color.

Furthermore, performance measurements were done using a PC with an Intel Core i5-6600 paired with a NVIDIA GTX 1070 graphics card and 16 GB RAM. Time measurements as well as the current frame rate dependent on the amount of data points being created are shown in Fig. 3. The time measurements in Fig. 3 (a)–(c) show a nearly linear scaling when increasing the amount of data points. The dependency of the frame rate in comparison to the amount of data points rendered by the graphics card can be seen in Fig. 3 (d). When rendering less than 1.6 million fiber points, the frame rate stays above 30 fps which is the main target. After that, a reciprocal decrease of the frame rate can be observed.

4   Discussion

By using the "FAConstructor" program, two synthetic fiber models have been efficiently and accurately created that can be used for simulation to better understand and improve the physical model of 3D PLI. Creating a replica of the fiber cup phantom took around 10 minutes for unexperienced users which indicates an user friendly environment which is easy to understand. Both synthetic fiber data sets show effects observed in data obtained from 3D-PLI measurements.

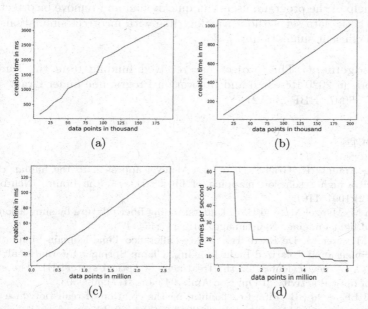

Fig. 3. Performance measurements for four scenarios during the fiber bundle creation process. The x-axis shows the amount of data points used for this measurement while the y-axis shows the passed time in ms. (a) Creating a fiber bundle with cubic spline interpolation, (b) Creating a helix with parametric functions, (c) Preparation of fiber data before rendering the scene, (d) Frame rate.

Just like in the real experiment crossing fiber sections show an orientation is based on the combined orientation of crossing fibers. The higher fiber density of the bundle in Fig. 3 (a) leads to an extinction of the signal of the crossing fibers. As a result, the bundle with a higher fiber density dominates the signal analysis. This also happens in the optic chiasm. In the central area, pixels are either darker or completely black indicating the extinction of signal caused by crossing fibers. Other parts are colored as expected and show the orientation present during the construction of fiber models.

Evaluating the performance of the developed tool shows that most processes have a nearly linear scaling with the amounts of data points used to describe the fiber models. The recorded frame rate shows that even big constructions still grant a stable frame rate. Models with less than 1.6 million data points retain a frame rate of more than 30 frames per second. Since the data generated here is only intended to represent partial sections of brain tissue for simulations, more than 1.6 million data points are rarely required. Therefore, a stable and fluent workflow is guaranteed. For comparison, the fiber cup phantom contains 426300 data points after filling the bundle while the original file contains 290 data points. This indicates that even big models are able to be rendered on similar hardware.

In summary, a fast and userfriendly program was implemented that enables the effective creation of synthetic fiber bundles for simulations with 3D-PLI. Created fiber bundles can be visualized simultaneously and edited interactively. With the help of the program, users can quickly find and remove incorrect parts of the synthetic data set without wasting time with incorrect simulations. This ensures an efficient simulation workflow.

Acknowledgement. This project has received funding from the European Unions Horizon 2020 Research and Innovation Programme under Grant Agreement No. 785907 (HBP SGA2).

References

1. Axer M, Amunts K, Grassel D, et al. A novel approach to the human connectome: ultra-high resolution mapping of fiber tracts in the brain. Neuroimage. 2011;54(2):1091–1101.
2. Dohmen M, Menzel M, et al HW. Understanding fiber mixture by simulation in 3D polarized light imaging. Neuroimage. 2015;111:464–475.
3. Menzel M, Axer M, De Raedt He. Finite-Difference Time-Domain Simulation for Three-Dimensional Polarized Light Imaging. Cham: Springer International; 2016.
4. Jones RC. A new calculus for the treatment of optical systemsIII. The sohncke theory of optical activity. J Opt Soc Am. 1941 Jul;31(7):500–503.
5. F NP, B LF, et al SB. Fiberfox: facilitating the creation of realistic white matter software phantoms. Magn Reson Med. 2013;72(5):1460–1470.
6. Fillard P, Descoteaux M, et al AG. Quantitative evaluation of 10 tractography algorithms on a realistic diffusion MR phantom. Neuroimage. 2011;56(1):220–234.

Resource-Efficient Nanoparticle Classification Using Frequency Domain Analysis

Mikail Yayla[1], Anas Toma[1], Jan Eric Lenssen[2], Victoria Shpacovitch[3], Kuan-Hsun Chen[1], Frank Weichert[2], Jian-Jia Chen[1]

[1]Department of Computer Science XII, TU Dortmund University, Germany
[2]Department of Computer Science VII, TU Dortmund University, Germany
[3]Leibniz-Institute for Analytical Science ISAS e.V.,Dortmund, Germany
mikail.yayla@tu-dortmund.de

Abstract. We present a method for resource-efficient classification of nanoparticles such as viruses in liquid or gas samples by analyzing Surface Plasmon Resonance (SPR) images using frequency domain features. The SPR images are obtained with the Plasmon Assisted Microscopy Of Nano-sized Objects (PAMONO) biosensor, which was developed as a mobile virus and particle detector. Convolutional neural network (CNN) solutions are available for the given task, but since the mobility of the sensor is an important factor, we provide a faster and less resource demanding alternative approach for the use in a small virus detection device.The execution time of our approach, which can be optimized further using low power hardware such as a digital signal processor (DSP), is at least 2.6 times faster than the current CNN solution while sacrificing only 1 to 2.5 percent points in accuracy.

1 Introduction

The evolution and emergence of viruses coupled with global travel and transport entail the risk of spreading epidemic diseases. Therefore there is a need for accessible mobile real-time virus detection, preferably in the size of a small mobile device. The PAMONO sensor is a viable candidate to perform such a task. It captures a sequence of images which need to be automatically analysed by an image analysis pipeline. Currently available solutions based on Convolutional neural networks (CNNs), i.e. proposed by Lenssen et al. [1], provide good classification and execution time performance on general purpose hardware. However, CNNs have complex architectures which require a considerable amount of resources, such as high-performance GPUs, to be evaluated [2, 3]. Research in developing dedicated hardware for CNN evaluation is ongoing [3, 4] but no general purpose low power solutions for mobile and embedded systems are currently available.

In this work, we modify the feature extraction and classification stages of the PAMONO image processing pipeline presented by Siedhoff et al. [5] to use frequency domain analysis. It allows us to build resource-efficient embedded systems for nanoparticle classification with high accuracy. The presented methods are able to utilize specialized low power hardware such as DSPs, which can be deployed in a small and mobile virus detection device.

2   Materials and methods

In the following we describe the workings of the PAMONO sensor, the framework used to deploy the image processing, and the image processing pipeline.

2.1   PAMONO sensor

The PAMONO sensor is an optical biosensor used to detect nanoparticles in liquid or gas samples [6, 7]. It utilizes Kretschmann's scheme [8] of plasmon excitation to visualize the binding of particles to antibodies that are applied to a gold surface. A camera observes the surface and produces image sequences to be analyzed. When a binding occurs, intesity steps can be observed. These steps appear on images as blob-like structures with wavelike excitations around them.

2.2   deepRacin

The framework deepRacin [9] is used in our implementation, which utilizes OpenCL to offload computations to accelerators. In deepRacin, computation graphs with tensor operations, such as trained deep neural networks or image processing pipelines, can be deployed. We implemented the spectral and wavelet transformations used in our frequency feature extraction in deepRacin and deployed them on a mobile GPU.

2.3   Modified image processing pipeline

Fig. 1 shows the modified image processing pipeline, which can be divided into four main stages: preprocessing, particle detection, feature extraction and classification. In this work we focus on the feature extraction and the classification stages which are highlighted by the dashed rectangle. The size of the raw input image is 1100×150 pixels. In the preprocessing stage, the constant background noise signal is removed from the raw sensor image using the model proposed in [5]. In the detection stage, the resulting image is segmented into smaller patches of size 48×48. Several techniques for the detection stage and their performance in generating patches are detailed in [1]. After the patch generation, we subsample 32×32 pixels images from the center of the generated patches and consider them as the input for our system. The images may contain particles in addition

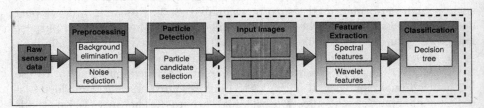

Fig. 1. The modified PAMONO image processing pipeline.

to the existing artefacts and non-constant noise. In the feature extraction stage, the images are loaded in our computation graph, which extracts features in the frequency domain. For the classification, we evaluate decision trees and random forests to decide whether excitations due to a particle binding were observed.

2.4   Spectral and wavelet feature extraction

We want to detect blob-like and periodic patterns in the images from the PA-MONO sensor. In Fig. 1 we can see positive and negative examples of input images in the first and second row, respectively. We can see that images with excitations due to particle binding show blob-like excitations with surrounding periodic patterns resembling sinusoidal waves. Therefore, we propose to use frequency analysis to classify particle bindings. As examples of frequency analysis techniques, we use the Fourier and wavelet transform to extract features.

We want to quantify differences between excitations with blob-like structures and without by computing the Fourier transform of the image to observe high magnitude bursts in halfcircles and lines in the frequency spectrum. For this application we implemented the 2D Fourier transform as a radix-2 out of place GPU accelerated fast Fourier transform (FFT) algorithm, but any other accelerators such as in DSPs can be used as well. Another frequency analysis technique, the two-dimensional wavelet transformation, derives from the correlation of the image with the wavelet ψ. Integrating over $\mathbb{R}^2$, the continuous two-dimensional wavelet transformation is defined as $W_f(\mathbf{t}, s, \theta) = \int f(\mathbf{p}) \psi^*_{\mathbf{t}, s, \theta}(\mathbf{p}) d\mathbf{p}$ where $\mathbf{t}$ represents the translation vector, s the scaling parameter, and θ the rotation angle. As an example of a wavelet function, we use the simplest form, the Haar wavelet. To extract the wavelet features, we calculate the energy of the wavelet transform with $E_{f_d} = \frac{1}{NM} \sum_{p_1=0}^{N-1} \sum_{p_2=0}^{M-1} |W_{f_d}(\mathbf{p})|$ with N and M as the image dimensions and $W_{f_d}(\mathbf{p})$ as the discrete Haar wavelet transform in position $\mathbf{p} = (p_1, p_2)^T$ in the image. Images with blob-like excitations have large energies in both low and middle frequencies, and the low frequency channels are dominant in smooth regions. We implemented the 2D Haar wavelet transform as a GPU accelerated fast Haar wavelet transform (FWT), but other accelerators can be used as well.

Spectral features For computing spectral (Fourier) features from the Fourier transformed image, we shift the zero-frequency components to the center and extract two ordered multisets of magnitude values, called S_{rad} and S_{ang}.

S_{rad} contains the sums of magnitudes over halfcircles for different radiuses r while S_{ang} consists of sums over magnitudes lying on straight lines between the image center and the outer half circle. We aim to capture dominant frequencies using values from S_{rad} and dominant periodic patterns using values from S_{ang}. From both sets S_{rad} and S_{ang} we extract the mean, the maximum, the argmax, the variance and the difference between minimum and maximum values, leading to a feature vector containing ten spectral features in total.

Wavelet features To extract the wavelet features we compute the level 3 Haar wavelet transform and calculate the wavelet energy. We then sum the energy values for each of the ten channels and normalize them, resulting in a feature vector consisting of ten extracted wavelet features.

2.5   Training and classification

We use the dataset provided by Lenssen et al. [1] consisting of 38871 image patches containing particles of sizes 100 nm and 200 nm. We use the provided train/test split, leading to 19526 images for training and 19345 for testing. All images are annotated with binary labels, indicating the existence or non-existence of a particle in the image patch.

For training the classifier using the spectral and wavelet features, we use the decision tree (DT) library in sk-learn [10]. After training the classifier model on features extracted from the training set, we extract the tree structure and split values of the tree from the trained model, convert them to deployable C code and append it to the image processing pipeline. The tree is executed after feature extraction with the spectral, the wavelet, or with both feature sets as input. The image processing pipeline with the decision tree at the end gives us a binary decision result for each extracted particle candidate.

3   Results

To evaluate the effectiveness of our classification, we measure the classification performance and the execution time of our approach, and compare it to the results of the CNN approach by Lenssen et al. [1]. For evaluating classification performance, we use precision, recall, and accuracy. The execution times are measured on Intel Core i7-4600U with integrated Intel HD Graphics 4400. We measure the time needed for computing all steps in the deepRacin computation graphs. All trees have a maximum depths no greater than 12. Since the execution time of the DT with depths less or equal to 12 is smaller than 1 μs, it is negligible for our comparison. Increasing the depth of the decision trees further does not increase classification performance by a large margin in our case.

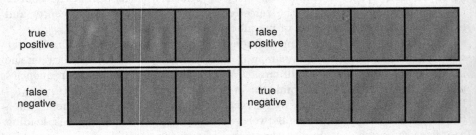

Fig. 2. TP, FP, FN, and TN for the approach with spectral and wavelet features.

Table 1. Comparisons between different classifiers using different feature compositions. DT stands for decision tree, RFn for random forest with n DTs.

Features	Measure	DT (%)	RF10 (%)	RF100 (%)
Spectral and wavelet	Precision	98.49	99.33	99.33
	Recall	97.04	97.19	97.76
Only spectral	Precision	97.78	98.50	98.66
	Recall	96.33	96.02	96.48
Only wavelet	Precision	96.77	97.59	97.66
	Recall	96.35	96.63	97.49

3.1 Classification performance

We can see in Tab. 1 that the classification has the best performance when using both spectral and wavelet features. When using only one set of features, the spectral features outperform the wavelet features by a small margin. Increasing the number of trees using a random forest increases the performance only slightly. In Fig. 2 a few classifications are shown. When excitations are not strong enough, the classification can miss it (FN). When vibrations or noise cause regular high frequency patterns, it can be mistaken as a particle binding (FP). Overall, for our approaches the precision and recall are above 96 % in all cases, and the accuracy is above 97 % except wavelet with one tree. The CNN [1] has a higher accuracy score of 99.5 % than both feature approaches in Tab. 2.

3.2 Execution time

In Tab. 2 we see that our spectral analysis approach is 2.63 times faster than the CNN solution. The wavelet approach is 1.83 times faster than the CNN. The Fourier transform and summing values take less than 0.2 ms in total, but the synchronization of GPU and CPU due to the kernel calls increase the total execution time of the computation graph. This overhead can be potentially further reduced when implementing the proposed approach on hardware like DSPs.

4 Discussion

The classification accuracy of our feature based approaches is sufficiently high for the task of virus detection, which indicates the usefulness of frequency analysis for this application. While the CNN approach performs better by approximately

Method	Time [ms]	Accuracy [%]
Spectral features	1.28	97.07
Wavelet features	1.50	96.57
Spectral and wavelet	2.78	97.78
CNN [1]	3.37	99.50

Table 2. Average execution time (Intel Core i7 4600U with integrated Intel HD Graphics 4400), and accuracy (with one DT for the feature based approaches).

2.5 percent points in accuracy, our approaches outperform it in execution time by a large factor. Using our proposed methods to build an embedded system for nanoparticle classification needs less resources than the CNN. Low power DSPs have specialized hardware for the FFT and are readily available for a low price, while applying CNNs in low power embedded systems is still in development [3].

With our contributions, we enrich the design space of nanoparticle classification systems with frequency analysis methods, which can be faster and more resource-efficient alternative to CNNs, and identified another way to utilize the trade-off between classification quality and execution time. In the future we plan to improve our feature extraction, include the classification of smaller particles, and build a small, fast, low power and low cost embedded system for nanoparticle classification using specialized hardware such as energy optimized DSPs.

Acknowledgement. This paper has been supported by DFG, as part of the Collaborative Research Center SFB876, subproject B2.

References

1. Lenssen JE, Toma A, Seebold A, et al. Real-time low SNR signal processing for nanoparticle analysis with deep neural networks. Biosignals. 2018; p. 36–47.
2. Ovtcharov K, Ruwase O, Kim JY, et al. Accelerating deep convolutional neural networks using specialized hardware. Microsoft Res. 2015;.
3. Andri R, Cavigelli L, Rossi D, et al. YodaNN: an ultra-low power convolutional neural network accelerator based on binary weights. ISVLSI. 2016; p. 236–241.
4. Qiao Y, Shen J, Xiao T, et al. FPGA-accelerated deep convolutional neural networks for high throughput and energy efficiency. Concurr Comput: Pract Exp. 2016;29(20):e3850.
5. Siedhoff D, Libuschewski P, Weichert F, et al. Modellierung und Optimierung eines Biosensors zur Detektion viraler Strukturen. Procs BVM. 2014; p. 108–113.
6. Shpacovitch V, Temchura V, Matrosovich M, et al. Application of surface plasmon resonance imaging technique for the detection of single spherical biological submicrometer particles. Anal Biochem. 2015;486:62 – 69.
7. Zybin A, Kuritsyn YA, Gurevich EL, et al. Real-time detection of single immobilized nanoparticles by surface plasmon resonance imaging. Plasmonics. 2010;5:31–35.
8. Kretschmann E. The determination of the optical constants of metals by excitation of surface plasmons. Eur Phys J A. 1971;241:313–324.
9. Github: deepRacin; Accessed 12/2018. "https://github.com/mrjel/deepracin".
10. Pedregosa F, Varoquaux G, Gramfort A, et al. Scikit-learn: machine learning in python. J Mach Learn Res. 2011;12:2825–2830.

Black-Box Hyperparameter Optimization for Nuclei Segmentation in Prostate Tissue Images

Thomas Wollmann[1], Patrick Bernhard[1], Manuel Gunkel[2], Delia M. Braun[3],
Jan Meiners[4], Ronald Simon[4], Guido Sauter[4], Holger Erfle[2], Karsten Rippe[3],
Karl Rohr[1]

[1] University of Heidelberg, BioQuant, IPMB, and DKFZ Heidelberg,
Biomedical Computer Vision Group
[2] High-Content Analysis of the Cell (HiCell) and Advanced Biological Screening
Facility, BioQuant, University of Heidelberg, Germany
[3] Division of Chromatin Networks, DKFZ and BioQuant, Heidelberg, Germany
[4] Department of Pathology, University Medical Center Hamburg-Eppendorf, Germany
thomas.wollmann@bioquant.uni-heidelberg.de

Abstract. Segmentation of cell nuclei is essential for analyzing high-content histological screens. Often, parameters of automatic approaches need to be optimized, which is tedious and difficult to perform manually. We propose a novel hyperparameter optimization framework, which formulates optimization as a combination of candidate sampling and an optimization strategy. We present a clustering based and a deep neural network based pipeline for nuclei segmentation, for which the parameters are optimized using state of the art optimizers as well as a novel optimizer. The pipelines were applied to challenging prostate cancer tissue images. We performed a quantitative evaluation using 28,388 parameter settings. It turned out that the deep neural network outperforms the clustering based pipeline, while the results for different optimizers vary slightly.

1   Introduction

The segmentation of cell nuclei in histological prostate tissue images is a crucial task to stratify prostate cancer. In particular, the properties of the microscopy data with regard to contrast, noise, cell clustering, edge information, shape variation, and intensity variation determine the complexity of the required segmentation pipeline. Generally, a complex pipeline is necessary for robustly segmenting heterogeneous data (Fig. 1), while the segmentation result highly depends on the used parameters. Since manual parameter optimization of complex algorithms is very time-consuming and difficult, automated parameter optimization is required. However, for complex pipelines the objective function is usually not fully differentiable, which prevents using first or higher order optimization methods. Instead, zero order optimization (black-box optimization) [1] can be performed without using further information of the objective function. Black-box optimization uses a limited number of evaluations of the objective function, and the non-convex optimization tries to determine the (local) optimum by finding the best parameters. For machine learning systems, black-box optimization can be used for automatically tuning hyperparameters as done for denoising algorithms [2], for simulated objective functions [3] or for cell segmentation in tissue images [4]. However, to our knowledge, a systematic evaluation on the applicability of automated black-box optimization has not been conducted for hyperparameter optimization of cell nuclei segmentation pipelines. Existing optimization frameworks like Spearmint [5], Hyperopt [6], Scikit-Optimize [7], or Google Vizier [8] do not satisfy the demands of cell nuclei segmentation as they have a low ease of use (e.g., mix of programming languages, workspace management), employ only few optimizers or only offer limited expandability. Furthermore, Google Vizier is not publicly available.

In this work, we introduce a novel black-box optimization framework, where hyperparameter optimization is formulated as a combination of candidate sampling and an optimization strategy. Our framework allows a modular design of new optimizers as well as quickly implementing state of the art optimizers. We applied our framework to a clustering based pipeline as well as a deep neural network based pipeline to segment cell nuclei in challenging prostate cell tissue images. We evaluated the pipelines using different optimizers and 28388 parameter settings. We provide insights into cell nuclei segmentation and suggest common practices for hyperparameter optimization in this application.

2   Methods

We investigated two nuclei segmentation pipelines, one based on K-means clustering and the other based on a U-Net convolutional neural network (CNN). The hyperparameters of the pipelines were optimized using our novel distributed black-box optimization framework.

2.1   Segmentation pipelines

Clustering based segmentation The pipeline involves several parameters (in the following highlighted in italic). An image is smoothed by a Gaussian filter (sigma) before performing K-means clustering using intensity values (cluster initialization method). Cluster initialization with a random seed value leads to a

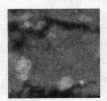 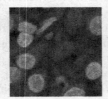 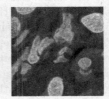 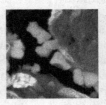

Fig. 1. Examples of prostate tissue images with various challenges for image analysis.(a) Strong background noise, (b) Low contrast, (c) Strong shape variation, (d) Strong intensity variation.

non-deterministic pipeline. To avoid this, we set the seed value to a fix value. Median filter and morphological closing of small holes are applied subsequently. By comparing a selected geometric feature of each cluster to the mean of all clusters, one cluster is assigned as foreground, whose labels are subsequently thresholded with regard to the geometric features area (upper and lower threshold) and solidity before using the foreground cluster as segmentation result.

CNN based segmentation We train a U-Net [9] on the respective training and validation datasets using the Adam optimizer and early stopping. For training we perform offline data augmentation using rotation, flipping, and elastic deformation. The local minimum found by Adam highly depends on the initialization of the network. Therefore, for a fair comparison we use the same seed value for sampling the initial network weights in all experiments. Small segmented objects are discarded using a threshold for the area. The parameters of this pipeline are the learning rate, batch size, and area threshold.

2.2   HyperHyper optimization framework

Our proposed distributed black-box optimization framework *HyperHyper* subdivides hyperparameter optimization in a hyperparameter candidate sampler and an optimization strategy. Candidate sampler and optimization strategy can be selected from a model zoo to form an optimizer for a specific application. Sequential model-based optimization (SMBO) is performed by sampling candidates and evaluating or dismissing them (Fig. 2). The candidate sampler employs a specified hyperparameter space definition as prior, which allows using numerical and categorical parameters with various distributions (e.g., discrete/continuous uniform, Gaussian, log Gaussian, exponential). The sampled hyperparameters are applied to the segmentation pipeline by a worker (compute node) and a performance score with respect to manually annotated ground truth is calculated. In our experiments, we use the Dice coefficient as performance measure. For each hyperparameter evaluation, a dedicated workspace is created and managed by the framework. The optimization can be performed by highly distributed computation. A database is used for distributing compute jobs including the hyperparameters as well as the compute pipeline, and collecting respective results. For each available compute cluster, a coordinator node manages the instantiation

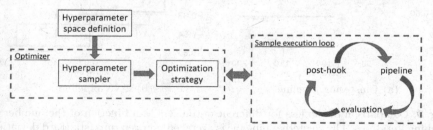

Fig. 2. Schematic representation of the black-box optimization framework.

of workers within the respective cluster. Since the used pipelines contain non-ordinal parameters, we decided to choose optimizers which can handle variables without a natural order. Besides random search (Random) we used sequential model-based algorithm configuration (SMAC) [10], which combines a random forest regression model and sampling from the prior, and represents a more sophisticated version of the general sequential model-based optimization (SMBO) framework [10]. We also modified SMAC by using the XGBoost [11] regression model (SMAC-XGBoost) instead of random forest (SMAC-RF), since XGBoost is currently one of the most popular decision tree based models. Alternatively, we use an evolutionary optimizer with a covariance matrix adaptation evolution strategy (CMA-ES), which is a generic population-based meta-heuristic based optimizer, where feature sets are assumed as "genomes", which undergo evolutionary processes like selection, recombination or mutation [12]. We further investigated the tree of parzen estimator (TPE) surrogate, which performs a nonparametric density approximation of a random variable [13].

3   Experimental results

We applied our hyperparameter optimization framework using multiple optimizers to two pipelines for cell segmentation in challenging prostate cancer tissue images (Fig. 1). The tissue microarray (TMA) images of varying sizes were divided into 256×256 pixel image patches before randomly splitting the dataset into 75 % for training and 25 % for testing. We used 60 ground truth images which were manually annotated by an expert. The clustering based pipeline includes six parameters, whereas the CNN based pipeline involves three parameters. As global optimum we used the result from extensive Grid Search. For each optimizer, 200 evaluations were performed on 20 compute nodes (clustering: 27280, CNN: 1108 parameter settings). The pipelines are deterministic, since we used a fix seed value. However, the hyperparameter optimization itself is stochastic. Therefore, we performed 10 runs per optimizer and report mean and standard deviation of the results for the clustering based pipeline (Tab. 1).

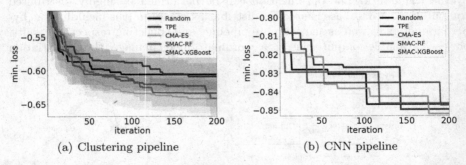

(a) Clustering pipeline   (b) CNN pipeline

Fig. 3. Comparison of the loss for different optimizers as a function of the number of training iterations. The clustering pipeline is averaged over ten runs (standard deviation highlighted).

Table 1. Results for different optimizers. Shown is the improvement Δ Dice after the warm-up phase and the absolute Dice value. Best results are highlighted in bold.

Pipeline	Optimizer	Δ Dice (Improvement)	Dice
Clustering	Random	0.030	0.606 ± 0.025
	TPE	0.045	$0.609 \pm \mathbf{0.020}$
	CMA-ES	0.077	$\mathbf{0.642} \pm 0.021$
	SMAC-RF	**0.094**	$\mathbf{0.642} \pm 0.026$
	SMAC-XGBoost	0.064	0.634 ± 0.021
	Grid Search	–	*0.654*
CNN	Random	0.019	0.847
	TPE	0.038	0.850
	CMA-ES	0.033	**0.852**
	SMAC-RF	0.017	0.846
	SMAC-XGBoost	**0.039**	0.847
	Grid Search	–	*0.864*

Due to computational resources needed for training deep neural networks, we ran the CNN based pipeline once per optimizer. In addition to Dice, we report the difference (Δ Dice) to the Dice value after the warm-up phase. The framework performs a warm-up phase for exploring the parameter space by evaluating 20 random samples before performing optimization. Thus, Δ Dice reflects the improvement achieved by the optimizer. For the clustering based pipeline, it turns out that SMAC-RF performs best regarding Δ Dice (Fig. 3), whereas for the CNN pipeline our proposed SMAC-XGBoost achieves the best value for Δ Dice (Fig. 4). Considering the absolute Dice value, CMA-ES and SMAC-RF perform best, deviating only 0.012 from the global minimum, whereas TPE yields the lowest standard deviation. SMAC-XGBoost achieves a slightly lower Dice value than the best performing SMAC-RF. However, SMAC-XGBoost outperforms SMAC-RF at the beginning of the training. For the CNN based pipeline, the CMA-ES achieves the best absolute Dice value. Overall, the CNN based pipeline significantly outperforms the clustering based pipeline.

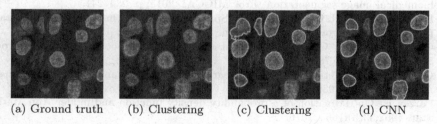

(a) Ground truth   (b) Clustering   (c) Clustering   (d) CNN

Fig. 4. Example image with ground truth (blue) and segmentation using SMAC-RF (red) and SMAC-XGBoost (green).

4 Conclusion

We presented a novel framework for hyperparameter optimization of nuclei segmentation pipelines. The framework allows implementing common optimizers as well, as designing novel optimizers. From our study using two pipelines for segmenting cell nuclei in prostate tissue images, it turned out that CMA-ES and SMAC derivatives perform best.

Acknowledgement. Support of the BMBF within the projects CancerTelSys (e:Med, #01ZX1602) and de.NBI (HD-HuB, #031A537C) is gratefully acknowledged.

References

1. Wang Y, Du S, Balakrishnan S, et al. Stochastic Zeroth-order Optimization in High Dimensions. arXiv:1710.10551; 2017.
2. Ramani S, Blu T, Unser M. Monte-carlo SURE: a black-box optimization of regularization parameters for general denoising algorithms. IEEE Trans Image Process. 2008;17(9):1540–1554.
3. Hansen N, Auger A, Ros R, et al.; ACM. Comparing results of 31 algorithms from the black-box optimization benchmarking BBOB-2009. Proc GECCO. 2010; p. 1689–1696.
4. Teodoro G, Kurç TM, Taveira LF, et al. Algorithm sensitivity analysis and parameter tuning for tissue image segmentation pipelines. Bioinformatics. 2016;33(7):1064–1072.
5. Snoek J, Larochelle H, Adams RP. Practical bayesian optimization of machine learning algorithms. Proc Adv Neural Inf Process Syst. 2012; p. 2951–2959.
6. Bergstra J, Yamins D, Cox DD; Citeseer. Hyperopt: a python library for optimizing the hyperparameters of machine learning algorithms. Proc SciPy. 2013; p. 13–20.
7. Komer B, Bergstra J, Eliasmith C. Hyperopt-sklearn: automatic hyperparameter configuration for scikit-learn. Proc ICML Workshop AutoML. 2014; p. 2825–2830.
8. Golovin D, Solnik B, Moitra S, et al.; ACM. Google vizier: a service for black-box optimization. Proc SIGKDD. 2017; p. 1487–1495.
9. Ronneberger O, Fischer P, Brox T; Springer. U-net: convolutional networks for biomedical image segmentation. Proc MICCAI. 2015; p. 234–241.
10. Hutter F, Hoos HH, Leyton-Brown K; Springer. Sequential model-based optimization for general algorithm configuration. Proc LION. 2011; p. 507–523.
11. Chen T, Guestrin C; ACM. Xgboost: a scalable tree boosting system. Proc SIGKDD. 2016; p. 785–794.
12. Goldberg DE. Genetic Algorithms in Search, Optimization, and Machine Learning. Addison-Wesley; 1989.
13. Parzen E. On estimation of a probability density function and mode. Ann Math Stat. 1962;33(3):1065–1076.

Kategorisierung der Beiträge

Autorenverzeichnis

Printed in the United States
By Bookmasters